Text Atlas of
Obstetric
Dermatology

Text Atlas of
Obstetric
Dermatology

EDITED BY

George Kroumpouzos, MD, PhD

Clinical Associate Professor of Dermatology
The Warren Alpert Medical School of Brown University
Department of Dermatology, Rhode Island Hospital
Providence, Rhode Island

. Wolters Kluwer | Lippincott Williams & Wilkins
Health

Philadelphia · Baltimore · New York · London
Buenos Aires · Hong Kong · Sydney · Tokyo

Executive Editor: Rebecca S. Gaertner
Senior Product Manager: Kristina Oberle
Developmental Editor: Louis Bierig
Production Manager: David Saltzberg
Senior Manufacturing Manager: Beth Welsh
Marketing Manager: Kimberly Schonberger
Senior Designer: Doug Smock
Production Service: Absolute Service, Inc.

© 2014 by LIPPINCOTT WILLIAMS & WILKINS, a WOLTERS KLUWER business
Two Commerce Square
2001 Market Street
Philadelphia, PA 19103 USA
LWW.com

Printed in China

Library of Congress Cataloging-in-Publication Data

Text atlas of obstetric dermatology / edited by George Kroumpouzos.
    p. ; cm.
 Includes bibliographical references and index.
 ISBN 978-1-4511-7674-2 (hardback : alk. paper)
 I. Kroumpouzos, George, editor of compilation, contributor.
 [DNLM: 1. Skin Diseases. 2. Pregnancy Complications. 3. Pregnancy. WR 140]
 RL73.W65
 616.5—dc23

                                                                        2013027004

Care has been taken to confirm the accuracy of the information presented and to describe generally accepted practices. However, the authors, editors, and publisher are not responsible for errors or
omissions or for any consequences from application of the information in this book and make no
warranty, expressed or implied, with respect to the currency, completeness, or accuracy of the contents
of the publication. Application of the information in a particular situation remains the professional
responsibility of the practitioner.

The authors, editors, and publisher have exerted every effort to ensure that drug selection and dosage
set forth in this text are in accordance with current recommendations and practice at the time of
publication. However, in view of ongoing research, changes in government regulations, and the constant flow of information relating to drug therapy and drug reactions, the reader is urged to check the
package insert for each drug for any change in indications and dosage and for added warnings and
precautions. This is particularly important when the recommended agent is a new or infrequently
employed drug.

Some drugs and medical devices presented in the publication have Food and Drug Administration
(FDA) clearance for limited use in restricted research settings. It is the responsibility of the health care
provider to ascertain the FDA status of each drug or device planned for use in their clinical practice.

To purchase additional copies of this book, call our customer service department at (800) 638-3030 or
fax orders to (301) 223-2320. International customers should call (301) 223-2300.

Visit Lippincott Williams & Wilkins on the Internet at LWW.com. Lippincott Williams & Wilkins
customer service representatives are available from 8:30 am to 6 pm, EST.

10 9 8 7 6 5 4 3 2 1

To my wife, Toula, for her invaluable advice, support, and encouragement.

To my daughters, Elena and Demi, for their endless patience and understanding throughout this project.

To my beloved father, In Memoriam.

To the contributing authors and my colleagues with deep appreciation.

To all my patients who make my work a sincere pleasure.

I thank you from the bottom of my heart and will always be indebted to you.

George Kroumpouzos

Many thanks to Teresa Exley, Project Manager, and Louise Bierig, Developmental Editor, for their enormous assistance.

My sincerest gratitude to Kristina Oberle, Senior Product Manager, and her dedicated team at LWW who brought this great endeavor to fruition.

CONTENTS

PREFACE

During gestation, the skin, hair, and nails may undergo numerous changes, some of which persist postpartum. Because these changes can have a significant effect on the pregnant patient, diagnosis, counseling, and treatment are of utmost importance. Pregnancy can also have profound effects on preexisting maternal skin disease, and healthcare providers should be familiar with the course of skin disease in pregnancy as well as safe management options.

It was more than 15 years ago that I published my first manuscript in the field of Obstetric Dermatology. Since then, I have always felt that this particular field could greatly benefit from a comprehensive textbook/atlas with rich pictorial content, also encompassing drug safety, skin surgery, cosmetics and skin care products, and dermato-ethics. My humble ambition was to create such a book that thoroughly covers all aspects of skin conditions in pregnancy and, furthermore, addresses the questions of the nondermatologist healthcare provider; I hope I have succeeded.

I am very pleased with the creation of the *Text Atlas of Obstetric Dermatology*. It was the result of a collaborative group effort, aimed to serve as a guide in diagnosing a wide spectrum of dermatologic conditions, including specific pregnancy dermatoses. Accompanied with over 400 impressive photos, I hope that this textbook will be an instrumental tool for dermatologists, gynecologists/obstetricians, family practitioners, internists, residents, and patients.

The completion of this work would not have been possible without the continuous support and encouragement of my colleagues and patients. A debt of gratitude goes to my peers; colleagues of the Department of Dermatology at the Warren Alpert Medical School of Brown University, especially Lionel Bercovitch, MD, and Charles J. McDonald, MD; and national and international experts for their assistance and vital contribution; also, to all my wonderful patients for sharing their stories and contributing essential and rare photos. This tremendous collaboration has made this endeavor a truly rewarding and unforgettable experience for me, and I will always be grateful.

George Kroumpouzos, MD, PhD

Iris K. Aronson, MD
Associate Head for Clinical Affairs
Associate Professor of Dermatology
University of Illinois
Chicago, Illinois

Lionel Bercovitch, MD
Professor of Dermatology
The Warren Alpert Medical School of Brown University
Rhode Island Hospital
Women and Infants' Hospital
Providence, Rhode Island

Joe Brooks, MD
Director
Arizona Vulvar Clinic
Phoenix, Arizona

Jeffrey P. Callen, MD
Professor of Medicine (Dermatology)
University of Louisville
Louisville, Kentucky

Kenneth K. Chen, MD
Assistant Professor of Medicine and Obstetrics and Gynecology
The Warren Alpert Medical School of Brown University
Division Director
Obstetric & Consultative Medicine
Staff Endocrinologist
Women & Infants' Hospital
Providence, Rhode Island

Jennie T. Clarke, MD
Associate Professor of Dermatology
Penn State Milton S. Hershey Medical Center
Hershey, Pennsylvania

Lisa M. Cohen, MD
Clinical Associate Professor
Department of Pathology
Massachusetts General Hospital
Harvard Medical School
Clinical Associate Professor
Department of Dermatology
Tufts Medical School
Boston, Massachusetts

Noah Craft, MD, PhD
Associate Professor of Dermatology
Division of Dermatology and Infectious Diseases
David Geffen School of Medicine at UCLA
Torrance, California

Paulo R. Cunha, MD, PhD
Professor and Chair of Dermatology
Jundiai Medical School, São Paulo, Brazil
Jundiai, São Paulo, Brazil

Zoe Draelos, MD
Consulting Professor of Dermatology
Duke University
High Point, North Carolina

Raymond Dufresne, MD
Professor and Interim Chair of Dermatology
The Warren Alpert Medical School of Brown University
Rhode Island Hospital
Providence, Rhode Island

Dirk Elston, MD
Managing Director
Ackerman Academy of Dermatopathology
New York, New York

Nicole Fett, MD
Assistant Professor
Department of Dermatology
University of Pennsylvania School of Medicine
Philadelphia VA Medical Center
Philadelphia, Pennsylvania

Galen Foulke, MD
Resident
Department of Dermatology
Penn State Milton S. Hershey Medical Center
Hershey, Pennsylvania

Victoria Geenes, MBBS
Academic Foundation Trainee
Maternal and Fetal Disease Group
Institute of Reproductive and Developmental Biology
Faculty of Medicine
Imperial College London
London, United Kingdom

Giampiero Girolomoni, MD
Professor of Dermatology
University of Verona
Verona, Italy

Aleksandr Itkin, MD
Division of Dermatology
Scripps Clinic
San Diego, California

Jennifer Jenkins, MD
Division of Dermatology
Dedham Medical Associates
Atrius Health
Dedham, Massachusetts

Farhan Khan, MD, MBA
Dermatology Clinical Research Fellow
University of Texas
Center for Clinical Studies
Webster, Texas

George Kroumpouzos, MD, PhD
Clinical Associate Professor of Dermatology
The Warren Alpert Medical School of Brown University
Department of Dermatology
Rhode Island Hospital
Providence, Rhode Island

Kachiu C. Lee, MD, MPH
Senior Resident
Department of Dermatology
The Warren Alpert Medical School of Brown University
Providence, Rhode Island

Elie B. Lowenstein, MD
Resident
Department of Dermatology
Mount Sinai Hospital and School of Medicine
New York, New York

Eve J. Lowenstein, MD, PhD
Chief of Dermatology
Brookdale University Hospital
Associate Professor of Dermatology
SUNY HSCB School of Medicine
Brooklyn, New York

Bonnie T. Mackool, MD, MSPH
Assistant Professor of Dermatology
Harvard Medical School
Director of Dermatology Consultation and Inpatient Services
Massachusetts General Hospital
Boston, Massachusetts

Rana M. Mays, MD
Dermatology Clinical Research Fellow
University of Texas
Center for Clinical Studies
Webster, Texas

Jessica J. Mercer, MD
Voluntary Assistant Professor of Dermatology
Miller School of Medicine
University of Miami
Miami, Florida

Jyoti P. Mundi, MD
Senior Resident
The Ronald O. Perelman Department of Dermatology
New York University Langone Medical Center
New York, New York

Jenny E. Murase, MD
Assistant Clinical Professor of Dermatology
University of California, San Francisco
San Francisco, California
Director of Phototherapy
Palo Alto Foundation Medical Group
Mountain View, California

Kudakwashe Mutyambizi, MD, MPhil
Medicine-Dermatology Resident
Harvard Medical School
Boston, Massachusetts

Kelly K. Park, MD, MSL
Resident
Division of Dermatology
Stritch School of Medicine
Loyola University Medical Center
Maywood, Illinois

Annalisa Patrizi, MD
Professor and Director of Dermatology
University of Bologna
Bologna, Italy

Miriam K. Pomeranz, MD
Assistant Professor, Clinical
The Ronald O. Perelman Department of Dermatology
New York University Langone Medical Center
New York, New York

Marcia Ramos-e-Silva, MD
Associate Professor and Head
Sector of Dermatology
University Hospital and School of Medicine
Federal University of Rio de Janeiro
Rio de Janeiro, Brazil

Leslie Robinson-Bostom, MD
Professor of Dermatology
The Warren Alpert Medical School of Brown University
Department of Dermatology
Rhode Island Hospital
Providence, Rhode Island

Gary Rogers, MD
Professor of Dermatology and Surgery
Director
Dermatologic Surgery and Oncology
Tufts University School of Medicine
Boston, Massachusetts

Richard K. Scher, MD
Professor of Clinical Dermatology
Weill Cornell Medical College
New York, New York

Zachary Schwager, BA
Department of Dermatology
The Warren Alpert Medical School of Brown University
Providence, Rhode Island

Emily Tierney, MD
Assistant Professor of Dermatology
Division of Dermatologic Surgery and Oncology
Department of Dermatology
Tufts University School of Medicine
Boston, Massachusetts

Stephen K. Tyring, MD, PhD
Clinical Professor of Dermatology
University of Texas
Center for Clinical Studies
Webster, Texas

Darshan C. Vaidya, MD
Senior Resident
Department of Dermatology
The Warren Alpert Medical School of Brown University
Providence, Rhode Island

Victoria P. Werth, MD
Professor
Department of Dermatology
University of Pennsylvania School of Medicine
Philadelphia VA Medical Center
Philadelphia, Pennsylvania

Catherine Williamson, MD
Professor of Obstetric Medicine
Maternal and Fetal Disease Group
Institute of Reproductive and Developmental Biology
Faculty of Medicine
Imperial College London
London, United Kingdom

Detlef Zillikens, MD
Professor and Chair
Department of Dermatology
University of Lübeck
Lübeck, Germany

George Kroumpouzos, from the Department of Dermatology, the Warren Alpert Medical School of Brown University, has assembled a world class array of medical experts in dermatology, dermatopathology, internal medicine, and obstetrics and gynecology to write an exceptionally comprehensive as well as excellent *Text Atlas of Obstetric Dermatology*. This textbook elaborates in great depth on every imaginable and recognizable dermatologic condition and/or disease known to occur during the period of gestation and in the postpartum period, as well as preexisting skin diseases that may be affected by pregnancy, and those physiologic changes that may occur during gestation and/or the postpartum period. This textbook should serve as an excellent resource for obstetricians, dermatologists, and those medical providers who have an interest in women's health.

Chapters 1 through 7 summarize those hormonal, immunologic, and physiologic changes that are unique to and tend to occur primarily during pregnancy. Chapters 8 through 16 review the vast array of preexisting skin diseases that may be affected by pregnancy. Diseases that may be characterized as specific to and dermatoses of pregnancy are discussed in Chapters 17 through 21. Additional useful features of this text include sections with detailed discussions on drug and cosmeceutical safety during pregnancy (Chapters 22 through 23), skin surgery during pregnancy (Chapter 24), and dermatoethics as related to pregnancy (Chapter 25).

The pictorial material of approximately 400 images, including many rare "before and after" photographs, is exceptional and will prove extremely useful to nondermatologists, resident trainees, medical students, and interested patients.

This text/atlas includes a comprehensive and up-to-date review of the management of skin problems in pregnancy. It also covers the postpartum course of skin disease, and discusses safe treatments in lactation. The detailed sections of etiology and the management of maternal/fetal risks can greatly assist healthcare providers in recognizing such risks and managing them effectively.

In conclusion, Dr. Kroumpouzos has successfully produced the most comprehensive text/atlas, in print, covering all aspects of dermatologic diseases and conditions that may occur during pregnancy and lactation. It should prove of great assistance in the diagnosis and treatment for dermatologists, obstetricians, and other healthcare providers. It is my belief that this text/atlas will ultimately become the standard reference resource in the field of obstetric dermatology.

Charles J. McDonald, MD
Professor of Medical Science
and Founding Chair, Department of Dermatology
The Warren Alpert Medical School of Brown University

Endocrine and Immunologic Changes

Kenneth K. Chen ■ George Kroumpouzos

INTRODUCTION

Profound hormonal and immunologic alterations occur in pregnancy,[1,2] which account for most physiologic skin changes[1] and effects on skin disease (see Ch. 2). These alterations are summarized in Table 1.1 and will be outlined throughout this chapter.

ENDOCRINE CHANGES

From an endocrine point of view, pregnancy may be divided into the *ovarian* and *placental periods*.[1] The first period typically parallels the first trimester and is characterized by the increasing production of human chorionic gonadotropin (hCG), estrogen, and progesterone by the corpus luteum. The second period is dominated by the increasing production of various hormones by the placenta, such as steroid hormones, and human placental lactogen (hPL) (Table 1.1). In the first few weeks of gestation, progesterone is produced exclusively by the corpus luteum, which is maintained by trophoblast-produced hCG. Around the seventh week, ovarian steroid hormone production declines while the production is taken over by the placenta (*luteal placental shift*). hCG level begins to rise and can be detected in maternal blood and urine 8 to 10 days after fertilization, peaks between 9 to 12 weeks gestation, and then declines quickly back to a low baseline level by 20 weeks gestation. hPL does not start to rise until weeks 7 to 8. Figure 1.1 illustrates this development.

Once pregnancy has been established, there are immediate effects on almost all endocrine axes. The anterior pituitary gland increases in weight and volume by more than twofold[3]; there is hyperplasia and proliferation of the lactotrophs, which causes an increase in prolactin secretion that continues through to the puerperium.[4] There is also increased output of gonadotropins, adrenocorticotropic hormone (ACTH),[5,6] and melanocyte-stimulating hormone (MSH).[7] Hypertrophy of the adrenal cortices occurs, which leads to an increased production of cortisol, aldosterone, and dehydroepiandrosterone ("physiologic" hypercortisolism).[8,9] Free cortisol levels increase 1.6-fold by the end of the third trimester (see Fig. 1.1).

Arginine vasopressin (AVP; also called antidiuretic hormone) is a hormone produced by the posterior pituitary whose metabolism changes significantly throughout pregnancy. A change in osmostat (the set point for plasma osmolality at which AVP is secreted) occurs from very early on in pregnancy—this results in a reduction in mean maternal plasma osmolality and in the osmolar threshold for thirst.[10] This leads to thirst at a lower osmolality, resulting in an increase in intravascular volume throughout pregnancy, which is important in maintaining blood flow to the fetoplacental unit.[10]

The alpha subunit of hCG is homologous to that of thyrotropin (TSH), and hCG exerts a TSH-like action on the thyroid gland. The rise in hCG in the first trimester results in a decrease in TSH secretion but is usually sufficient to stimulate an excess secretion of total thyroid hormone; free thyroxine (FT4) rises slightly and peaks at 8 weeks (Fig. 1.1).[11] An increased production of circulating estrogen, first from the ovary and later the placenta, stimulates a compensatory increase in the production of thyroxine-binding globulin so that the free thyroid hormone concentrations remain relatively stable throughout the rest of gestation.[11]

Although the mother has a huge reserve of calcium in her own skeleton, it is now recognized that fetal demands for calcium associated with fetal growth are typically met by increasing the maternal absorption of calcium rather than mobilizing her bony reserves.[12] This is mainly achieved through the action of 1,25-dihydroxyvitamin D, whereas parathormone levels remain relatively stable.[12] Changes in glucose tolerance in pregnancy mainly relate to the increased secretion of hPL and cortisol in increasing insulin resistance.[13]

An area of renewed interest is the complex physiology of relaxin. With close structural homology to insulin, the original understanding was that relaxin was a peptide hormone involved in the remodeling of maternal joints as well as the cervix to facilitate both carriage and passage of the fetus through the birth canal; it also acts synergistically with progesterone to reduce contractility of the uterine myometrium. As it weakens collagen and elastin, it may contribute to vascular distention and varicose vein formation. More recently, it has been reported that it maintains hypervolemia in late pregnancy as it stimulates AVP secretion and drinking; it also alters breast tissue to promote lactation, reduces connective tissue fibrosis and the severity of allergic reactions, and enhances wound healing.[14]

TABLE 1.1	Summary of Endocrine and Immunologic Changes*
Endocrine Changes	
Corpus luteum (*ovarian period*)	Estrogen, progesterone
Fetal–placental unit (*placental period*)	Estrogen, progesterone, androgens, GnRH, CRH, TRH, peptides (hCG, hPL, inhibin, relaxin), insulin-like growth factors I & II
Anterior pituitary gland	Gonadotropins, ACTH, MSH, prolactin
Posterior pituitary gland	Arginine vasopressin, oxytocin
Adrenal gland	Cortisol, aldosterone, dehydroepiandrosterone
Thyroid gland	Thyroid hormones (slight increase in first trimester)
Immunologic Changes	
Cellular immunity	↓ numbers of CD3, CD4, CD8, CD20; ↓ IL-2, TNF-α, IFN-γ
Humoral immunity	IL-4, IL-10, asymmetric antibodies, pregnancy-specific glycoproteins
Placental HLA antigens	HLA-G antigen, absence of HLA class II (trophoblast), HLA null (villous trophoblast)

* All hormones, cytokines, antigens, and other immune response modulators increase unless otherwise indicated.

ACTH, adrenocorticotropic hormone; CD, clusters of differentiation; CRH, corticotropin-releasing hormone; GnRH, gonadotropin-releasing hormone; hCG, human chorionic gonadotropin; HLA, human leukocyte antigen; hPL, human placental lactogen; IFN, interferon; IL, interleukin; MSH, melanocyte-stimulating hormone; TNF, tumor necrosis factor; TRH, thyrotropin-releasing hormone.

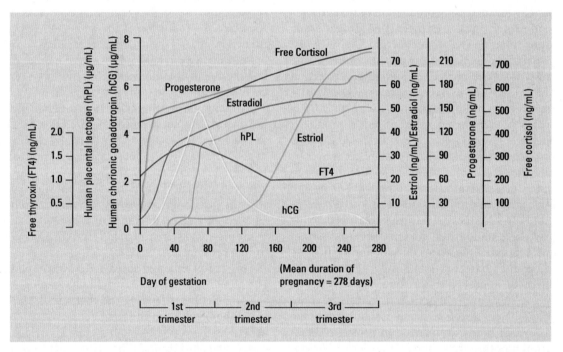

Figure 1.1. Hormonal changes in pregnancy. hCG (human chorionic gonadotropin) and FT4 peak in the first trimester, whereas free cortisol, progesterone, estradiol, hPL (human placental lactogen), and estriol levels increase progressively throughout gestation and peak in the third trimester. (Figure substantially modified from Black MM, Ambros-Rudolph C, Edwards L, et al., eds. *Obstetric and Gynecologic Dermatology.* 3rd ed. Philadelphia, PA: Mosby Elsevier; 2008. Data on free cortisol and FT4 were obtained from References 7 and 12, respectively.)

IMMUNOLOGIC CHANGES

Following conception, a state of maternal immune tolerance to the fetus develops that aims to prevent the rejection of the fetus. This tolerance is a result of the properties of the fetoplacental unit and changes in the maternal immune system.[2] The production of asymmetric antibodies, a characteristic of pregnancy, may protect the woman from a destructive maternal immune response to paternal antigens.[15] At the maternal–fetal interface, the extra-villous trophoblast inhibits fetal rejection by maternal lymphocytes[16] and expresses regulatory proteins, which protect against the action of maternal complement[17]; this may contribute to fetal tolerance. The placenta produces a number of proteins and steroids (hPL, hCG, estrogen, progesterone) that nonspecifically suppress the local immune response, contributing to maternal tolerance to the fetus. Finally, the trophoblast lacks an expression of human leukocyte antigen (HLA) class II while it expresses special HLAs, which protect it from maternal immune-mediated cytotoxicity, such as HLA G[16]; the altered HLA profile has been implicated in maternal tolerance during pregnancy.[18]

The absolute numbers of peripheral T cells, such as CD4 and CD8, slightly decline during the first 2 trimesters, rise in the third trimester, and reach prepartum levels in the postpartum period[19]; however, the significance of the finding is uncertain. The most important finding is a shift in T-cell response from T-helper 1 (Th1) to T-helper 2 (Th2) (Fig. 1.2).[20] This is mainly due to production of Th2 cytokines, especially interleukin (IL) 10, 4, 5, 6, and 13.[15] Additionally, pregnancy-specific glycoproteins have been shown to induce Th2 cytokines in vitro.[15] A number of studies have shown that the success of pregnancy is associated with the production of IL-4 and IL-10 at the maternal–fetal interface. Also, progesterone decreases IL-12 with a subsequent reduction of cytotoxic natural killer activity that favors a normal pregnancy outcome.[21] Other authors, however, indicate that a failure of the Th1/Th2 shift is a marker of an unsuccessful pregnancy but not a cause on its own.[15] Th2 cytokines fall abruptly in the postpartum period.[20] At this time, the levels of Th1 cytokines (IL-2, IL-1, interferon [IFN]-γ, and tumor necrosis factor [TNF]-α) rise abruptly and the T-cell response shifts back from Th2 to Th1.

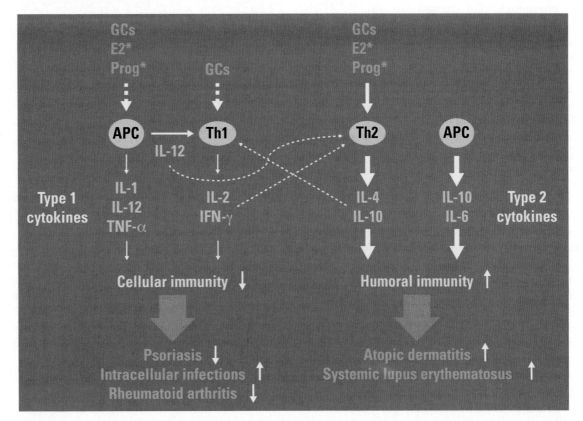

Figure 1.2. The effects of estrogen, progesterone, and glucocorticoids on type 1 (proinflammatory) and type 2 (anti-inflammatory) cytokine production are shown. Note the mutual inhibition of Th1 and Th2 pathways. A change in Th1/Th2 balance results in improvement of diseases that were mediated through cellular responses, such as psoriasis and rheumatoid arthritis, and worsening of diseases that are mediated through humoral responses, such as atopic dermatitis and systemic lupus erythematosus. (Figure substantially modified from Elenkov IJ. Neuroendocrine effects on immune system. In: Chrousos G, ed. *Adrenal Physiology and Diseases*. Endotext.com Web site. http://www.endotext.org/adrenal/adrenal28/adrenal28.htm. Accessed March 4, 2013.) APC, antigen presenting cell; E2, estradiol; GCs, glucocorticoids; IFN, interferon; IL, interleukin; Prog, progesterone; TNF, tumor necrosis factor; ↓, decreases; ↑, increases. Solid lines represent stimulation and dashed lines represent inhibition.

The Interplay between the Endocrine and Immunologic Systems

The interplay between the endocrine and immunologic systems is illustrated in Figure 1.2. Estrogen promotes Th2 responses and suppresses the production of Th1 cytokines (see Fig. 1.2) in a multitude of ways,[22,23] including the modulation of antigen-presenting cells and the inhibition of IL-2 at the transcriptional level as well as of the IL-2 receptor.[24] Progesterone increases the production of IL-4 and has been shown to decrease steady state levels of TNF-α; however, it does not affect levels of IL-10.[22] Raised serum glucocorticoids inhibit the production of Th1 cytokines, such as TNF-α and IFN-γ, while stimulating the synthesis of Th2 cytokines, such as IL-4, IL-10, and IL-13, by lymphocytes both at the systemic level and the maternal–fetal interface.[25]

THE RELEVANCE TO PHYSIOLOGIC SKIN CHANGES AND SKIN DISEASE

Endocrine and immunologic alterations are responsible for most physiologic skin changes (see Ch. 2).[1] High estrogen levels increase tyrosinase activity, which along with increased MSH levels, contributes to pigmentary changes such as hyperpigmentation and melasma. An increase in adrenocortical hormones has been associated with striae and facial plethora. Changes in glucose tolerance, mediated via increased hPL and cortisol levels, are associated with an exacerbation of acanthosis nigricans and the development of pseudoacanthotic changes during pregnancy.[26] Estrogens, hCG, ACTH-like substance, and thyrotropin-releasing hormone (TRH) have dramatic effects on the vascular system, accounting for an impressive vascular increase in the dermis and a wide spectrum of vascular mucocutaneous changes.[27] The proliferative effects of high estrogen levels on vascular and connective tissues account for the development of a number of benign skin tumors during gestation. Effects of estrogen on the hair cycle manifest with hair changes during pregnancy and the postpartum period, such as telogen effluvium. Finally, both estrogen and progesterone have cholestatic effects, thus playing a crucial role in pruritus and obstetric cholestasis.[28]

Skin disease is significantly affected by the endocrine and immunologic changes of gestation. The effects of high estrogen levels on the maternal immune system, including a decrease of cellular-mediated immunity, may account for an increased susceptibility to intracellular infections such as mycobacterial infections and chlamydia. Some diseases, such as porphyria cutanea tarda, are adversely affected by estrogen. Estrogen may also be implicated in flares of pustular psoriasis in pregnancy (*impetigo herpetiformis*). On the other hand, the improvement of autoimmune progesterone dermatitis may be attributed to a gradual increase in progesterone levels that may result in desensitization.

Pregnancy may trigger the development of autoimmune disease through the phenomenon of microchimerism (i.e., the migration of fetal DNA to maternal circulation, which may trigger an inflammatory response in the skin of the mother after gestation).[29]

The most clinically relevant immunologic alteration during gestation is the Th1/Th2 shift, which results in a Th2-biased immunity. Skin diseases that are Th2-mediated, such as autoimmune disorders and atopic dermatitis, tend to exacerbate during gestation, and atopic dermatitis may develop for the first time in pregnancy.[24,30] However, Th1-mediated processes, such as psoriasis and rheumatoid arthritis, tend to improve.[31] Despite T-cell suppression in the pregnant patient, which aims at preventing rejection of the fetal allograft, a consistent effect of the Th1/Th2 shift on T-cell recognition of tumor antigen has not been shown. Pregnancy does not seem to have a significant effect on the course of malignant skin tumors.

KEY POINTS

- Corpus luteum produces estrogen and progesterone during the first trimester; the placenta takes over production of these hormones around the seventh to eighth week (*luteal placental shift*) and starts to produce other hormones, such as hPL and relaxin.

- Other important endocrine alterations include an increase in ACTH, resulting in raised free serum cortisol and increases in prolactin and AVP; FT4 increases slightly in the first trimester.

- Maternal tolerance to the fetus is a result of various immunologic mechanisms, including the hormone-mediated suppression of immune responses at the maternal–fetal boundary, the lack of expression of HLA class II, and the expression of HLA G by the trophoblast.

- An important immunologic finding is the shift in Th1 to Th2 cytokine production that results from an interplay between hormones and the immune system; skin diseases that are Th2 mediated, such as autoimmune disorders and atopic dermatitis, tend to exacerbate, whereas Th1-mediated processes, such as psoriasis and rheumatoid arthritis, tend to improve during gestation.

REFERENCES

1. Ingber A. Endocrine and immunologic alterations during pregnancy. In: Ingber A, ed. *Obstetric Dermatology, A Practical Guide*. Berlin, Germany: Springer-Verlag; 2009:1–5.
2. Yip L, McCluskey J, Sinclair R. Immunological aspects of pregnancy. *Clin Dermatol*. 2006;24:84–87.
3. Dinç H, Esen F, Demirci A, et al. Pituitary dimensions and volume measurements in pregnancy and post partum. MR assessment. *Acta Radiol*. 1998;39:64–69.

4. Tyson JE, Hwang P, Guyda H, et al. Studies of prolactin secretion in human pregnancy. *Am J Obstet Gynecol*. 1972;113:14–20.

5. Carr BR, Parker CR Jr, Madden JE, et al. Maternal plasma adrenocorticotropin and cortisol relationships throughout pregnancy. *Am J Obstet Gynecol*. 1981;139:416–422.

6. Jung C, Ho JT, Torpy DJ, et al. A longitudinal study of plasma and urinary cortisol in pregnancy and postpartum. *J Clin Endocrinol Metab*. 2011;96:1533–1540.

7. Wilson JF. Levels of alpha-melanotrophin in the human fetal pituitary gland throughout gestation, in adult pituitary gland and in human placenta. *Clin Endocrinol*. 1982;17:233–242.

8. Lindsay JR, Nieman LK. The hypothalamic-pituitary-adrenal axis in pregnancy: Challenges in disease detection and treatment. *Endocr Rev*. 2005;26:775–799.

9. Elsheikh A, Creatsas G, Mastorakos G, et al. The renin-aldosterone system during normal and hypertensive pregnancy. *Arch Gynecol Obstet*. 2001;264:182–185.

10. Lindheimer MD, Barron WM, Davison JM. Osmotic and volume control of vasopressin release in pregnancy. *Am J Kidney Dis*. 1991;17:105–111.

11. Galofre JC, Davies TF. Autoimmune thyroid disease in pregnancy: A review. *J Womens Health (Larchmt)*. 2009;18: 1847–1856.

12. Kovacs CS. Calcium and bone disorders during pregnancy and lactation. *Endocrinol Metab Clin N Am*. 2011;40:795–826.

13. McIntyre HD, Chang AM, Callaway LK, et al. Hormonal and metabolic factors associated with variations in insulin sensitivity in human pregnancy. *Diabetes Care*. 2010;33:356–360.

14. Sherwood OD. Relaxin's physiological roles and other diverse actions. *Endocr Rev*. 2004;25:205–234.

15. Zenclussen AC. Adaptive immune responses during pregnancy. *Am J Reprod Immunol*. 2013;69(4):291–303.

16. Redman CW, McMichael AJ, Stirrat GM, et al. Class I major histocompatibility complex antigens on human extra-villous trophoblast. *Immunology*. 1984;52:457–468.

17. Girardi G, Bulla R, Salmon JE, et al. The complement system in the pathophysiology of pregnancy. *Mol Immunol*. 2006;43: 68–77.

18. Moreau P, Paul P, Rouas-Freiss N, et al. Molecular and immunologic aspects of the non-classical HLA class I antigen HLA-G: Evidence for an important role in the maternal tolerance of the fetal allograft. *Am J Reprod Immunol*. 1998;40:136–144.

19. Burns DN, Nourjah P, Minkoff H, et al. Changes in CD4+ and CD8+ cell levels during pregnancy and post-partum in women seropositive and seronegative for human immunodeficiency virus-1. *Am J Obstet Gynecol*. 1996;174:1461–1468.

20. Marzi M, Vigano A, Trabattoni D, et al. Characterization of type 1 and type 2 cytokine production profile in physiologic and pathologic human pregnancy. *Clin Exp Immunol*. 1996;106:127–133.

21. Szekeres-Bartho J, Polgar B, Kozma N, et al. Progesterone-dependent immunomodulation. In: Markert UR, ed. *Immunology of Pregnancy*. Basel, Switzerland: Karger; 2005:118–125.

22. Elenkov IJ. Neuroendocrine effects on immune system. In: Chrousos G, ed. *Adrenal Physiology and Diseases*. Endotext .com Web site. http://www.endotext.org/adrenal/adrenal28/ adrenal28.htm. Accessed March 4, 2013.

23. Salem ML. Estrogen, a double-edged sword: modulation of TH1- and TH2-mediated inflammations by differential regulation of TH1/TH2 cytokine production. *Curr Drug Targets Inflamm Allergy*. 2004;3:97–104.

24. McMurray RW, Ndebele K, Hardy KJ, et al. 17-beta-estradiol suppresses IL-2 and IL-2 receptor. *Cytokine*. 2001;14:324–333.

25. Ramirez F, Fowell DJ, Puklavee M, et al. Glucocorticoids promote a Th2 cytokine response by CD4+ T cells in vivo. *J Immunol*. 1996;156:2406–2412.

26. Kroumpouzos G, Avgerinou G, Granter SR. Acanthosis nigricans without diabetes during pregnancy. *Br J Dermatol*. 2002;146: 925–928.

27. Elling SV, Powell FC. Physiological changes in the skin during pregnancy. *Clin Dermatol*. 1997;15:35–43.

28. Geenes V, Williamson C. Intrahepatic cholestasis of pregnancy. *World J Gastroenterol*. 2009;15:2049–2066.

29. Nelson JL. Microchimerism and autoimmune disease. *N Engl J Med*. 1998;338:1224–1225.

30. Koutroulis I, Papoutsis J, Kroumpouzos G. Atopic dermatitis in pregnancy: current status and challenges. *Obstet Gynecol Surv*. 2011;66:654–663.

31. Doria A, Iaccarino L, Arienti S, et al. Th2 immune deviation induced by pregnancy: The two faces of autoimmune rheumatic diseases. *Reprod Toxicol*. 2006;22:234–241.

CHAPTER 2

Introduction to Physiologic Skin Changes and Skin Disease in Pregnancy

George Kroumpouzos

INTRODUCTION

During pregnancy, the skin undergoes changes that are caused by the profound endocrine, immunologic, vascular, and metabolic alterations of the gestational period.[1] This results in a wide spectrum of physiologic changes (Table 2.1) and effects on skin disease. Physiologic changes usually resolve postpartum but can be a source of significant distress to the patient.[2–5] Infections, as well as rheumatic, metabolic, and connective tissue skin disease, genodermatoses, and miscellaneous disease can be affected by pregnancy.[6,7] This chapter introduces the physiologic changes of pregnancy discussed in Chapters 3 through 7 and skin diseases primarily affected by gestation, which are discussed in Chapters 8 through 16.

PHYSIOLOGIC SKIN CHANGES

Prevalence

Pigmentary physiologic changes are the most common, followed by vascular changes in Caucasians and connective tissue changes in Indian patients; glandular, hair, and nail changes follow. Pigmentary changes are encountered in up to 90% of Caucasians[3] and their prevalence is approximately the same in Indian[8,9] and Pakistani pregnant women.[10] A significant variation in the prevalence of melasma exists in different studies. It has been traditionally reported in 50% to 70% of Caucasians,[3] but a low prevalence (5%) was reported by a small European study.[11] Recent studies showed a prevalence (51%) in Indian[8] and in Pakistani populations (31%),[10] which was not confirmed by a smaller study in an Indian population (2.5%).[9] These discrepancies may reflect differences in data collection as well as population and racial differences.

Connective tissue changes, the most common being *striae gravidarum*, are approximately as common in Caucasian as in Indian and Pakistani pregnant women; *striae gravidarum* was reported in 62%,[11] 64% to 80%,[8,9] and 77%,[10] respectively. There have been inconsistent results in various studies regarding the effect of skin type on *striae gravidarum*.[12,13] Vascular changes are more common in Caucasians (83%)[11] than in patients of Indian (26%)[8]

and Pakistani descent (34%)[10] and in African Americans.[14] The lower prevalence of vascular lesions in non-Caucasian populations may be due to the fact that these lesions become less noticeable in skin of color. There is a lack of good epidemiologic data in Caucasians on hair, including telogen effluvium, and nail changes. Hair changes, including hirsutism, were surprisingly uncommon (3.4%) in a large study in Indian patients[8]; the prevalence of telogen effluvium was not reported. Epidemiologic studies show a low prevalence (2.1%) of nail changes in Indian and Pakistani populations,[8,10] whereas toenail changes were very common (>50%) in a study in a predominantly African American population.[15]

Onset

The onset of common physiologic changes is shown in Figure 2.1. The earliest changes in gestation are mucosal (Chadwick and Jacquemier signs), vascular (gingival hyperemia/edema, spider angiomas, palmar erythema), and glandular (Montgomery tubercles, increased sweating), which develop in the first trimester.[4] Pigmentary changes start usually in the second trimester and pruritus starts in the late second or third trimester. Hair and nail changes as well as connective tissue changes (*striae gravidarum, molluscum fibrosum gravidarum*) commonly start in the third trimester. Vascular changes such as edema, purpura/petechiae, and hemangiomas are more likely to occur in the third trimester.

Course and Duration

Most physiologic changes resolve spontaneously at delivery or in the early postpartum period. Nevertheless, pigmentary changes, such as melasma, can persist postpartum. Hair changes can also persist, and although telogen effluvium is expected to resolve, hair may not be as thick as it was prior to pregnancy.[3] Vascular changes such as varicosities may also persist. Benign tumors that develop in pregnancy, such as skin tags (*molluscum fibrosum gravidarum*), hemangiomas, and seborrheic keratoses may not regress postpartum. Addressing the course of these changes and introducing postpartum treatment options can help alleviate patient anxiety.

TABLE 2.1	Physiologic Skin Changes of Pregnancy

Pigmentary[a]
Hyperpigmentation
Melasma
Pigmentation of scars and benign skin lesions
Darkening of preexisting pigmentation
Less common pigmentary changes

Vascular
Palmar erythema
Vascular spiders
Edema
Varicosities
Thrombosis
Cutis marmorata
Purpura
Hemangiomas
Granuloma gravidarum

Mucosal
Gingival edema/gingivitis
Other mucosal changes (pelvic organs, nasal mucosa)

Connective Tissue
Striae gravidarum
Skin tags
Hypertrophic scars
Keloids

Hair Changes
Hirsutism
Scalp hair loss/thinning
Improvement in scalp hair
Telogen effluvium
Male pattern–like alopecia

Nail Changes
Brittleness
Faster growth
Rough texture
Nail curvature
Distal onycholysis
Transverse grooving
Subungual hyperkeratosis
Longitudinal melanonychia

Glandular
Hypertrophy of the areolar sebaceous glands (Montgomery tubercles)
↑ sebaceous gland activity (third trimester)[b]
↑ eccrine gland activity (third trimester)
↓ apocrine gland activity

[a] More detailed overview shown in Table 3.1.
[b] Inconsistent change.
↑, increased; ↓, decreased.

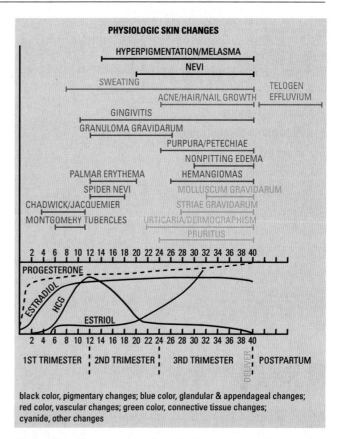

Figure 2.1. The onset of physiologic changes and respective hormonal levels during gestation. (Modified from Elling SV, Powell FC. Physiological changes in the skin during pregnancy. *Clin Dermatol.* 1997;15:35–43.)

SKIN DISEASE IN PREGNANCY

Effects of Pregnancy on Skin Disease

Pregnancy has profound effects on the endocrine and immune systems, and consequently, most diseases can be affected by gestation.[6] The vast majority of skin diseases worsens or remains stable in pregnancy. Diseases that may improve are shown in Table 2.2.[1] However, the course of these diseases is not predictable, and exacerbations during gestation are not uncommon, as is the case with atopic dermatitis and acne vulgaris.

The most common skin diseases encountered in pregnancy are shown in Table 2.3. Atopic dermatitis warrants special attention because it is the most common pregnancy dermatosis and can develop for the first time in gestation.[16] Physicians should be familiar with the presentation and management of atopic dermatitis and other inflammatory and glandular skin diseases, such as psoriasis and acne. Candida vaginitis shows a high prevalence in pregnancy and should be diagnosed and treated promptly[17]; symptomatic bacterial vaginosis also requires prompt treatment.[18] An accurate diagnosis as well as knowledge of possible risks from pharmacologic treatment (see Chs. 22 and 23) are paramount in management and patient counseling.

TABLE 2.2	Diseases That May Improve in Pregnancy
Acne vulgaris	
Atopic dermatitis	
Autoimmune progesterone dermatitis	
Behçet disease	
Chronic plaque psoriasis	
Fox–Fordyce disease	
Hidradenitis suppurativa	
Linear IgA dermatosis	
Rheumatoid arthritis	
Sarcoidosis	
Urticaria	

IgA, immunoglobulin A.

Effects of Skin Disease on Maternal and Fetal Outcomes

Maternal and fetal risks associated with skin disease in gestation are outlined in Chapters 11 through 16. Major maternal–fetal risks are encountered with psoriasis, especially generalized pustular psoriasis of pregnancy (*impetigo herpetiformis*).[19] Rheumatic skin diseases with substantial maternal and fetal risks include systemic and neonatal lupus erythematosus, systemic sclerosis, dermatomyositis, and antiphospholipid syndrome.[20] Bullous and metabolic disorders such as pemphigus vulgaris and acrodermatitis enteropathica, respectively, have also been associated with maternal and fetal risks.[1] Furthermore, infectious diseases, such as leprosy,[21] have been associated with maternal and fetal adverse effects. Major fetal risks have been reported with most viral and sexually

TABLE 2.3	Most Common Skin Diseases in Pregnancy	
Disease Category	**Most Common Skin Disease**	
Inflammatory	Atopic dermatitis	
Rheumatic	Lupus erythematosus	
Metabolic	Porphyria cutanea tarda	
Bullous	Pemphigus vulgaris	
Infectious	Infectious vaginitis	
Adnexal	Acne vulgaris	
Tumors	Benign tumors	
Genodermatoses	Neurofibromatosis type 1	

transmitted diseases (see Ch. 14), especially syphilis.[22] Prompt management of these infections is of utmost importance in decreasing such risks. Advanced melanoma is linked to serious maternal risks and can metastasize to the placenta and fetus.[23] Genodermatoses such as Ehlers Danlos syndrome, hereditary hemorrhagic telangiectasia, Marfan syndrome, and tuberous sclerosis have been associated with major complications for both the mother and fetus.[24,25]

Healthcare providers should be well aware of these risks because early recognition is crucial to improving outcomes. Planning pregnancy when the disease is inactive or well-controlled, as in systemic lupus erythematosus and leprosy, helps prevent maternal and fetal complications. A multidisciplinary management approach is of great importance in order to minimize maternal and fetal risks.

KEY POINTS

- Most common physiologic changes are pigmentary, connective tissue, and vascular, with glandular, hair, and nail changes being less common; to help alleviate unnecessary stress, the patient should be advised about their onset, course, and duration.

- Most skin diseases can worsen in gestation; the most commonly encountered diseases are atopic dermatitis, acne vulgaris, psoriasis, and infectious vaginitis; the development of benign skin tumors is also common.

- Diseases that may improve in pregnancy include acne vulgaris, autoimmune progesterone dermatitis, chronic plaque psoriasis, Behçet disease, Fox–Fordyce disease, hidradenitis suppurativa, and sarcoidosis.

- Maternal and fetal risks are encountered with a plethora of skin disease, especially infectious, rheumatic, and genodermatoses; early recognition and a multidisciplinary management approach are crucial to improving outcomes.

REFERENCES

1. Kroumpouzos G, Cohen LM. Dermatoses of pregnancy. *J Am Acad Dermatol.* 2001;45:1–19.
2. Parmley T, O'Brien TJ. Skin changes during pregnancy. *Clin Obstet Gynecol.* 1990;33:713–717.
3. Wong RC, Ellis CN. Physiologic skin changes in pregnancy. *J Am Acad Dermatol.* 1984;10:929–940.
4. Elling SV, Powell FC. Physiological changes in the skin during pregnancy. *Clin Dermatol.* 1997;15:35–43.
5. Muallem MM, Rubeiz NG. Physiological and biological skin changes in pregnancy. *Clin Dermatol.* 2006;24:80–83.
6. Winton GB. Skin diseases aggravated by pregnancy. *J Am Acad Dermatol.* 1989;20:1–13.
7. Oumeish OY, Al-Fouzan AW. Miscellaneous diseases affected by pregnancy. *Clin Dermatol.* 2006;24:113–117.

8. Rathore SP, Gupta S, Gupta V. Pattern and prevalence of physiological cutaneous changes in pregnancy: a study of 2000 antenatal women. *Indian J Dermatol Venereol Leprol.* 2011;77(3): 402.

9. Kumari R, Jaisankar TJ, Thappa DM. A clinical study of skin changes in pregnancy. *Indian J Dermatol Venereol Leprol.* 2007; 73:141.

10. Muzaffar F, Hussain I, Haroon TS. Physiologic skin changes during pregnancy: a study of 140 cases. *Int J Dermatol.* 1998;37: 429–431.

11. Estève E, Saudeau L, Pierre F, et al. Physiological cutaneous signs in normal pregnancy: a study of 60 pregnant women. *Ann Dermatol Venereol.* 1994;121:227–231.

12. Chang AL, Agredano YZ, Kimball AB. Risk factors associated with striae gravidarum. *J Am Acad Dermatol.* 2004;51:881–885.

13. Murphy KW, Dunphy B, O'Herlihy C. Increased maternal age protects against striae gravidarum. *J Obstet Gynecol.* 1992;12: 297–300.

14. Bean W, Cogswell R, Dexter M. Vascular changes of the skin in pregnancy: vascular spiders and palmar erythema. *Surg Gynecol Obstet.* 1949;88:739–752.

15. Ponnapula D, Boberg JS. Lower extremity changes experienced during pregnancy. *J Foot Ankle Surg.* 2010;49:452–458.

16. Koutroulis I, Papoutsis J, Kroumpouzos G. Atopic dermatitis in pregnancy: current status and challenges. *Obstet Gynecol Surv.* 2011;66:654–663.

17. Parveen N, Munir AA, Din I, et al. Frequency of vaginal candidiasis in pregnant women attending routine antenatal clinic. *J Coll Physicians Surg Pak.* 2008;18:154–157.

18. Centers for Disease Control and Prevention. Sexually transmitted disease treatment guidelines, 2010. *Morb Mort Wkly Rep.* 2010;17(59):1–110.

19. Vaidya D, Kroumpouzos G, Bercovitch L. Recurrent postpartum impetigo herpetiformis presenting after a "skip" pregnancy. *Acta Derm Venereol.* 2013;93:102–103.

20. Kroumpouzos G. Skin disease. In: James DK, Steer PJ, Weiner CP, et al., eds. *High-Risk Pregnancy: Management Options.* 4th ed. Philadelphia, PA: Elsevier Saunders; 2011:929–949.

21. Duncan ME. An historical and clinical review of the interaction of leprosy and pregnancy: a cycle to be broken. *Soc Sci Med.* 1993;37:457–572.

22. Winton G, Lewis C. Dermatoses of pregnancy. *J Am Acad Dermatol.* 1982;6:977–998.

23. Jhaveri MB, Driscoll MS, Grant-Kels JM. Melanoma in pregnancy. *Clin Obstet Gynecol.* 2011;54:537–545.

24. Chetty SP, Shaffer BL, Norton ME. Management of pregnancy in women with genetic disorders, Part 1: Disorders of the connective tissue, muscle, vascular, and skeletal systems. *Obstet Gynecol Surv.* 2011;66:699–709.

25. King JA, Stamilio DM. Maternal and fetal tuberous sclerosis complicating pregnancy: a case report and overview of the literature. *Am J Perinatol.* 2005;22:103–108.

CHAPTER 3

Pigmentary Changes

Jessica J. Mercer ■ Marcia Ramos-e-Silva ■ George Kroumpouzos

INTRODUCTION

Pigmentary changes are the most common physiologic changes in pregnancy and are seen in up to 90% of patients[1] (Table 3.1); this prevalence does not vary significantly among different races.[1,2] They may present as the development of pigmentation in normopigmented skin areas, the accentuation of naturally hyperpigmented skin areas, darkening of benign skin lesions, and the development of hormone-induced pigmented lesions. The most common pigmentary changes of pregnancy are melasma and hyperpigmentation, but less common pigmentary patterns can also be seen. The clinical features, pathogenesis, and treatment of these entities are highlighted in this chapter.

COMMON PIGMENTARY CHANGES

Melasma

Melasma, also referred to as chloasma or mask of pregnancy, is a hypermelanosis that presents with light to dark brown or blue-gray symmetric patches most commonly located on the face. Melasma has traditionally been reported in up to 75% of Caucasian pregnant women,[2] but its prevalence varies among different races and populations (e.g., 31% in a Pakistani population)[1] (see Ch. 2, "Prevalence"). Although onset is reported mostly in the second trimester,[1,2] onset in the first trimester is not uncommon.[1] It is thought to be associated with the hormonal changes of gestation.[2] The areas of hyperpigmentation are distributed into three common patterns: the centrofacial, which is the most common pattern and involves the entire central face (Fig. 3.1); the malar, which involves the cheeks and nose (Fig. 3.2); and the mandibular, which involves the ramus of the mandible (Fig. 3.3).[3] Mandibular melasma starts in the late reproductive years or around the onset of menopause. Partial patterns or a combination of patterns is not unusual (Fig. 3.4). Extrafacial melasma (Fig. 3.5), usually on the upper extremities and less commonly on the chest, occurs less often because it tends to be observed in older women; the vast majority of cases have been reported in postmenopausal women.

Melasma can be classified into four types based on the location of pigment within the skin when viewed under a Wood lamp: epidermal (most common type[1,2]), dermal, mixed, and indeterminate. Lesions that are enhanced when viewed with a Wood lamp predominantly contain epidermal pigment, and those that are not enhanced are predominantly dermal. Melasma is considered mixed when melanin is located in both the epidermis and the dermis. In fact, the mixed type is much more common than previously thought because recent histopathologic studies have shown that dermal melanin deposition can be seen in a significant percentage of cases of the epidermal type.[4] Therefore, correlation between Wood lamp examinations and histopathologic findings may not be as accurate. Indeterminate melasma is seen in patients with very dark skin.

Melasma typically improves spontaneously in the postpartum period but may recur in subsequent pregnancies or secondary to hormonal therapies. Application of a broad-spectrum sunscreen in pregnancy is essential because melasma worsens with exposure to ultraviolet and visible light. Treatment of melasma in pregnancy is not recommended, and camouflage can be used for cosmetic reasons. When therapeutic intervention is indicated postpartum, the depth of pigment deposition must be taken into consideration because the dermal type of melasma is more resistant to treatment than the epidermal. Topical medications that have been evaluated in randomized controlled trials (RCTs) and that can be used postpartum are listed in Table 3.2.[5] Hydroquinone is the current standard[5,6] and is often combined with a topical retinoid and a mild topical steroid[7,8] or with other topical agents such as glycolic or kojic acid.[9,10] A triple combination cream consisting of 4% hydroquinone, 0.01% fluocinolone acetonide, and 0.05% tretinoin is often the recommended initial treatment.[7,8] Azelaic acid may be helpful in mild melasma and is safe in pregnant and nursing mothers (pregnancy category B).[9,10] For challenging cases, such as recalcitrant dermal or mixed melasma, postpartum treatment with cosmetic procedures is typically required (those evaluated in RCTs are listed in Table 3.3). Chemical peels[10–12] (Fig. 3.6) and device-based therapies,[13–18] including laser and intense pulsed light, may be effective in resistant cases but must be utilized with caution in patients at risk for dyschromia, such as dark-skinned individuals, because they may cause hyper- or hypopigmentation. Device-based therapies have shown mild to modest efficacy. Outcomes are better when the previous procedures are combined with topical hydroquinone and/or other topical medications. Dermabrasion[19] and microdermabrasion[20] have been used with some success but have not been evaluated in RCTs. The safety of these topical medications and procedures during lactation is discussed in Chapters 23 and 25.

TABLE 3.1	Patterns of Pigmentary Changes in Pregnancy

Common Pigmentary Changes
- Melasma
- Hyperpigmentation

Less Common Pigmentary Changes
- Pseudoacanthosis nigricans
- Confluent and reticulated papillomatosis of Gougerot and Carteaud-like pigmentation
- Localized reticulate pigmentation
- Dermal melanocytosis
- Idiopathic eruptive macular pigmentation
- Nevoid hyperkeratosis of the nipple and/or areola
- Verrucous areolar pigmentation

Darkening of Preexisting Pigmentation
- Acanthosis nigricans
- Pigmentary demarcation lines

Darkening of Benign Skin Lesions
- Melanocytic nevi
- Skin tags
- Seborrheic keratoses
- Scars

Postinflammatory Pigmentation

Jaundice

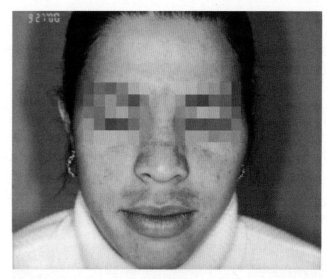

Figure 3.1. The centrofacial pattern of melasma with accentuation on the nose and upper lip; the philtrum is relatively spared.

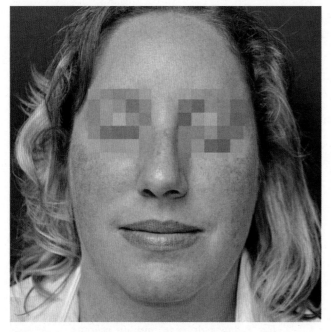

Figure 3.2. The malar pattern of melasma with accentuation on the cheeks and nose.

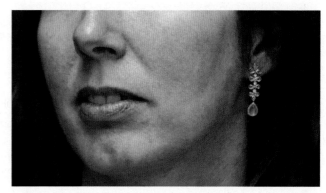

Figure 3.3. The mandibular pattern of melasma showing pigmentation of mandibular ramus. (Courtesy of Dr. Mariana Soirefmann.)

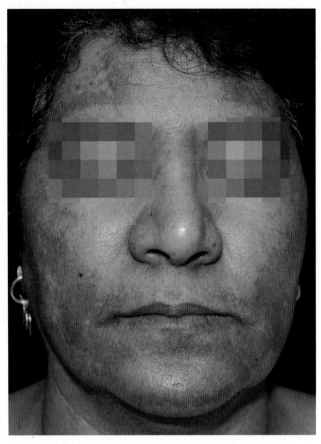

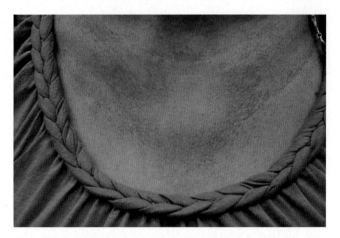

Figure 3.5. Extrafacial melasma on the upper chest.

Figure 3.4. The mixed pattern of melasma with accentuation on the lateral forehead, the lateral cheeks, and the chin.

TABLE 3.2	Topical Medications for Melasma in Randomized Controlled Trials (Postpartum Options)	
Agent	**Mechanism of Action**	**Special Considerations**
Hydroquinone 2, 4%[6–10]	Inhibits tyrosinase leading to decreased production of melanin	Typically combined with tretinoin and steroid; overuse may result in skin darkening (ochronosis)
Azelaic acid 20%[35,36]	Dicarboxylic acid inhibits tyrosinase	Successfully combined with adapalene ± glycolic acid peels; no potential for significant AEs
Kojic acid[10]	Inactivates tyrosinase by chelation of copper	Typically combined with hydroquinone; potential for sensitization
Retinoic acid 0.025%, 0.05%, 0.1%[6]	Influences melanosome transfer	Typically combined with hydroquinone and topical steroid
Topical steroid[7]	Influences melanocyte cellular functions	Overuse may result in topical adverse effects, such as atrophy, telangiectasia, and acne
Ellagic acid 1%[37]	Antioxidant that acts as tyrosinase substrate potentially inhibiting melanogenesis pathway	Naturally derived from plant extracts or synthetically produced, both of which demonstrate improvement in hyperpigmentation
Rucinol 0.1, 0.3%[38]	Resorcinol derivative that inhibits tyrosinase and tyrosinase-related protein-1	Demonstrated efficacy but risk of mild irritation (i.e., redness, dryness, burning, pruritus)
Arbutin 1%[37]	Hydroquinone derivative from bearberry plant; inhibits tyrosinase	Considered to have fewer AEs than hydroquinone
Oligopeptide[39]	Inhibits tyrosinase	Promising topical with favorable cytotoxicity and efficacy profile when compared to hydroquinone

AEs, adverse effects.

TABLE 3.3	Procedures for Melasma Evaluated in Randomized Controlled Trials (Postpartum Options)	
Agent/Device	**Mechanism of Action**	**Special Considerations**
Chemical Peels		
Glycolic acid 20%–70%[11,16]	Promotes exfoliation of stratum corneum and dispersion of melanin pigment	Risk of PIH
Salicylic acid 20%–30%[17]	Exhibits keratolytic, anti-inflammatory, and comedolytic properties	Risk of PIH
Trichloroacetic acid 20%[10]	Precipitates epidermal proteins and cell necrosis	Risk of PIH
Jessner solution (salicylic acid, lactic acid, resorcinol)[10,17]	Disrupts corneocyte cohesion	Risk of PIH
Amino fruit acid 20%–60%[16]	Carboxylated acidic amino acids with antioxidant and exfoliating effects	Promising in Rx of photopigmentation
Lasers		
Ablative -CO2[18,19] -Erbium[20]	Ablative skin resurfacing	Risk of PIH or hypopigmentation
Q-switched -Alexandrite[18,19] -Nd:YAG[21]	Disrupts pigment using short pulse, high power delivery	Nd:YAG may carry smaller risk of dyspigmentation as AE
Fractionated[22]	Produces microscopic areas of thermal necrosis	Increased efficacy when used in combination with tyrosinase inhibitor
Other Devices		
Intense pulsed light[23]	Converts light energy to heat energy to heat and destroy melanin	Risk of dyspigmentation, blistering, and scarring

AE, adverse effect; CO2, carbon dioxide; Nd:YAG, neodymium-doped yttrium aluminum garnet; PIH, postinflammatory hyperpigmentation; Rx, treatment.

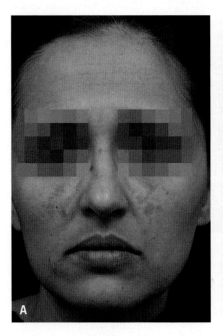 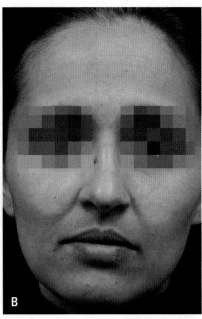

Figure 3.6. Melasma, malar type. (**A**) Before chemical peels. (**B**) After a series of monthly trichloroacetic acid peels in combination with twice daily application of a triple combination cream consisting of 4% hydroquinone, 0.01% fluocinolone acetonide, and 0.05% tretinoin. (Courtesy of Dr. Jason Michaels.)

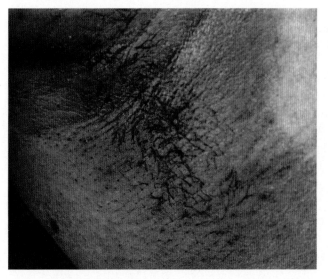

Figure 3.7. Hyperpigmentation of the axilla.

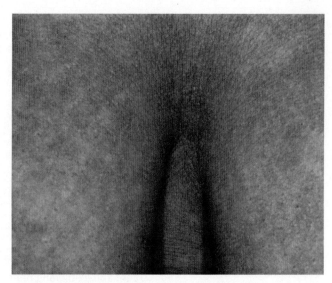

Figure 3.9. Hyperpigmentation of the chest.

Hyperpigmentation

Hyperpigmentation commonly occurs during pregnancy and may be seen in up to 90% of women.[2] Hyperpigmentation may manifest as an accentuation of naturally pigmented areas such as the nipples, areolae, genital skin, axillae, and inner thighs (Figs. 3.7 and 3.8). Additionally, observed skin findings include pigmentation of normopigmented skin (Figs. 3.9 and 3.10) as well as generalized hypermelanosis. When normopigmented skin is involved, there is the occasional development of specific patterns of darkening. Examples of this phenomenon include *linea nigra* (Fig. 3.11), which results from pigmentation of *linea alba* and manifests as a longitudinal band of hyperpigmentation from the xiphoid process to the symphysis pubis, and secondary areolae (Fig. 3.12), which is the darkening of the skin adjacent to the areolae. **Vulvar melanosis**, also known as vulvar lentiginosis, presents as pigmented macules on the vulvar mucosa and may

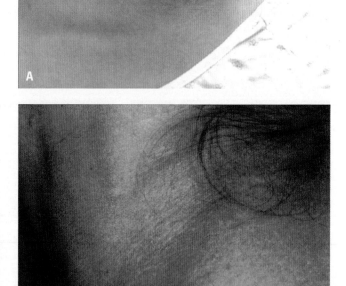

Figure 3.10. Hyperpigmentation of the neck. (**A**) Spotty on the lower neck, and (**B**) mild, confluent.

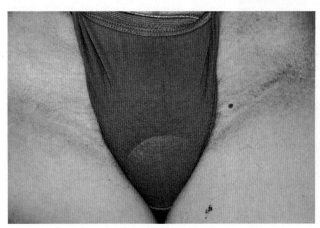

Figure 3.8. Hyperpigmentation of the inguinal folds.

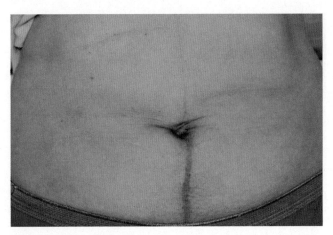

Figure 3.11. *Linea nigra* is a very common pigmentary change of pregnancy.

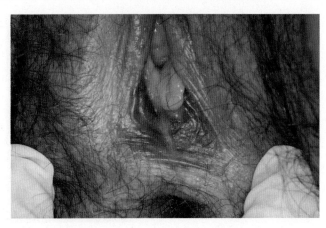

Figure 3.13. Vulvar melanosis that developed in pregnancy. In cases in which the association with pregnancy is not clear, vulvar melanosis may require a biopsy in order to rule out atypical melanocytic lesions. (Courtesy of Dr. Joe Brooks.)

also develop during gestation (Fig. 3.13). The physiology of hyperpigmentation may be related to elevated serum levels of melanocyte-stimulating hormone, estrogen, and possibly progesterone.[21] Pigmentation typically normalizes in the postpartum period.

LESS COMMON PIGMENTARY CHANGES

Worsening of acanthosis nigricans in pregnancy secondary to gestational diabetes and/or glucose intolerance has been reported. **Pseudoacanthosis nigricans (pseudoacanthotic changes)** has been shown to arise without evidence of glucose intolerance.[22] Clinically, pseudoacanthosis nigricans presents with symmetric, hyperpigmented, velvety plaques on any skin site, but most commonly on the posterolateral neck, axillae,

groin, and antecubital and popliteal fossae (Figs. 3.14 and 3.15A). The increase in estrogen levels during pregnancy is thought to be implicated in the pathogenesis of this pigmentary abnormality. High estrogen levels stimulate melanogenesis, thus accounting for the pigmentary changes.[21] The velvety skin changes seen in pseudoacanthosis nigricans have been associated with decreased extracellular matrix viscosity in the setting of weakened or altered glycosaminoglycans; these glycosaminoglycans can be secondary to high estrogen levels.[23] Pseudoacanthotic changes have been reported to resolve in the postpartum period when estrogen levels return to prepregnancy levels (Fig. 3.15).[22] **Confluent and reticulated papillomatosis of Gougerot and Carteaud-like pigmentary changes** have been observed in pregnancy (Fig. 3.16). A case of **localized reticulate hyperpigmentation** has been reported.[24]

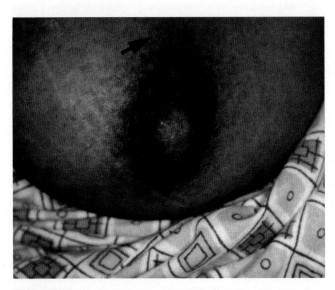

Figure 3.12. Hyperpigmentation of the areola and secondary areola *(arrow)*.

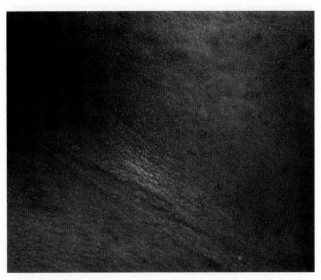

Figure 3.14. Pseudoacanthotic changes: confluent, velvety, hyperpigmented plaques on the neck in an Asian patient.

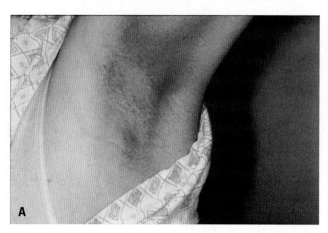
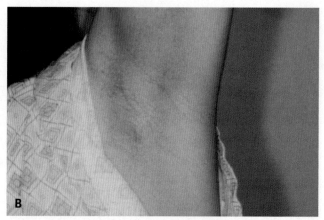

Figure 3.15. Pseudoacanthotic changes of the axilla. **(A)** During pregnancy, and **(B)** spontaneous postpartum improvement. (Reproduced from Kroumpouzos G, Avgerinou G, Granter SR. Acanthosis nigricans without diabetes during pregnancy. *Br J Dermatol.* 2002;146:925–928.)

Acquired dermal melanocytosis presents with the development of asymptomatic brown to gray to blue macules on the trunk or extremities (Fig. 3.17). Skin lesions in the acquired variant share the same histologic feature of melanocytes in the dermis as their congenital counterparts: Mongolian spots, nevi of Ito, and nevi of Ota. The pathogenesis of acquired dermal melanocytosis in pregnancy may be related to the activation of preexisting immature melanocytes due to estrogen or progesterone.[25] It is believed that there is a faulty migration of melanocytes from the neural crest to the epidermis leading to misplaced dermal melanocytes, which become activated from a dormant state when exposed to high hormone levels of pregnancy.[26]

Idiopathic eruptive macular pigmentation is a rare condition that presents with brownish, nonconfluent, asymptomatic macules involving the trunk, neck, and proximal extremities in children or adolescents (Fig. 3.18) in the absence of preceding inflammatory lesions and previous drug exposure. Histopathologic features include basal cell layer hyperpigmentation, prominent dermal melanophages without basal cell layer damage or lichenoid inflammatory infiltrate, and a normal mast cell count.[27] Both the development and a worsening of the existing disease has been associated with pregnancy.[28,29] Because of the usual onset in adolescence and the reported associations with pregnancy, hormonal factors are thought to play a key role. Pigmented lesions usually resolve spontaneously within months to a few years.

Nevoid hyperkeratosis of the nipple and/or areola is an asymptomatic, hyperpigmented, verrucous thickening of the nipple and/or areola (see Ch. 5, Fig. 5.11).

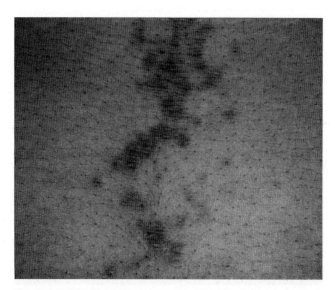

Figure 3.16. Confluent and reticulated papillomatosis of Gougerot and Carteaud-like pigmentation of the abdomen that developed in pregnancy.

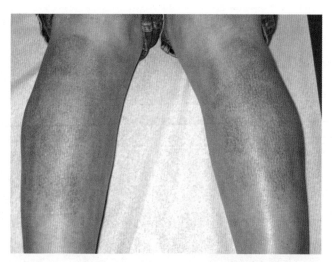

Figure 3.17. Dermal melanocytosis on the shins developed in pregnancy. (Reproduced from Kroumpouzos G. Skin disease. In: James DK, Steer PJ, Weiner CP, et al., eds. *High-Risk Pregnancy: Management Options.* 4th ed. Philadelphia, PA: Elsevier Saunders; 2011:929–949.)

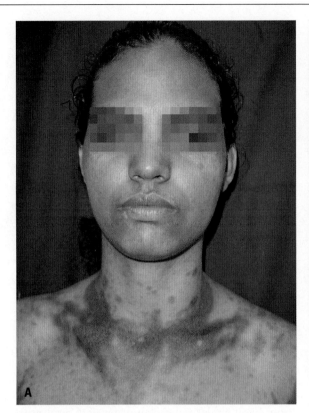 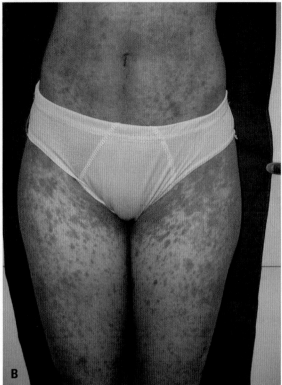

Figure 3.18. Idiopathic eruptive macular pigmentation in a Brazilian woman that developed in pregnancy. **(A)** On the face, neck, and chest. **(B)** On the abdomen and proximal lower extremities. (Courtesy of Dr. Dominique Fausto de Souza.)

Several cases have demonstrated an association with changing estrogen levels (i.e., the development of lesions *de novo* with both puberty and pregnancy, progression from unilateral to bilateral involvement in pregnancy, and spontaneous resolution of lesions postpartum).[30] A case of **verrucous areolar hyperpigmentation** has been reported; however, it is uncertain whether this entity represents a form of nevoid hyperkeratosis of the areola.[31]

DARKENING OF PREEXISTING PIGMENTATION

Pigmentary demarcation lines (PDLs), also called Voigt or Futcher lines, are boundaries of abrupt transition between lighter pigmented skin and darker pigmented skin occurring due to differences in melanocyte distribution. PDLs may develop or darken during gestation. Type B PDLs, noticed on the posteromedial aspect of the lower extremities (Fig. 3.19), and type A PDLs, located

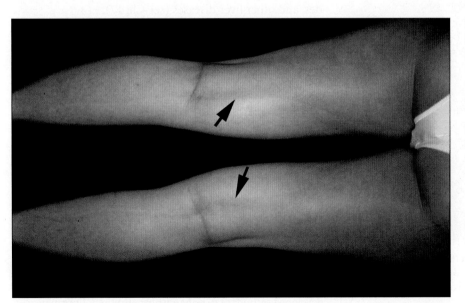

Figure 3.19. Type B pigmentary demarcation lines along the posteromedial aspect of the lower extremities *(arrows)* developed in this 28-year-old Caucasian female during the third to fourth month of her first pregnancy. They disappeared on the thighs within 3 to 4 months postpartum but persisted on the legs, although barely noticeable. (Courtesy of Dr. Annalisa Patrizi.)

on the lateral upper arms, have been observed in pregnancy. In most cases, PDLs appear in the third trimester and spontaneously regress or become barely noticeable within months of the delivery.[32,33] Because type A and B PDLs correspond to Voigt lines, which demarcate the distribution of peripheral nerves, it has been suggested that clinically inconspicuous melanocytes are present within the boundaries of specific nerves, and hyperpigmentation of these areas is triggered by an increase in hormones during pregnancy.[32] Also, because PDLs are occasionally associated with erythema, the potential for neurogenic inflammation and the obstruction of cutaneous vasculature by an enlarged uterus during pregnancy has been suggested to play a role in the pathogenesis.[34]

PIGMENTATION OF BENIGN TUMORS

Nevi, **seborrheic keratoses**, **skin tags**, **lentigines**, and **scars** may become hyperpigmented during pregnancy (Fig. 3.20). Nevi may also enlarge, especially if they are located on areas of skin distention such as the abdomen.[1] Darkening and enlargement of nevi can be explained by the upregulation of estrogen and progesterone receptors on the surface of nevus cells. Scar darkening, particularly pigmentation of the lower segment of a cesarean section, is also often reported (Fig. 3.21).

POSTINFLAMMATORY HYPERPIGMENTATION

Inflammatory dermatoses occurring in pregnancy, such as polymorphic eruption of pregnancy, pemphigoid gestationis, impetigo herpetiformis, atopic dermatitis, and

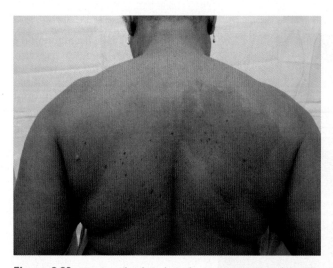

Figure 3.20. Nevi and seborrheic keratoses increased in size and became more pigmented in this Brazilian pregnant female. Dermatosis papulosa nigra also worsened in pregnancy. (Courtesy of Dr. Tania Cestari.)

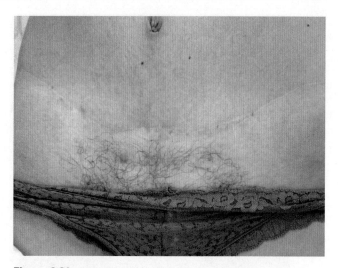

Figure 3.21. Pigmentation of the lower segment cesarean section in pregnancy. (Courtesy of Dr. Jenny Murase.)

others, may cause **postinflammatory hyperpigmentation** (Fig. 3.22). In some instances, hypopigmentation, rather than hyperpigmentation, follows the inflammatory process. Inflammation may cause a loss of melanin from basal epidermal melanocytes with accumulation in the melanophages of the upper dermis, or it may induce melanocytes to increase their pigment production. Treatment of the underlying condition often halts progression of the dyspigmentation.

JAUNDICE

Jaundice, the yellowish discoloration of the skin, conjunctiva, and mucous membranes due to hyperbilirubinemia, may be seen in cholestasis of pregnancy, acute fatty liver of pregnancy, preeclampsia-associated HELLP (hemolysis, elevated liver enzymes, low platelets) syndrome, hepatitides, and other liver diseases (see Ch. 17).

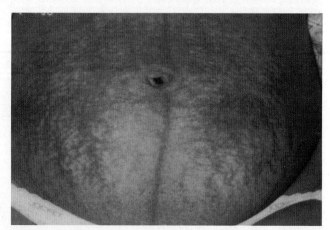

Figure 3.22. Extensive postinflammatory hyperpigmentation developed secondary to polymorphic eruption of pregnancy.

- Pigmentary abnormalities are not associated with maternal or fetal risks but may be a source of concern and distress for the pregnant patient; therefore, recognition is essential.

- Pigmentary changes can be seen in up to 90% of pregnant women; the most common are hyperpigmentation and melasma.

- Melasma is classified by distribution (centrofacial, malar, mandibular), or by depth of pigment (predominantly epidermal versus predominantly dermal), but a combination of types may occur.

- Less common pigmentary patterns that can develop in pregnancy include, among others, pseudoacanthosis nigricans, dermal melanocytosis, pigmentary demarcation lines, idiopathic eruptive macular pigmentation, and nevoid hyperkeratosis of the nipple and/or areola.

- Pigmentary abnormalities often resolve once estrogen and progesterone return to prepregnancy levels; for persistent cases, dermatologists should be familiar with topical medications and procedures that can be employed postpartum and should be able to counsel the patient appropriately.

REFERENCES

1. Muzaffar F, Hussain I, Haroon TS. Physiologic skin changes during pregnancy: a study of 140 cases. *Int J Dermatol.* 1998;37: 429–431.
2. Wong RC, Ellis CN. Physiologic skin changes in pregnancy. *J Am Acad Dermatol.* 1984;10:929–940.
3. Sheth VM, Pandya AG. Melasma: a comprehensive update: part I. *J Am Acad Dermatol.* 2011;65:689–697.
4. Grimes PE, Yamada N, Bhawan J. Light microscopic, immuno-histochemical, and ultrastructural alterations in patients with melasma. *Am J Dermatopathol.* 2005;27:96–101.
5. Ball Arefiev KL, Hantash BM. Advances in the treatment of melasma: a review of the recent literature. *Derm Surg.* 2012;38: 971–984.
6. Haddad AL, Matos LF, Brunstein F, et al. A clinical, prospective, randomized, double-blind trial comparing skin whitening complex with hydroquinone vs. placebo in the treatment of melasma. *Int J Dermatol.* 2003;42:153–156.
7. Ferreira CT, Hassun K, Sittart A, et al. A comparison of triple combination cream and hydroquinone 4% cream for the treatment of moderate to severe facial melasma. *J Cosmet Dermatol.* 2007;6:36–39.
8. Taylor SC, Torok H, Jones T, et al. Efficacy and safety of a new triple-combination agent for the treatment of facial melasma. *Cutis.* 2003;72:67–72.
9. Garcia A, Fulton JE. The combination of glycolic acid and hydroquinone or kojic acid for the treatment of melasma and related conditions. *Dermatol Surg.* 1996;22:443–447.
10. Azzam OA, Leheta TM, Nagui NA, et al. Different therapeutic modalities for treatment of melasma. *J Cosmet Dermatol.* 2009;8:275–281.
11. Ilknur T, Biçak MU, Demirtaşoğlu M, et al. Glycolic acid peels versus amino fruit acid peels in the treatment of melasma. *Dermatol Surg.* 2010;36:490–495.
12. Ejaz A, Raza N, Iftikhar N, et al. Comparison of 30% salicylic acid with Jessner's solution for superficial chemical peeling in epidermal melasma. *J Coll Physicians Surg Pak.* 2008;18:205–208.
13. Nouri K, Bowes L, Chartier T, et al. Combination treatment of melasma with pulsed CO2 laser followed by Q-switched alexandrite laser: a pilot study. *Dermatol Surg.* 1999;25:494–497.
14. Angsuwarangsee S, Polnikorn N. Combined ultrapulse CO2 laser and Q-switched alexandrite laser compared with Q-switched alexandrite laser alone for refractory melasma: split-face design. *Dermatol Surg.* 2003;29:59–64.
15. Manaloto RM, Alster T. Erbium:YAG laser resurfacing for refractory melasma. *Dermatol Surg.* 1999;25:121–123.
16. Wattanakrai P, Mornchan R, Eimpunth S. Low-fluence Q-switched neodymium-doped yttrium aluminum garnet (1,064 nm) laser for the treatment of facial melasma in Asians. *Dermatol Surg.* 2010;36:76–87.
17. Trelles MA, Velez M, Gold MH. The treatment of melasma with topical creams alone, CO2 fractional ablative resurfacing alone, or a combination of the two: a comparative study. *J Drugs Dermatol.* 2010;9:315–322.
18. Goldman MP, Gold MH, Palm MD, et al. Sequential treatment with triple combination cream and intense pulsed light is more efficacious than sequential treatment with an inactive (control) cream and intense pulsed light in patients with moderate to severe melasma. *Dermatol Surg.* 2011;37:224–233.
19. Kunachak S, Leelaudomlipi P, Wongwaisayawan S. Dermabrasion: a curative treatment for melasma. *Aesthetic Plast Surg.* 2001;25:114–117.
20. Kauvar AN. Successful treatment of melasma using a combination of microdermabrasion and Q-switched Nd:YAG lasers. *Lasers Surg Med.* 2012;44:117–124.
21. Snell RS, Bischitz PG. The effect of large doses of estrogen and estrogen and progesterone on melanin pigmentation. *J Invest Dermatol.* 1960;35:73–82.
22. Kroumpouzos G, Avgerinou G, Granter SR. Acanthosis nigricans without diabetes during pregnancy. *Br J Dermatol.* 2002; 146:925–928.
23. Stone OJ. Acanthosis nigricans—decreased extracellular matrix viscosity: cancer, obesity, diabetes, corticosteroids, somatotrophin. *Med Hypotheses.* 1993;40:154–157.
24. Schiller M, Kütting B, Luger T, et al. Localized reticulate hyperpigmentation. *Hautarzt.* 1999;50:580–585.
25. Mizoguchi M, Murakami F, Ito M, et al. Clinical, pathological, and etiologic aspects of acquired dermal melanocytosis. *Pigment Cell Res.* 1997;10:176–183.
26. Mizushima J, Nogita T, Higaki Y, et al. Dormant melanocytes in the dermis: do dermal melanocytes of acquired dermal melanocytosis exist from birth? [letter]. *Br J Dermatol.* 1998;139:349–350.
27. Sanz de Galdeano C, Leaute-Labreze C, Bioulac-Sage P, et al. Idiopathic eruptive macular pigmentation: report of five patients. *Pediatr Dermatol.* 1996;13:274–277.
28. de Souza DF, Cunha AC, Pineiro-Maceira J, et al. Idiopathic eruptive macular pigmentation associated with pregnancy. *Int J Dermatol.* 2010;49:810–812.
29. Milobratovic D, Djordjevic S, Vukicevic J, et al. Idiopathic eruptive macular pigmentation associated with pregnancy and Hashimoto thyroiditis. *J Am Acad Dermatol.* 2005;52:919–921.
30. Krishnan RS, Angel TA, Roark TR, et al. Nevoid hyperkeratosis of the nipple and/or areola: a report of two cases and a review of the literature. *Int J Dermatol.* 2002;41:775–777.

31. Garcia RL. Verrucose areolar hyperpigmentation of pregnancy. *Arch Dermatol.* 1973;107:774.

32. Nakama T, Hashikawa K, Higuchi M, et al. Pigmentary demarcation lines associated with pregnancy. *Clin Exp Dermatol.* 2009;34:e573–576.

33. James WD, Meltzer MS, Guill MA, et al. Pigmentary demarcation lines associated with pregnancy. *J Am Acad Dermatol.* 1984;11:438–440.

34. Ozawa H, Rokugo M, Aoyama H. Pigmentary demarcation lines of pregnancy with erythema. *Dermatology.* 1993;187: 134–136.

35. Erbil H, Sezer E, Taştan B, et al. Efficacy and safety of serial glycolic acid peels and a topical regimen in the treatment of recalcitrant melasma. *J Dermatol.* 2007;34:25–30.

36. Balina LM, Graupe K. The treatment of melasma. 20% azelaic acid versus 4% hydroquinone cream. *Int J Dermatol.* 1991;30: 893–895.

37. Ertam I, Mutlu B, Unal I, et al. Efficiency of ellagic acid and arbutin in melasma: a randomized, prospective, open-label study. *J Dermatol.* 2008;35:570–574.

38. Khemis A, Kaiafa A, Queille-Roussel C, et al. Evaluation of efficacy and safety of rucinol serum in patients with melasma: a randomized controlled trial. *Br J Dermatol.* 2007;156: 997–1004.

39. Hantash BM, Jimenez F. A split-face, double-blind, randomized and placebo-controlled pilot evaluation of a novel oligopeptide for the treatment of recalcitrant melasma. *J Drugs Dermatol.* 2009;8:732–735.

CHAPTER 4

Vascular Changes

Jyoti P. Mundi ■ Miriam K. Pomeranz

INTRODUCTION

Vascular changes have been reported as being more common in Caucasian (83%)[1] than in Indian (26%),[2] Pakistani (34%),[3] and African American pregnant women.[4] They occur secondarily to the production of placental hormones, such as human chorionic gonadotropin, adrenocorticotropic-like substance, and thyrotropin-releasing hormone, as well as maternal hormones. Plasma volume increases to 149% of normal levels by the end of gestation, and blood flow to skin increases 4 to 16 times in the first 2 months of pregnancy and doubles again during the third month.[5] A microscopic evaluation of nail fold capillaries (capillaroscopy) shows a gradually enlarging pericapillary papilla reflecting water retention in the interstitial tissue. Additionally, increases in capillary blood flow velocity in the first trimester and viscosity at low shear rates at the end of pregnancy have been noted.[6] This dramatic vascular increase in the dermis accounts for significant blood loss with an incision in the skin of a pregnant woman, especially with major procedures such as cesarean section. The altered circulatory milieu may manifest with a number of cutaneous and mucosal changes. The course and management of these changes are highlighted in this chapter (Table 4.1).

SPIDER ANGIOMAS

Spider angiomas (spider nevi, nevi aranei, vascular spiders, arterial spiders) are dilated capillaries radiating from a central pulsatile punctum, representing an afferent arteriole, with surrounding erythema that may extend several millimeters beyond the visible vessels (Figs. 4.1 and 4.2). Pressure of the punctum produces blanching. Lesions may be warm to the touch. Their presence has been attributed to high levels of estrogens and angiogenesis factors during gestation. Spider angiomas occur in approximately 67% of pregnant Caucasian women[4] versus 10% to 15% of healthy, nonpregnant patients.[7] However, they are only reported in about 11% of pregnant African American women[4] and 1.4% of Pakistani patients,[3] possibly because they are less noticeable in patients of color.[4] Spider angiomas tend to appear in the second to fifth months and increase in size and number until parturition. They are most notable in areas drained by the superior vena cava such as the neck, face (particularly around the eyes), upper chest, arms, and hands. Approximately 75% of lesions fade by the seventh week postpartum.[4] Spider angiomas rarely disappear completely, and recurrences and enlargement during subsequent pregnancies have been reported.[7]

A pulsed dye laser (PDL) is the treatment of choice for persistent lesions (Fig. 4.3). The use of 577-nm PDL in the treatment of spider telangiectasia was first reported by Polla, Tan, and Garden, where all six cases treated had >75% clearance after an average of two treatments.[8] Geronemus treated 12 children with facial spider telangiectases with a 585-nm PDL, producing complete resolution without adverse effects after one treatment in 11 children[9]; similar results were reported in an Australian study.[10] Spider nevi with an elevated central point require a higher fluence, more treatments, and can recur.[11] Treatment can be complicated by transient purpura, blistering, scab formation,[10] and transient hyperpigmentation.[9] Intense pulsed light is another effective treatment modality.[12] Fine needle electrodessication at low voltage can be applied to the center of the punctum until the vessel blanches; radiating tributaries may be obliterated in the same manner.[13] Still, treatment can be complicated by pain, purpura, bleeding, altered pigmentation, and scarring.[14] Cryosurgery is another alternative to fine needle electrodessication for people with pale complexions, especially those with diffuse lesions with multiple feeding vessels.[15] However, it can be complicated by pain, edema/blister formation, hyper- or hypopigmentation, and scar formation.

PALMAR ERYTHEMA

Palmar erythema has been reported in approximately 63% of Caucasian, 35% of African American,[3] and 12% to 19% of Indian/Pakistani pregnant patients.[2,3] It develops by the second month of pregnancy in one-third of Caucasian patients, usually before vascular spiders appear, and resolves by the seventh week postpartum in 91% of cases.[4] Palmar erythema occurs in pregnancy in two distinct clinical presentations: (1) diffuse erythema of the entire palm with accompanying cyanosis and pallor (Fig. 4.4), similar to that observed in patients with cirrhosis and hyperthyroidism and (2) mottled erythema that is most pronounced over the thenar and hypothenar eminences, near the metacarpophalangeal joints, and the fleshy tips of the fingers. The former is more common. It may be intermittently accompanied by a burning sensation.[14]

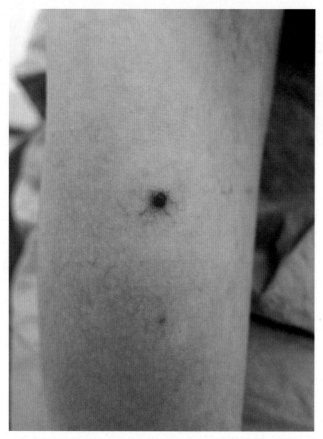

Figure 4.1. A spider angioma in pregnancy: A red papule with radiating branches and surrounding erythema on the arm.

EDEMA

Nonpitting edema of the extremities and face may develop in 70% and 50% of patients, respectively, usually during the last trimester.[7] It presents as firm, pinkish puffiness (Figs. 4.5 and 4.6). It is more pronounced in the morning and improves with activity throughout

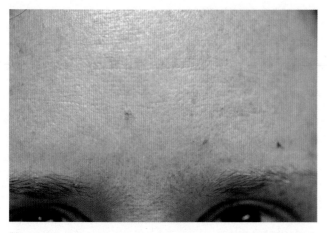

Figure 4.2. Spider angiomas in pregnancy: Small red telangiectatic macules on the forehead. Distribution around the eyes is common. (Courtesy of Dr. George Kroumpouzos.)

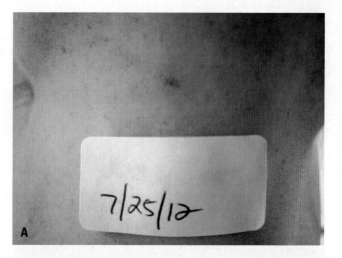

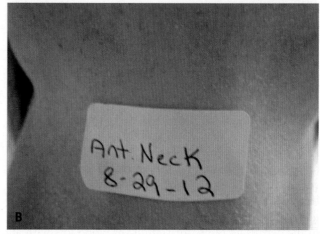

Figure 4.3. A spider angioma on the anterior neck of a pregnant patient. (**A**) Prior to treatment. (**B**) One month after treatment with a pulsed dye laser (Vbeam, Candela; 595 nm, 10-mm spot size, 1.5-msec pulse duration, fluence 8 J/cm²), the lesion resolved. (Courtesy of Dr. Julie K. Karen.)

the day.[14] Transient physiologic hypercortisolism and increased estrogen levels result in salt and water retention, vascular expansion, and increased capillary permeability. Elevated estrogen levels induce nitric oxide–mediated vasodilatation, which compounds the edematous effect. Additionally, pitting edema resulting from fluid retention may develop in dependent areas. The prolonged gravid uterine compression of pelvic and femoral vessels elevates hydrostatic pressures and impairs venous return, thus contributing to fluid retention in the lower extremities. Cardiac and renal abnormalities as well as eclampsia/preeclampsia must be excluded. Edema can result in compression neuropathies, such as carpal tunnel syndrome,[16] thus causing significant discomfort; these changes resolve postpartum. Measures to decrease edema[17] are summarized in Table 4.1.

    The vulva can be affected by the hemodynamic changes during pregnancy because it has a thin epithelium and loose connective tissue. However, massive vulvar edema[18,19] deserves special attention because it can signify impending

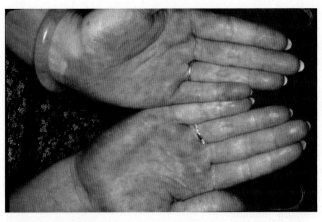

Figure 4.4. Palmar erythema in pregnancy: Diffuse mottling of the entire palm with a speckling of pale or cyanotic areas. (Courtesy of Dr. Lisa M. Cohen.)

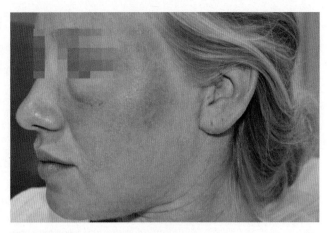

Figure 4.6. Facial edema in a pregnant patient. Note the puffiness of the upper and lower eyelids.

cardiovascular collapse and maternal death, especially if accompanied by fever and leukocytosis. It is important to promptly evaluate the patient's circulatory status. Preeclampsia, characterized by hypertension, proteinuria, and generalized edema, is a potential cause of massive vulvar edema. The differential diagnosis also includes infectious, neoplastic, inflammatory, and posttraumatic disorders. A history and physical examination and laboratory studies including a complete blood count, liver and renal function tests, urinary evaluation, an infectious workup, and imaging studies are needed.

VENOUS ABNORMALITIES

Varicosities have been reported in up to 40% of pregnancies in Western populations.[7] Their prevalence is much lower (2.8%) in Pakistani patients, which was attributed to work habits (sitting position).[3] Enlarged and tortuous veins may be visible on the lower extremities (Fig. 4.7A), perianal area (hemorrhoids), or in the vulvar region (Fig. 4.7B). An increase in iliac blood volume and flow, impaired venous

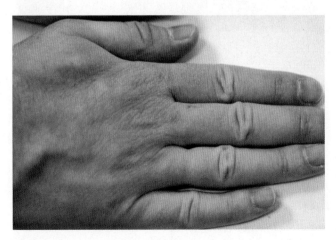

Figure 4.5. Edema of the upper extremity in pregnancy: Note the indentation due to edema upon removal of a ring.

return, and secondary valvular incompetence contribute to their development. However, varicosities can develop in the third month of gestation, prior to a significant increase in intrapelvic pressures. Patients may have a familial predisposition.[7] Relaxin, an estrogen-dependent hormone, weakens collagen and elastin and may contribute to vascular distention and fragility. Increased maternal age and parity also result in a loss of valvular patency and may predispose a patient to varicosities.[17] Prolonged sitting and standing, elastic garters, and panty girdles contribute to venous return obstruction and may be exacerbating factors.[7]

Varicosities may cause pain. Thrombosis occurs in less than 10% of pregnant women,[20] and thromboembolic events are more common during the first trimester. Plasma levels of fibrinogen and coagulation factors, such as those produced by the liver (VII, VIII, IX, and X), are usually elevated in pregnancy.[16] Hemorrhoids can cause pain and bleeding and, in contrast to leg varicosities, often produce thrombi during pregnancy.[7] Occasionally, phlebitis may occur.[14] *Phlegmasia alba dolens*, an edematous swelling of the leg following childbirth due to iliofemoral thrombosis, and *phlegmasia cerulea dolens*, which manifests with severe pain, edema, and cyanosis of a limb due to massive venous occlusion, are rare complications.[20] Vaginal and perineal varicosities may cause difficulties with delivery.[16] Varicosities tend to regress postpartum but, often, not completely.[7]

Intrapartum treatment options for varicose veins and hemorrhoids are summarized in Table 4.1. It is recommended that pregnant patients wait until at least 6 to 12 months after pregnancy before treating persistent varicosities. Postpartum treatment options include surgery, sclerotherapy (Fig. 4.8), and laser or radiofrequency endoluminal ablation.[21]

VASOMOTOR INSTABILITY

Increased estrogen levels may trigger hypothalamic fluctuations, thus resulting in vasomotor instability. Signs of vasomotor instability include flushing, pallor, hot and

TABLE 4.1	**Summary of Management Options**	
Entity	**Therapeutic Recommendation During Pregnancy**	**Therapeutic Options Postpartum**
Spider angiomas and hemangiomas	Observation and reassurance	Pulsed dye laser,[8–11] intense pulsed light,[12] electrodessication,[13,14] cryosurgery[15]
Palmar erythema	Observation and reassurance, no effective treatment[7]	See left
Edema	Reassurance regarding transient nature of problem; avoid tight-fitting clothing; lying in the left lateral decubitus position, sleeping in a Trendelenburg position; immersion in water; lower extremity elevation and compression; a sodium-controlled diet; exercise[7,17]	See left
Varicose veins	Measures similar to those used for edema (previous); for distended vulvar veins, supportive pantyhose and pressure pads[7,16,17]	Surgery, liquid or foam sclerotherapy, laser or radiofrequency endoluminal ablation[21]
Hemorrhoids	Hot sitz baths, laxatives, suppositories, topical anesthetics, astringent compresses[7]	Conservative measures as indicated on the left; consider referral to anorectal specialist for more aggressive management
Cutis marmorata	Observation and reassurance, transient vasomotor instability[7]	If persistent, evaluation for connective tissue disease, intravascular or vessel wall pathology, and vascular obstruction[7]
Gingival hyperemia and hyperplasia	Reassurance, proper dental hygiene, avoidance of trauma, strong astringents; dental surgery such as supragingival scaling and subgingival curettage if chewing causes significant bleeding, ulceration, or pain[7]	See left
Pyogenic granuloma	Observation and reassurance, removal of local irritants; surgical removal by standard scalpel techniques, electrocoagulation, cryotherapy, and/or laser[24,28–31] if ulcerated and painful or if interfering with eating	See left
Glomus tumor	Complete excision and close observation[35,36]	See left

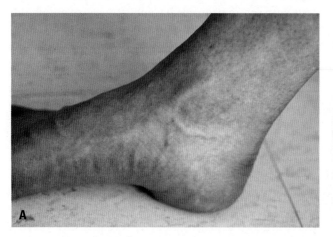
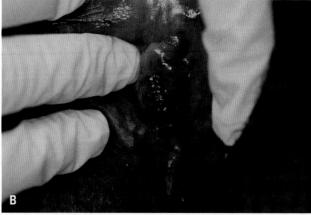

Figure 4.7. (**A**) Varicose veins on the foot. (**B**) Large vulvar varicosities. (Courtesy of Dr. Joe Brooks.)

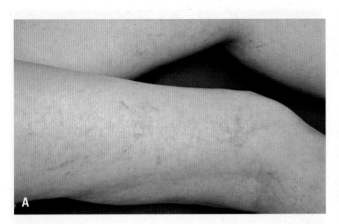 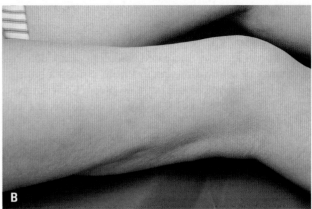

Figure 4.8. **(A)** Reticular and spider veins in the early postpartum period. **(B)** Three months after postpartum treatment with 0.25% Sotradecol solution, the veins have resolved. (Courtesy of Dr. George Kroumpouzos.)

cold sensations, and *cutis marmorata*.[7] **Cutis marmorata** ("marble skin") is a transient bluish mottling of the skin of the lower extremities upon exposure to cold (Fig. 4.9). Persistent postpartum livedoid changes should trigger an evaluation for etiologies of livedo reticularis, such as collagen vascular and neoplastic disorders and blood dyscrasias.[7] **Purpura** and **petechiae** are common over the lower extremities, especially during the second half of pregnancy, and develop secondary to increased capillary fragility/permeability and elevated hydrostatic pressures. The Rumpel-Leede tourniquet test is positive in the legs in up to 80% of pregnant women. Purpura and petechiae usually resolve spontaneously postpartum.[16]

Benign parturient purpura is due to intermittent increased intravascular pressure of the Valsalva maneuver during the second stage of labor (**Valsalva purpura**). It is suggested by a triad of petechiae distributed on the upper chest, upper back, upper arms, neck, and face, especially on the relatively loose tissues of the face and neck; vigorous pushing during the second stage of labor; and normal platelet count. Valsalva purpura can also develop after prolonged coughing or vomiting (Fig. 4.10). Blood may leak from vessels because of increased intravascular pressure, inadequate support, and/or increased fragility of vessels. It is important to distinguish this petechial eruption from that of disseminated intravascular coagulation.[22]

MUCOUS MEMBRANE CHANGES

Increased vascularity and softening of the vaginal portion of the cervical mucosa, called the Goodell sign, may be noted as early as the fourth week of pregnancy. Distention and congestion of vaginal vasculature may impart a violaceous hue, termed the Jacquemier-Chadwick sign, visible by the eighth week.[7] These signs are noted in virtually all patients. Nasal congestion is often noted and results from mucosal edema and relaxation of smooth muscles.[16]

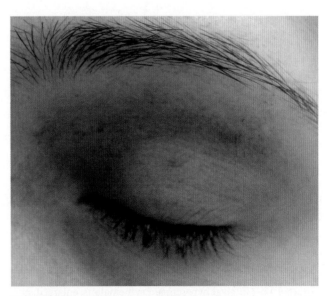

Figure 4.9. Cutis marmorata on the lower extremities in pregnancy.

Figure 4.10. Valsalva purpura in pregnancy secondary to vomiting. (Courtesy of Dr. Mayra Ianhez.)

GINGIVAL HYPEREMIA

Gingival edema and *hyperemia* occur in approximately 80% of pregnancies.[20] Increased vascularity is evident by the change in color of the gingiva from pink to a bluish-red, and a tendency of the gums to bleed. Concomitant inflammation, or gingivitis, occurs in response to local irritants, poor oral hygiene, and nutritional deficiencies,[7] such as vitamin C.[23] The prevalence of gingivitis was only 16.4% in a Pakistani population in which vitamin C deficiency is rare.[3] Altered tissue metabolism in pregnancy may heighten the local response to irritants.[16] Both a deficiency of estrogen in the gingival tissues and estrogen stimulation are possible causes of gingivitis. High progesterone levels may stimulate vascular proliferation at sites of microtrauma.[7] Pregnancy gingivitis starts between the second and fourth months of gestation and worsens until delivery. There is enlargement and blunting of the interdental papillae, which are more prominent along the lower front teeth, and mucosal friability (Fig. 4.11). The gingival margins appear pink to dark red, depending on vascularity. They become swollen, smooth, and glossy and have a mottled appearance.[7,16] Mild pain and ulceration are common. Granuloma gravidarum can develop within the hypertrophic gum (see the following). Interestingly, pregnancy gingivitis does not usually progress to periodontitis. Regression may not occur until 1 to 2 months postpartum. Treatment options are summarized in Table 4.1.

GRANULOMA GRAVIDARUM

Pyogenic granuloma (PG) of pregnancy, also referred to as *granuloma gravidarum*, pregnancy tumor, or epulis of pregnancy, can develop usually in association with pregnancy gingivitis. It is a soft or semifirm, pedunculated,

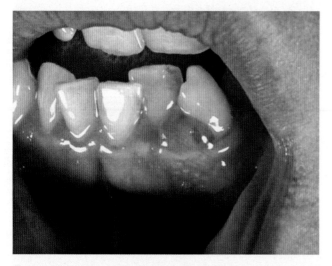

Figure 4.11. Gingival hyperemia: Erythematous, enlarged, and blunt interdental papillae. The gingival margins look swollen, smooth, and glossy and have a mottled appearance.

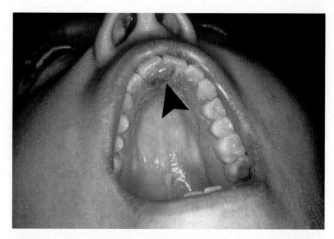

Figure 4.12. Granuloma gravidarum: A pyogenic granuloma on the lingual surface of the gingiva. (Reprinted from Kroumpouzos G, Cohen LM. Dermatoses of pregnancy. *J Am Acad Dermatol.* 2001;45[1]:1–19, with permission from Elsevier.)

or sessile; deep red or purple; friable nodule that arises from the gingiva in approximately 2% of pregnant patients (Fig. 4.12). Although typically located along the interdental papillae, it can also be located along the buccal or lingual surfaces of the gingiva as well as the lingual, palatal, and buccal mucosa. The lesion appears between the second and fifth months of pregnancy and continuously grows during gestation (Fig. 4.13).[16,20] Similar lesions have also been noted on extraoral locations, such as the face (see Fig. 4.13), hands (*epulis gravidarum manum*) (Fig. 4.14),[24] and nail apparatus (see Ch. 6, Fig. 6.12).

Marked immunoreactivity for estrogen receptors in both endothelium and mucosal surfaces has been shown in PGs of pregnancy, indicating that the hyperestrogenism of pregnancy may play a role in the development of PG.[25] Estrogen enhances vascular endothelial growth factor production in macrophages, which may contribute to the development of PGs during pregnancy through a downregulation of apoptosis of vascular and fibroblastic cells of the tumor.[26] In addition, high levels of progesterone have been shown in inflamed tissues during pregnancy and may inhibit an acute inflammatory response. This hormonal milieu may lead to the establishment of a chronic healing environment that may provide the matrix for granuloma formation in the setting of antecedent trauma.[27]

PGs can bleed (see Fig. 4.13B) and ulcerate (see Fig. 4.14) easily with minor trauma, cause pain, and can interfere with eating. Tumors on extraoral locations, such as the hands, may often persist postpartum, necessitating removal.[24] PG often regresses spontaneously weeks to months postpartum and does not warrant intervention unless it becomes very symptomatic and/or bleeds profusely. Surgical removal by standard scalpel techniques, such as shave removal (see Ch. 24, Fig. 24.3), cryotherapy,[28] electrocoagulation, and therapy using neodymium-doped yttrium aluminum garnet (Nd:YAG) laser,[29] a CO2 laser,[30]

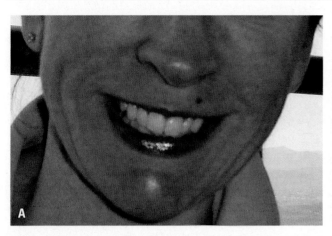
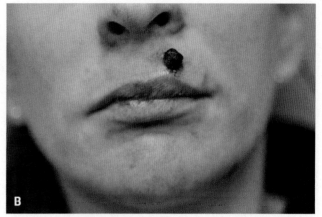

Figure 4.13. (**A**) A pyogenic granuloma: A vascular papule on the left side of the upper lip at 10 weeks' gestation. (**B**) At 26 weeks, the lesion was triple in size and started to bleed profusely. (Courtesy of Dr. George Kroumpouzos.)

or 585-nm PDL,[31] are therapeutic modalities. PG treated by surgical excision during pregnancy may recur due to incomplete excision or inadequate oral hygiene.[32]

OTHER VASCULAR PROLIFERATIONS

Vascular proliferations such as *hemangiomas*, *hemangioendotheliomas*, and *glomangiomas* can develop. Hemangiomas develop in up to 5% of pregnancies as small superficial or subcutaneous lesions, usually by the end of the first trimester. They are frequently located on the head and neck, and occasionally on oral mucosa. Hemangiomas enlarge slowly until delivery and usually regress postpartum.[33] Arteriovenous shunting resulting in high-output cardiac failure has been reported with large hemangiomas.[16] If postpartum involution is incomplete, lesions can be treated with PDL or intense pulsed light. Subcutaneous hemangioendotheliomas

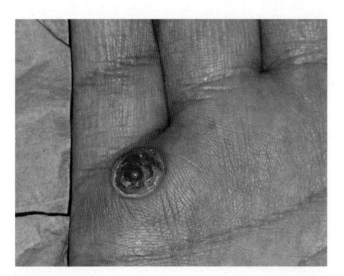

Figure 4.14. A pyogenic granuloma: A deep red ulcerated nodule on the volar aspect of the hand.

may occur in periorbital areas, on the breasts, or in the umbilical region.[16] Intraskeletal, presacral, intracranial, hepatic, and cardiac hemangioendotheliomas have been reported.[34] A glomus tumor is classically located in the subungual region and presents as a reddish blue, occasionally painful nodule. A complete excision and close follow-up are recommended because approximately 1% of cases are malignant. Both benign and malignant variants have been reported in pregnancies.[35,36] Glomangiomas can develop in gestation, with new lesions appearing in successive pregnancies.[20]

UNILATERAL NEVOID TELANGIECTASIA SYNDROME

Unilateral nevoid telangiectasia syndrome (UNTS) is a rare entity that can be congenital or acquired. It is characterized by multiple, unilateral, linearly arranged blanching telangiectasias in a dermatomal or Blaschkoid pattern (Fig. 4.15).[37] UNTS occurs most frequently in the trigeminal, cervical, and upper thoracic dermatomes. Sites of predilection hence include the face, neck, shoulder, upper extremities, and thorax. A pale ring around the telangiectasias, referred to as anemic halo, may be observed. The majority of cases reported to date have occurred during pregnancy, with the onset of puberty, or in patients with hepatic disease, suggesting a strong association with hyperestrogenism. The association with hyperestrogenism, dermatomes of distribution, and the presence of anemic halos suggest a relationship with spider angiomas. Some authors suggest that angiogenic molecules may play a role because it has been also suggested for spider angiomas. Others indicate that a congenitally determined, abnormal distribution of estrogen-sensitive target end organs may be involved. Finally, others purport that there is a localized increase in estrogen receptors in dermatomal distribution, possibly due to chromosomal mosaicism, which is unmasked

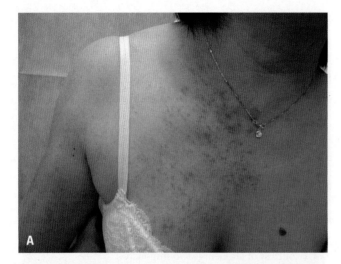

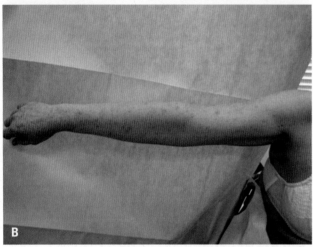

Figure 4.15. Unilateral nevoid telangiectasia syndrome in a nonpregnant patient presenting with bright red, telangiectatic macules. (**A**) The right side of the chest. (**B**) Continuous distribution onto cervical dermatomes 5–7 of the right upper extremity.

at times of estrogen excess. Cases occurring in pregnancy often wane or resolve postpartum. A 585-nm PDL is effective at improving the patient's cosmetic appearance; however, the response is short-lived and lesions tend to recur.[37–39]

MANAGEMENT OPTIONS

Most vascular changes spontaneously resolve postpartum. These changes are not usually harmful to the pregnant patient or fetus but can be a source of significant distress. Patient education can help alleviate anxiety. Additionally, most therapeutic devices are not tested in pregnant patients, and the effects on the fetus are unknown. Therefore, a conservative approach of observation is recommended unless more aggressive intervention is medically necessary, in which case the risks and benefits of a particular procedure must be thoroughly reviewed with the patient.

- Physiologic vascular changes are a consequence of the altered hormonal environment of pregnancy and occur as early as the fourth week of pregnancy with increased vascularity and softening of the vaginal portion of the cervical mucosa.
- Patients often develop spider angiomas and other vascular proliferations, palmar erythema, edema of the extremities and face, venous abnormalities, vasomotor instability, gingival edema/hyperemia, and, occasionally, pyogenic granulomas.
- Granuloma gravidarum is a soft, pedunculated, deep red or purple vascular growth that arises from the gingiva in approximately 2% of patients; it can ulcerate, cause pain, bleed profusely, and interfere with eating, thus necessitating removal.
- Most vascular changes fade or resolve spontaneously postpartum; these changes are not usually harmful to the pregnant woman and are not associated with fetal risks.
- A conservative management approach of observation and reassurance is recommended unless intervention is medically necessary.

REFERENCES

1. Estève E, Saudeau L, Pierre F, et al. Physiological cutaneous signs in normal pregnancy: a study of 60 pregnant women. *Ann Dermatol Venereol.* 1994;121:227–231.
2. Rathore SP, Gupta S, Gupta V. Pattern and prevalence of physiological cutaneous changes in pregnancy: a study of 2000 antenatal women. *Indian J Dermatol Venereol Leprol.* 2011;77(3):402.
3. Muzaffar F, Hussain I, Haroon TS. Physiologic skin changes during pregnancy: a study of 140 cases. *Int J Dermatol.* 1998;37:429–431.
4. Bean W, Cogswell R, Dexter M. Vascular changes of the skin in pregnancy: vascular spiders and palmar erythema. *Surg Gynecol Obstet.* 1949;88:739–752.
5. Papoutsis J, Kroumpouzos G. Dermatologic disorders. In: Gabbe SG, Niebyl JR, Simpson JL, et al., eds. *Obstetrics: Normal and Problem Pregnancies.* 5th ed. Philadelphia, PA: Churchill Livingstone Elsevier; 2007:1178–1192.
6. Linder H, Reinhart W, Hanggi W. Peripheral capillaroscopic findings and blood rheology during normal pregnancy. *Eur J Obstetr Gynecol Reprod Biol.* 1995;58:141–145.
7. Wong R, Ellis C. Physiologic skin changes in pregnancy. *J Am Acad Dermatol.* 1984;10:929–940.
8. Polla L, Tan Q, Garden J. Tunable pulsed dye laser for the treatment of benign cutaneous vascular ectasia. *Dermatologica.* 1987;174:11–17.
9. Geronemus R. Treatment of spider telangiectasias in children using the flashlamp-pumped pulsed dye laser. *Pediatr Dermatol.* 1991;8:61–63.
10. Tan E, Vinciullo C. Pulsed dye laser treatment of spider telangiectasia. *Austral J Dermatol.* 1997;38:22–25.

11. Scheepers J, Quaba A. Treatment of nevi aranei with the pulsed tunable dye laser at 585 nm. *J Pediatr Surg.* 1995;30:101–104.

12. Schroeter C, Neumann H. An intense light source. The photoderm VL-flashlamp as a new treatment possibility for vascular skin lesions. *Dermatol Surg.* 1998;24:743–748.

13. Robinson J. Electrodessication of nevi aranei ("spiders") and senile angiomas. *J Dermatol Surg Oncol.* 1980;6:794–795.

14. Henry F, Quatresooz P, Valverde-Lopez J. Blood vessel changes during pregnancy: a review. *Am J Clin Dermatol.* 2006;7:65–69.

15. Thai K, Sinclair R. Cryotherapy of benign skin lesions. *Australian J Dermatol.* 1999;40:175–184.

16. Ingber A. Physiologic vascular changes during pregnancy. In: Ingber A, ed. *Obstetric Dermatology, A Practical Guide.* Berlin, Germany: Springer-Verlag; 2009:33–44.

17. Ponnapula P, Boberg J. Lower extremity changes experienced during pregnancy. *J Foot Ankle Surg.* 2010;49:452–458.

18. Hernandez C, Lynn R. Massive antepartum labial edema. *Cutis.* 2010;86:148–152.

19. Guven E, Guven S, Durukan T. Massive vulvar oedema complicating pregnancy. *Obstet Gynaecol.* 2005;25:216–218.

20. Winton G, Lewis C. Dermatoses of pregnancy. *J Am Acad Dermatol.* 1982;6:977–998.

21. Murad M, Coto-Yglesias F, Zumaeta-Garcia M. A systematic review and meta-analysis of the treatments of varicose veins. *J Vascular Surgery.* 2011;53:49S–65S.

22. Wilkin J. Benign parturient purpura. *JAMA.* 1978;239:930.

23. Muallem M, Rubiez N. Physiological and biological skin changes in pregnancy. *Clin Dermatol.* 2006;24:80–83.

24. Rader C, Piorkowski J, Bass D. Epulis gravidarum manum: pyogenic granuloma of the hand occurring in pregnant women. *J Hand Surg Am.* 2008;33:263–265.

25. Whitaker S, Bouquot J, Alimario A. Identification and semiquantification of estrogen and progesterone receptors in pyogenic granulomas of pregnancy. *Oral Surg Oral Med Oral Pathol.* 1994;78:755.

26. Kanda N, Watanabe S. Regulatory roles of sex hormones in cutaneous biology and immunology. *J Dermatol Sci.* 2005;38:1–7.

27. Manus D, Sherbert D, Jackson I. Management considerations for the granuloma of pregnancy. *Plast Reconstr Surg.* 1995;95:1045–1050.

28. Cohen P. Pregnancy-associated pyogenic granuloma of the lip: successful management using cryotherapy. *J Gt Houst Dent Soc.* 1996;67:18–19.

29. Powell J, Bailey C, Coopland A. Nd:YAG laser excision of a giant gingival pyogenic granuloma of pregnancy. *Lasers Surg Med.* 1994;14:178–183.

30. Lindenmuller I, Noll P, Mameghani T. CO_2 laser-assisted treatment of a giant pyogenic granuloma of the gingiva. *Int J Dent Hyg.* 2010;8:249–252.

31. Khandpur S, Sharma V. Successful treatment of multiple gingival pyogenic granulomas with pulsed-dye laser. *Indian J Dermatol Venereol Leprol.* 2008;74:275–277.

32. Jafarzadeh H, Sanatkhani M, Mohtasham N. Oral pyogenic granuloma: a review. *J Oral Sci.* 2006;48:167–175.

33. Letterman G, Schurter M. Cutaneous hemangiomas of the face in pregnancy. *Plast Reconstr Surg Transplant Bull.* 1962;29:293–300.

34. Lutgendorf M, Magann E, Yousef M. Hepatic epithelial hemangioendothelioma in pregnancy. *Gynecol Obstet Invest.* 2009;67:238–240.

35. Cibull T, Gleason B, O'Malley D. Malignant cutaneous glomus tumor presenting as a rapidly growing leg mass in a pregnant woman. *J Cutan Pathol.* 2008;35:765–769.

36. Laymon C, Peterson W Jr. Glomangioma (glomus tumor). *Arch Dermatol.* 1965;92:509–514.

37. Wenson S, Jan F, Sepehr A. Unilateral nevoid telangiectasia syndrome: a case report and review of the literature. *Dermatol Online J.* 2011;17:2.

38. Dadlani C, Kamino H, Walters R. Unilateral nevoid telangiectasia. *Dermatol Online J.* 2008;14:3.

39. Cliff S, Harland C. Recurrence of unilateral naevoid telangiectatic syndrome following treatment with the pulsed dye laser. *J Cutan Laser Ther.* 1999;1:105–107.

CHAPTER 5

Connective Tissue Changes

Kelly K. Park ■ Jenny E. Murase

INTRODUCTION

Nearly 65% of pregnant patients develop connective tissue changes, which include, in decreasing order of incidence, *striae gravidarum*, skin tags, keloids, and hypertrophic scars.[1] In this chapter, common connective tissue changes in pregnancy and their prevention and management are described.

STRIAE GRAVIDARUM

Striae distensae (stretch marks) are atrophic scars of the dermis that are common in the general population. The characteristic form appearing during pregnancy is referred to as *striae gravidarum* (SG, or *linear gravidarum*) and is observed in 50% to 90% of pregnancies.[1–3] Although SG can appear in primigravidas, they can also develop for the first time in subsequent pregnancies. Onset is typically in the late second trimester and the early third trimester; however, 43% of women have onset prior to week 24.[1,2,4] SG predominantly occur on the abdomen, favoring the lower half (92.7% of cases) and breasts, but may also occur on the upper arms, lower back, hips, buttocks, inguinal regions, and thighs (Fig. 5.1).[1]

When SG first appear, they appear as *striae rubra* (immature striae), which are initially flat, pink red, and become raised, violaceous red, longer, and wider with time (Fig. 5.2). They fade to become *striae alba* (mature striae), which are characterized as scarlike, wrinkled, white, atrophic, and parallel to skin tension lines (Figs. 5.3 and 5.4). SG may cause symptoms such as pruritus, burning, and discomfort. They can also be disfiguring and impact clothing choice and personal relationships, which can subsequently lead to a decreased quality of life.

The identified risk factors for the development of striae in pregnancy include a maternal and family history of striae; the presence of breast or thigh striae; young maternal age (in particular, teenagers); being in the third trimester of pregnancy; premature birth; newborn weight, height, and head measurements; local body modifications (e.g., piercing, implants); decreased water intake; and alcohol intake. Changes between maternal baseline and delivery weight and anthropometry are controversial.[2–8] An association with non-Caucasian race (Fig. 5.5),[4] has not been confirmed.[2,3,5] Although the exact pathogenesis

of SG is unclear, it is thought that genetic factors as well as gestational hormones play a role in their development.[3] There are twice as many estrogen receptors and increased levels of androgen and glucocorticoid receptors in striae compared to healthy skin.[9] This hormonal milieu is thought to be responsible for making connective tissue susceptible to SG when the skin is stretched or strained.

The histologic appearance of striae is dependent on lesion age. As they mature, the epidermis flattens and becomes atrophic with blunted rete ridges. The dermis thins and collagen in the upper dermis decreases. Collagen bundles become attenuated and are arranged in a parallel or perpendicular fashion compared to striae direction. There is a significant increase in glycosaminoglycans, whereas there is a decrease in elastic fiber content, papillary dermis, and fibrillin microfibrils in striae compared to adjacent normal skin.[10] The elastin and fibrillin fibers in the deep dermis are parallel to the dermal–epidermal junction compared to their normal perpendicular orientation.[10]

Prevention

Existing data for SG prevention is limited. Trofolastin cream, containing *Centella asiatica* extract, alpha tocopherol, and collagen-elastin hydrolysates, may help prevent stretch mark development, but only in patients who previously had SG.[11] There is less evidence that verum ointment, whose active ingredients include vitamin E, panthenol, hyaluronic acid, elastin, and menthol, in combination with massage may prevent striae because the results may have reflected the benefits of massage alone.[11] Alphastria cream, which contains hyaluronic acid, allantoin, vitamin A, vitamin E, and dexpanthenol, may prevent SG compared to placebo, perhaps due to the effects of hyaluronic acid.[12]

Postpartum Management

Treatment should be instituted during the active stages of SG rather than when striae have matured (Table 5.1). Homeopathic and alternative therapies empirically utilize various fruit and vegetable oils and emollients based on their ability to hydrate the skin, but recommendations for usage are limited by lack of reliable evidence. Lifestyle changes through diet and/or exercise leading to

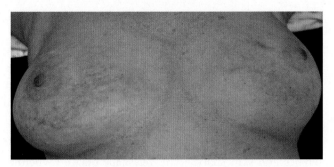

Figure 5.1. Striae of breasts during pregnancy.

weight loss do not seem to alter striae, particularly in obese women.[13]

Topical Treatments

Tretinoin 0.1% cream has been shown to improve SG.[14] Glycolic acid (GA) is an alpha hydroxy acid that likely works by collagen stimulation. Topical 20% GA combined with either 10% L-ascorbic acid or 0.05% tretinoin were found to improve the appearance of *striae alba*.[15] Trichloroacetic acid (TCA) is thought to be useful for SG treatment due to its keratolytic activity. Low concentrations of 15% to 20% TCA at 1-month intervals may

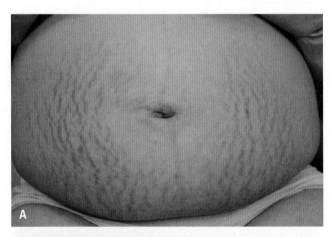

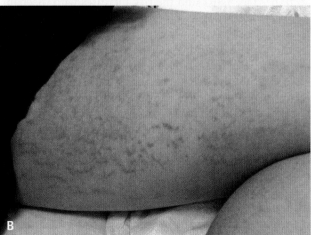

Figure 5.2. (A) *Striae rubra* (immature red stretch marks) of the abdomen in a Hispanic female. **(B)** *Striae rubra* on the thigh.

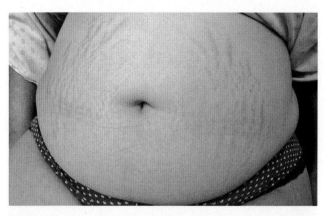

Figure 5.3. *Striae alba* on the abdomen at 16 weeks' gestation.

improve the color and texture of scars and wrinkles by chemexfoliation.[16] Microdermabrasion is useful for the improvement of striae, with better outcomes in *striae rubra*.[17]

Lasers and Light Treatments

A variety of lasers have shown efficacy in the treatment of striae. The 1,550-nm erbium-doped fiber fractionated laser is a nonablative resurfacing laser that is used for photothermolysis, which has been shown to improve the overall appearance, dyschromia, and texture of both *striae alba* and *rubra* (Fig. 5.6).[18] The 10,600-nm ablative carbon dioxide (CO_2) fractional laser is effective for scars and has a satisfactory therapeutic effect on *striae alba*.[19] The noncoherent, nonlaser, filtered intense pulsed light (IPL) flashlamp, which emits broadband visible light, improves white atrophic striae in women with skin types III to IV.[20] The 1,064-nm neodymium-doped yttrium aluminum garnet (Nd:YAG) laser increases dermal collagen density and improves the appearance of *striae rubra* after a single treatment, with best clinical results after three treatment sessions.[21] The 585-nm pulsed dye laser (PDL) has been purported to increase the amount of collagen in the extracellular

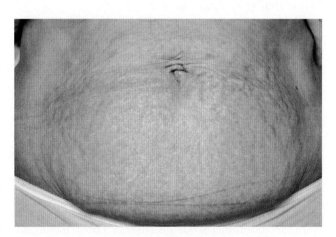

Figure 5.4. Postpartum *striae alba* (mature white stretch marks) of the abdomen and excessive skin laxity.

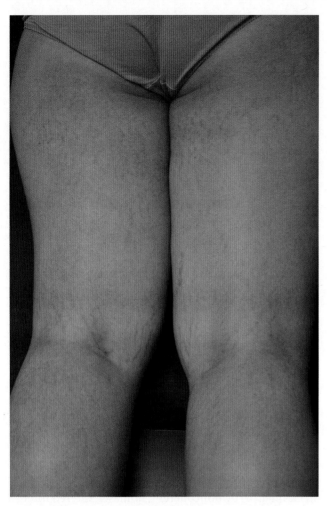

Figure 5.5. Extensive postpartum hyperpigmentation along gestational striae on the lower extremities in an Asian female.

matrix. Overall, the laser was found to moderately improve the appearance of *striae rubra* by reducing erythema (Fig. 5.7).[22] The copper bromide (CuBr) laser (577-511 nm) has been used for stretch marks in women with skin types II to III. The majority of patients had positive clinical results, which were maintained at 1- and 2-year follow-up intervals.[23]

The targeted narrowband ultraviolet light B/ultraviolet light A1 (UVB/UVA1) device (MultiClear, Curelight Ltd., Israel) provides short-term repigmentation of *striae alba* in patients with skin types II through VI.[24] The 308-nm xenon chloride (XeCl) excimer laser is a targeted "super narrowband" form of phototherapy that is effective in the repigmentation of mature *striae alba*.[25] However, it is limited by pigment splaying and the need for maintenance treatment every 1 to 4 months.[25]

Radiofrequency (RF) is a nonablative method of skin rejuvenation that is used for tightening and decreasing wrinkles by changing the electrical charge of the skin. Bipolar RF was found to clinically and histologically improve abdominal *striae distensae*.[26] The TriPollar RF device was observed to improve the appearance of striae in skin types IV and V.[27]

SKIN LAXITY AFTER PREGNANCY

Excessive skin laxity, commonly appearing as loose abdominal or flank skin, along with localized fat deposits after pregnancy, is not uncommon (see Fig. 5.4). Noninvasive postpartum body contouring can be performed with RF monotherapy or as part of combination treatment (see Table 5.1). The ThermaCool TC device (Solta Medical Inc., Hayward, CA) uses monopolar RF to decrease waist circumference and skin laxity.[28] The Velashape device (Syneron Medical Ltd., Israel), which uses a combination of infrared light, bipolar RF, and vacuum and mechanical massage, was studied specifically in the postpartum population and was found to cause significant circumferential reduction and tightening of skin.[29] Well-established surgical options are shown in Table 5.1.

WOUND HEALING IN PREGNANCY

Wound healing is altered in pregnancy, which is likely due to a combination of physiologic changes and other maternal, fetal, environmental, and exogenous factors. Microchimerism, which is fetal cell migration into the maternal circulation, may help repair maternal deficiencies in wound healing.[30]

HYPERTROPHIC SCARS AND KELOIDS

Hypertrophic scars and keloids are related to abnormal wound healing. During pregnancy, preexisting scars can grow or tear (Fig. 5.8A).[31] Keloid formation is due to both genetic and external factors. Keloids most commonly develop in individuals with a familial predisposition; in ages 10 to 30; and in African Americans, Hispanics, and Asians. They often affect areas with high melanocyte density, such as the chest, shoulders, upper back, nape of the neck, and earlobes, whereas they rarely occur on the palms and soles. Keloid formation can occur at surgical sites (e.g., cesarean section) (Fig. 5.8B), and the risk increases with mechanical force or tension on surgical wounds, susceptible body locations, infections, and foreign body reactions. There is a higher incidence of keloids in pregnancy that may be due to abnormal wound healing due to hormonal changes and neoangiogenesis.[32] In a prospective study of cesarean sections, keloids occurred in 0.5% of Caucasians, 1.6% of Hispanics, 5.2% of Asians, and 7.1% of African Americans; those with keloids went on to have a greater incidence of postsurgical intra-abdominal adhesions.[33]

Prevention

Although hypertrophic scars and keloids cannot be wholly prevented, there are ways to reduce the risk of occurrence. In pregnancy-related surgery, the surgical technique should be atraumatic and precise; incisions should follow skin lines and be perpendicular to joint surfaces in

TABLE 5.1	Summary of Postpartum Management Options
Treatment	**Comment**
Striae Gravidarum	
Tretinoin 0.1% cream	Daily application[14]
Glycolic acid peel 15%–20%	Daily application ± 10% L-ascorbic acid or tretinoin 0.05%[15]
Trichloroacetic acid peel 10%–35%	Monthly application[16]
Microdermabrasion	Utilizing aluminum oxide, particularly effective for *striae rubra*[17]
Erbium-doped fiber fractional laser, 1,550 nm	Effective for *striae alba* and *rubra*[18]
Carbon dioxide fractional laser, 16,600 nm	Useful for *striae alba*[19]
Intense pulsed light	Useful for *striae alba*[20]
Neodymium-doped yttrium aluminum garnet (Nd:YAG) laser, 1,064 nm	Best results after three treatment sessions[21]
Pulsed dye laser, 585 nm	Effective in *strie rubra*; avoid in skin types IV through VI due to risk of postinflammatory hypopigmentation[22]
Radiofrequency	Bipolar and tripolar[26,27]
Combination ultraviolet A/ultraviolet B (UVA/UVB) light	For short-term repigmentation of *striae alba*[24]
Excimer laser, 308 nm	Useful for *striae alba*, maintenance treatment every 1–4 months[25]
Copper bromide laser, 577–511 nm	Results maintained ≤2 years[23]
Skin Laxity	
ThermaCool TC	Monopolar radiofrequency[28]
Velashape	Combination infrared light, bipolar radiofrequency, and vacuum and mechanical massage[29]
Surgical options	Liposuction, abdominoplasty, and brachioplasty
Keloids and Hypertrophic Scars	
Intralesional triamcinolone acetate	Keloids: First-line therapy, use 10–40 mg/ml mixed with 2% lidocaine for three injections every 1–2 months[37,40] Hypertrophic scars: Second-line therapy, use 5–10 mg/ml and inject every 3–6 weeks[37] Both: After surgical excision, combined with intraoperative local injection, repeat injections weekly for 2–5 weeks, then every month for 4–6 months[37,40]
Topical silicone gel sheeting	Apply daily ≥12 hours daily for ≥2 months[37]
Pressure therapy	8–24 hours daily for 6 months[37]
Cryosurgery utilizing nitrous oxide (−86°C) ± liquid nitrogen (−196°C)	≥3 treatments of 30 seconds each, applied once monthly using the contact method; not recommended for darker skin types[41]
Surgical resection	± postexcisional intralesional steroids or radiation[37,39]
Simple excision and primary closure	Hypertrophic scars: If due to complicated wound or delayed closure, Z- or W-plasty can be used for cosmetically sensitive areas, ± skin graft[37]
Pulsed dye laser, 595 nm	Hypertrophic scars: Moderate efficacy[42]
Carbon dioxide fractional laser, 10,600 nm	Hypertrophic scars: Moderate efficacy[42]
Erbium:YAG laser, 2,940 nm	Hypertrophic scars: Moderate efficacy[42]

(continued)

TABLE 5.1	Summary of Postpartum Management Options *(continued)*
Treatment	**Comment**
Keloids and Hypertrophic Scars *(continued)*	
Fractional nonablative laser, 1,540 m	Hypertrophic scars: Moderate efficacy[42]
Pulsed dye laser, 585 nm	Keloids: Effective; can be performed after CO2 laser vaporization, or combined with intralesional triamcinolone, or 5-fluorouracil[43]
Molluscum Gravidarum (Skin Tags)	
Scissor excision, electrodessication, radiofrequency, and cryosurgery	All procedures safe in pregnancy
Nevoid Hyperkeratosis of the Nipple and/or Areola	
Tretinoin 0.025% cream or isotretinoin gel	Varying responses; recurrence after drug cessation[44]
Lactic acid 12% lotion	Moderate response (one case)[44]
Keratolytics (i.e., 6% salicylic acid gel)	Varying responses[44]
Topical calcipotriol ± low-dose acitretin	Satisfactory responses, short follow-up in cases treated with: calcipotriol alone[44]
Surgical options (cryosurgery, shave excision, surgical removal, carbon dioxide laser, and radiofrequency ablation)	Immediate results, satisfactory duration of improvement[44]
Pregnancy-Associated Hyperkeratosis of the Nipple	
Tretinoin 0.025% cream	Mild-to-moderate efficacy[45]
Emollients (i.e., 12% ammonium lactate cream or 12% lactic acid lotion)	Mild efficacy[45]
Surgical options (curettage)	Effective (one case)[45]

order to decrease wound tension.[34] Hemostasis and closure using skin edge eversion is warranted. It has been reported that women who underwent a cesarean section with absorbable subcuticular stitch closure had better cosmetic results and less pain at 6 weeks compared to

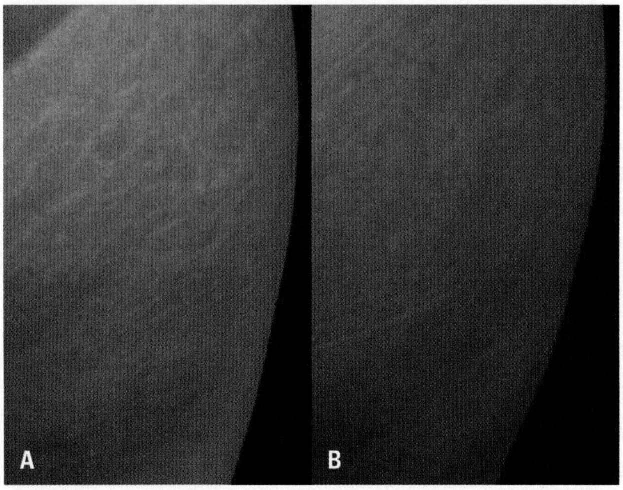

Figure 5.6. *Striae gravidarum.* (**A**) Before treatment. (**B**) After treatment with the 1,550-nm erbium-doped fiber fractionated laser. (Courtesy of Tina Alster, MD, Washington DC.)

surgical staple closure, although the latter was associated with decreased operating times.[35] Otherwise, bilayered closures of the trunk and extremities (moderate and high tensions sites) have a better overall appearance and have less erythema when using subcuticular running polyglactin 910 sutures that are left in place.[36] Infections should be avoided at all costs, and proper wound care and debridement should be performed. After wound closure, avoiding tension and stretching of the areas should be practiced. The use of massage, greasy ointments, and occlusive materials such as bandages, compressive garments, silicone gel sheeting, and taping may be used.[37]

Obesity is a risk factor for complicated wound infections after a cesarean section. To minimize risk, there is some evidence to support the use of prophylactic antibiotics, the closure of any subcutaneous space over 2 cm, and the maintenance of procedural normothermia. Primary or secondary wound closure is encouraged over healing by a secondary intention.[38]

Management

The treatment of both hypertrophic scars and keloids is challenging, with variable efficacy and a high risk of recurrence (see Table 5.1). Intralesional corticosteroids

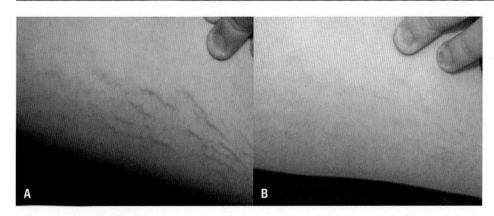

Figure 5.7. *Striae gravidarum.* (**A**) Before treatment. (**B**) After treatment with 585-595-nm pulsed dye laser. (Courtesy of Tina Alster, MD, Washington DC.)

can soften and flatten scars, making them less noticeable. They are first-line therapies for keloids and second-line therapies for hypertrophic scars when other treatments, including silicone gel sheeting and lasers, have failed.[39] There is a mixed response rate of 50% to 100% and a high recurrence rate of 9% to 50% with corticosteroid monotherapy.[37,40]

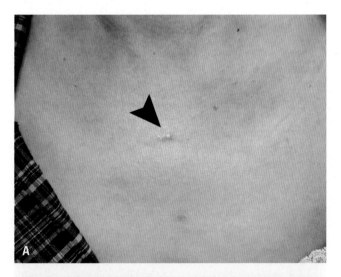

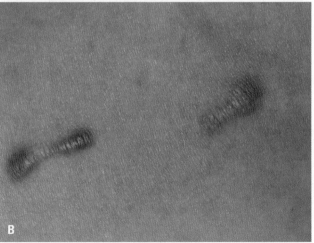

Figure 5.8. (**A**) Keloid *(arrow)* increasing in size during pregnancy. (**B**) Keloids at the surgical sites of a cesarean section.

Topical silicone gel sheeting can be used prophylactically in patients who are prone to hypertrophic scar formation. It can be used for both hypertrophic scars and keloids as soon as reepithelialization is complete. Pressure therapy should be started immediately after reepithelialization, but its efficacy depends on patient compliance,[39] especially since its use can be associated with discomfort secondary to heat or perspiration. It is a first-line treatment for hypertrophic scars caused by burns. Cryosurgery is a treatment option by which the majority of patients have good-to-excellent results.[41] Hypertrophic scars respond better than keloids and lesions less than 2 years old than older scars. Its use in darker skin types is not recommended due to the side effect of hypopigmentation.

Complete surgical resection is used for keloids to debulk the scar tissue and to attempt to alleviate related symptoms; however, as monotherapy, it has a high recurrence rate of 45% to 100%. After surgery, intralesional steroids can decrease recurrence to less than 50%, and, if combined with surgery, it is recommended that sutures be left in place for 3 to 5 days longer than usual to prevent wound dehiscence.[37,40] Surgically, hypertrophic scars may be treated with revision: an excision and primary closure can be performed if they were due to complicated wounds (e.g., infected) or delayed closure. In cosmetically sensitive areas, Z- or W-plasty can hide scar sites within skin tension lines.[37] When scar excision wounds cannot be closed, skin grafts allow for closure with minimal tension.

Both ablative and nonablative lasers have been used for the treatment of hypertrophic scars. The fractional nonablative laser (1,540 nm), the 595-nm PDL (Fig. 5.9), the CO_2 laser (10,600 nm), and the erbium:YAG laser (2,940 nm) have each been found to moderately improve hypertrophic scars; the 585-nm PDL has shown low efficacy.[42] For keloids, the 585-nm flashlamp PDL is preferred.[43]

MOLLUSCUM FIBROSUM GRAVIDARUM (SKIN TAGS)

Skin tags (acrochordons) are common benign pedunculated outgrowths of skin that are typically found on friction-prone surfaces, such as the neck, axillae, and inguinal areas.

Figure 5.9. A hypertrophic scar on a cesarean section. (**A**) Before treatment. (**B**) After treatment with 585-595-nm pulsed dye laser. (Courtesy of Tina Alster, MD, Washington DC.)

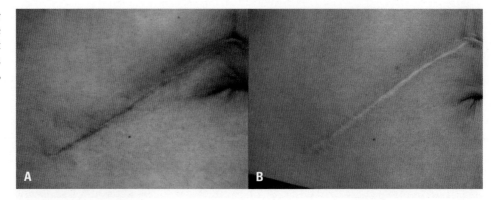

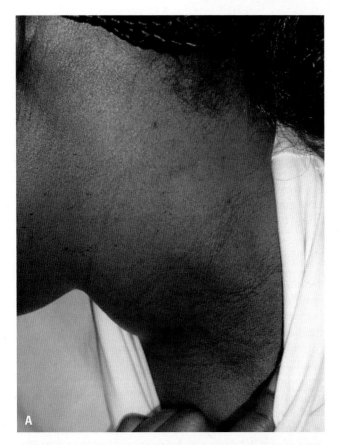

Histologic features include collagenous stroma with a core of blood vessels. Skin tags may proliferate in the second half of pregnancy but often regress after delivery. New skin tags that appear in pregnancy are referred to as *molluscum fibrosum gravidarum*. They vary in size from that of the size of a pinhead to that of a pea and may form in the inframammary areas, the sides of the face, the neck (Fig. 5.10A), the upper chest, and occasionally at less common sites such as the nipple (Fig. 5.10B). Treatment options are shown in Table 5.1.

NIPPLE AND AREOLAR CHANGES

Physiologic pigmentary and glandular changes of the nipple and areola are discussed in Chapters 3 and 7, respectively.

Nevoid Hyperkeratosis of the Nipple and/or Areola

Nevoid hyperkeratosis of the nipple and/or areola (NHNA) is a rare idiopathic condition that occurs in both genders with a significant female predominance.[44] It may develop or worsen in pregnancy. Lesions are most commonly bilateral and typically hyperkeratotic and hyperpigmented but can occasionally be verrucous (Fig. 5.11), yellowish,

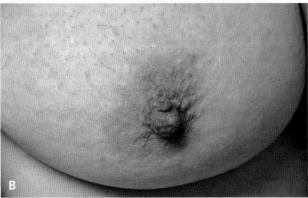

Figure 5.10. Skin tags appeared during pregnancy. (**A**) On the neck. (Courtesy of Bellevue Dermatology Department Collection, New York University.) (**B**) On the nipple.

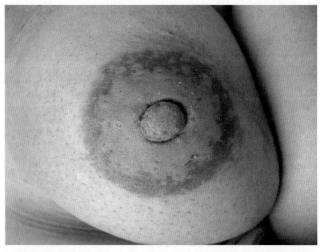

Figure 5.11. Unilateral nevoid hyperkeratosis of the nipple and areola presenting as a verrucous plaque with mild inflammatory changes and desquamation. (Courtesy of Dr. Milan Anadkat.)

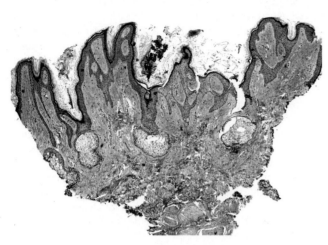

Figure 5.12. Histopathologic features of nevoid hyperkeratosis of the nipple and/or areola include orthokeratotic hyperkeratosis, ramifying epidermal hyperplasia with marked elongation of rete ridges, and variable papillomatosis.

or desquamate. The histopathologic features include orthokeratotic hyperkeratosis, ramifying epidermal hyperplasia with marked elongation of rete ridges (Fig. 5.12), and variable papillomatosis; basal layer hyperpigmentation, keratotic plugging, and horned pseudocysts are occasionally seen. NHNA is typically asymptomatic but can occasionally cause pruritus. Management includes topical medications and surgical modalities (see Table 5.1).

Pregnancy-Associated Hyperkeratosis of the Nipple

This recently reported clinicopathologic entity may be considered a physiologic change of pregnancy (Fig. 5.13).[45] Lesions involve the apex of the nipple bilaterally and can be associated with tenderness or discomfort, sensitivity to touch, and/or discomfort with breastfeeding. The majority of patients have lesions that persist postpartum. Histopathologic findings include conspicuous orthokeratotic hyperkeratosis, mild or absent papillomatosis, and an absence of acanthosis; the histopathologic features of NHNA are not seen. Topical medications and emollients have provided only mild-to-moderate relief (see Table 5.1).[45]

- *Striae gravidarum* are stretch marks appearing during pregnancy that may be due to hormonal changes and influenced by maternal and family history, race, ethnicity, genetics, and lifestyle factors.
- There is some evidence that Trofolastin cream and, to a lesser extent, verum ointment may prevent *striae gravidarum*; tretinoin, glycolic acid peels, microdermabrasion, radiofrequency, ultraviolet light, and a number of ablative and nonablative lasers can improve the appearance of *striae gravidarum* postpartum.
- Skin laxity and localized fat deposition can be treated postpartum with radiofrequency or surgery.
- Abnormal wound healing in pregnancy may account for hypertrophic scar and keloid formation and/or exacerbation.
- The prevention of hypertrophic scars and keloids includes atraumatic and precise surgical technique and proper wound care; hypertrophic scars and keloids can be treated postpartum with intralesional corticosteroids, surgery, silicone gel sheeting, pressure therapy, cryosurgery, or laser surgery.
- *Molluscum gravidarum* is the appearance of skin tags in the second or third trimesters.
- Nevoid hyperkeratosis of the nipple and/or areola is a rare condition that may develop or worsen in pregnancy.
- Pregnancy-associated hyperkeratosis of the nipple is typically bilateral, can be symptomatic, and commonly persists postpartum.

REFERENCES

1. Rathore SP, Gupta S, Gupta V. Pattern and prevalence of physiological cutaneous changes in pregnancy: a study of 2000 antenatal women. *Indian J Dermatol Venereol Leprol*. 2011;77(3):402.
2. Ghasemi A, Gorouhi F, Rashighi-Firoozabadi M, et al. Striae gravidarum: associated factors. *J Eur Acad Dermatol Venereol*. 2007;21:743–746.
3. Murphy KW, Dunphy B, O'Herlihy C. Increased maternal age protects against striae gravidarum. *J Obstet Gynecol*. 1992;12:297–300.

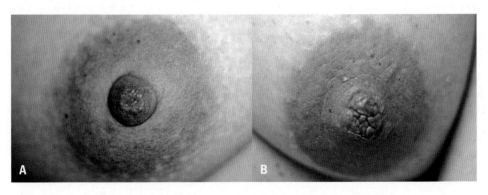

Figure 5.13. Pregnancy-associated hyperkeratosis of the nipple. (**A**) Focal, mild hyperkeratosis of the apex of the nipple. (**B**) Florid hyperkeratosis presenting as tan to mildly pigmented, warty papules covering the entire apex of the nipple. (Courtesy of Dr. George Kroumpouzos.)

4. Chang AL, Agredano YZ, Kimball AB. Risk factors associated with striae gravidarum. *J Am Acad Dermatol.* 2004;51:881–885.

5. Atwal GS, Manku LK, Griffiths CE, et al. Striae gravidarum in primiparae. *Br J Dermatol.* 2006;155:965–969.

6. Kelekci KH, Kelekci S, Destegul E, et al. Prematurity: is it a risk factor for striae distensae? *Int J Dermatol.* 2011;50:1240–1245.

7. J-Orh R, Titapant V, Chuenwattana P, et al. Prevalence and associate factors for striae gravidarum. *J Med Assoc Thai.* 2008;91:445–451.

8. Kluger N. Body art and pregnancy. *Eur J Obstet Gynecol Reprod Biol.* 2010;153:3–7.

9. Cordeiro RC, Zecchin KG, de Moraes AM. Expression of estrogen, androgen, and glucocorticoid receptors in recent striae distensae. *Int J Dermatol.* 2010;49:30–32.

10. Watson RE, Parry EJ, Humphries JD, et al. Fibrillin microfibrils are reduced in skin exhibiting striae distensae. *Br J Dermatol.* 1998;138:931–937.

11. Young GL, Jewell D. Creams for preventing stretch marks in pregnancy. *Cochrane Database Syst Rev.* 2000;(2):CD000066.

12. De-Bauman M, Walther M, De-Weck R. Effectiveness of alphastria cream in the prevention of pregnancy stretch marks (striae distensae). Results of a double-blind study. *Gynakologische Rundschau.* 1987;27:79–84.

13. Schwingel AC, Shimura Y, Nataka Y, et al. Exercise and striae distensae in obese women. *Med Sci Sports Exerc.* 2003;35:S33.

14. Rangel O, Arias I, Garcia E, et al. Topical tretinoin 0.1% for pregnancy-related abdominal striae: an open-label, multicenter, prospective study. *Adv Ther.* 2001;18:181–186.

15. Ash K, Lord J, Zukowski M, et al. Comparison of topical therapy for striae alba (20% glycolic acid/0.05% tretinoin versus 20% glycolic acid/10% L-ascorbic acid). *Dermatol Surg.* 1998;24:849–856.

16. Obagi ZE, Obagi S, Alaiti S, et al. TCA-based blue peel: a standardized procedure with depth control. *Dermatol Surg.* 1999;25:773–780.

17. Abdel-Latif AM, Elbendary AS. Treatment of striae distensae with microdermabrasion: a clinical and molecular study. *J Egypt Wom Dermatol Soc.* 2008;5:24–30.

18. Stotland M, Chapas AM, Brightman L, et al. The safety and efficacy of fractional photothermolysis for the correction of striae distensae. *J Drugs Dermatol.* 2008;7:857–861.

19. Lee SE, Kim JH, Lee SJ, et al. Treatment of striae distensae using an ablative 10,600-nm carbon dioxide fractional laser: a retrospective review of 27 participants. *Dermatol Surg.* 2010;36:1683–1690.

20. Hernandez-Perez E, Colombo-Charrier E, Valencia-Ibiett E. Intense pulsed light in the treatment of striae distensae. *Dermatol Surg.* 2002;28:1124–1130.

21. Goldman A, Rossato F, Prati C. Stretch marks: treatment using the 1,064-nm Nd:YAG laser. *Dermatol Surg.* 2008;34:686–691.

22. Jimenez GP, Flores F, Berman B, et al. Treatment of striae rubra and striae alba with the 585-nm pulsed-dye laser. *Dermatol Surg.* 2003;29:362–365.

23. Longo L, Postiglione MG, Marangoni O, et al. Two-year follow-up results of copper bromide laser treatment of striae. *J Clin Laser Med Surg.* 2003;21:157–160.

24. Sadick NS, Magro C, Hoenig A. Prospective clinical and histological study to evaluate the efficacy and safety of a targeted high-intensity narrow band UVB/UVA1 therapy for striae alba. *J Cosmet Laser Ther.* 2007;9:79–83.

25. Alexiades-Armenakas MR, Bernstein LJ, Friedman PM, et al. The safety and efficacy of the 308-nm excimer laser for pigment correction of hypopigmented scars and striae alba. *Arch Dermatol.* 2004;140:955–960.

26. Montesi G, Calvieri S, Balzani A, et al. Bipolar radiofrequency in the treatment of dermatologic imperfections: clinicopathological and immunohistochemical aspects. *J Drugs Dermatol.* 2007;6:890–896.

27. Manuskiatti W, Boonthaweeyuwat E, Varothai S. Treatment of striae distensae with a TriPollar radiofrequency device: a pilot study. *J Dermatolog Treat.* 2009;20:359–364.

28. Anolik R, Chapas AM, Brightman LA, et al. Radiofrequency devices for body shaping: a review and study of 12 patients. *Semin Cutan Med Surg.* 2009;28:236–243.

29. Brightman L, Weiss E, Chapas AM, et al. Improvement in arm and post-partum abdominal and flank subcutaneous fat deposits and skin laxity using a bipolar radiofrequency, infrared, vacuum and mechanical massage device. *Lasers Surgery Med.* 2009;41:791–798.

30. Droitcourt C, Khosrotehrani K, Girot R, et al. Healing of sickle cell ulcers during pregnancy: a favourable effect of foetal cell transfer? *J Eur Acad Dermatol Venereol.* 2008;22:1256–1257.

31. Webb JC, Baack BR, Osler TM, et al. A pregnancy complicated by mature abdominal burn scarring and its surgical solution: a case report. *J Burn Care Rehabil.* 1995;16:276–279.

32. Oluwasanmi JO. Keloids in the African. *Clin Plast Surg.* 1974;1:179–195.

33. Tulandi T, Al-Sannan B, Akbar G, et al. Prospective study of intraabdominal adhesions among women of different races with or without keloids. *Am J Obstet Gynecol.* 2011;204:132.e1–132.e4.

34. Broughton G, Janis JE, Attinger CE. Wound healing: an overview. *Plast Reconstr Surg.* 2006;117:1e-S–32e-S.

35. Alderdice F, McKenna D, Dornan J. Techniques and materials for skin closure in caesarean section. *Cochrane Database Syst Rev.* 2003;(2):CD003577.

36. Alam M, Posten W, Martini MC, et al. Aesthetic and functional efficacy of subcuticular running epidermal closures of the trunk and extremity: a rater-blinded randomized control trial. *Arch Dermatol.* 2006;142:1272–1278.

37. Wolfram D, Tzankov A, Pülzl P, et al. Hypertrophic scars and keloids—a review of their pathophysiology, risk factors, and therapeutic management. *Dermatol Surg.* 2009;35:171–181.

38. Tipton AM, Cohen SA, Chelmow D. Wound infection in the obese pregnant woman. *Semin Perinatol.* 2011;35:345–349.

39. Atiyeh BS. Nonsurgical management of hypertrophic scars: Evidence-based therapies, standard practices, and emerging methods. *Aesthetic Plast Surg.* 2007;31:468–492.

40. Al-Attar A, Mess S, Thomassen JM, et al. Keloid pathogenesis and treatment. *Plast Reconstr Surg.* 2006;117:286–300.

41. Zouboulis CC, Blume U, Buttner P, et al. Outcomes of cryosurgery in keloids and hypertrophic scars: a prospective consecutive trial of case series. *Arch Dermatol.* 1993;129:1146–1151.

42. Vrijman C, van Drooge AM, Limpens J, et al. Laser and intense pulsed light therapy for the treatment of hypertrophic scars: a systematic review. *Br J Dermatol.* 2011;165:934–942.

43. Alster TS. Laser treatment of hypertrophic scars, keloids, and striae. *Dermatol Clin.* 1997;15:419–429.

44. Kartal Durmazlar SP, Eskioglu F, Bodur Z. Hyperkeratosis of the nipple and areola: 2 years of remission with low-dose acitretin and topical calcipotriol therapy. *J Dermatolog Treat.* 2008;19:337–340.

45. Higgins HW, Jenkins J, Horn TD, et al. Pregnancy-associated hyperkeratosis of the nipple: a report of 25 cases. *JAMA Dermatol.* 2013;149:722–726.

CHAPTER 6

Hair and Nail Changes

George Kroumpouzos ■ Richard K. Scher

INTRODUCTION

Hair cycle and growth changes are common in pregnancy and the immediate postpartum period. Changes in hair growth during pregnancy have been reported in 2.6% to 12.8% of patients, with many women noticing vigorous growth and thickening of scalp hair.[1-3] Mild hirsutism can be noticed in most pregnant women, and postpartum shedding of scalp hair (telogen effluvium) is common. Nail changes are less common, seen in 0.66% to 2.1% of patients.[1,2] This chapter reviews these changes and focuses on etiology and management options.

HAIR CHANGES

Large-scale studies with a focus on hair changes in pregnancy are missing, and the studies noted, which follow, have not provided consistent results. In a study of 2,000 pregnant women, hair changes were observed in 3.4% of patients, 1.6% showed increased scalp hair growth, 1% showed male pattern alopecia, and 0.8% showed hirsutism.[1] Muzaffar, Hussain, and Haroon reported hair changes in 12.8% of patients.[2] Of those, 50% reported lengthening/improvement in scalp hair, 39% reported thinning, 5.5% reported frontoparietal recession, and 5.5% reported hypertrichosis. Nevertheless, scalp hair loss was reported more often (1.8%) than improvement (0.82%) by pregnant women in the study by Kumari, Jaisankar, and Thappa.[3]

Hair Cycle and Growth Changes

The hair cycle consists of three phases: (1) the anagen (growth) phase (85% of scalp hair, lasts 2 to 5 years on the vertex); (2) the catagen (transition) phase that lasts 2 to 3 weeks; and (3) finally, the telogen (resting) phase, which lasts 3 months and ends with hair shedding. Scalp hair changes during gestation include an increase in percentage of anagen and thick hairs.[4] Estrogens prolong the anagen phase,[5] as indicated also by early animal studies on pregnant rats.[6] Nissimov and Elchalal showed an increase in scalp hair diameter during pregnancy.[7] A study of the trichogram of pregnant women showed an increase in the percentage of anagen hairs during pregnancy, with 81%

occurring during the first trimester, 90% during the second trimester, and 94% during the third trimester, when compared with 84% anagen in nonpregnant women.[4] Lynfield reported 95% anagen and 5% telogen hairs during both second and third trimesters.[8] Pecoraro, Astore, and Barman showed that during the second and third trimesters, when anagen percentages are higher than during the first trimester, the hair density of the parietal scalp is lower than in nonpregnant women; there are no differences regarding the frontal, coronal, and occipital scalp areas.[4] The authors suggested that a more rapid shedding of telogen hairs may occur in pregnancy rather than a prolongation of the anagen phase. The results of the aforementioned studies need to be reproduced by human scalp biopsy data in order to reach final conclusions about the actual follicular changes during pregnancy.

Hirsutism

Hirsutism, defined as the presence of terminal hairs in a male pattern, starts early in pregnancy. Minor degrees of hirsutism can be noticed in most pregnant women.[9] Hirsutism is more prominent in women with dark hair and/or abundant body hair at the outset.[10] Facial areas, such as the upper lip, chin, cheeks and jaw lines, are predominantly affected (Fig. 6.1) but the arms, legs, back, and genital areas may also be involved. Hair growth along the suprapubic midline, consistent with a male-pattern distribution, is often observed (Fig. 6.2). Acne is often an accompanying feature (see Fig. 6.1). Interestingly, a significant increase in anagen hair follicles during pregnancy, such as that reported in the scalp, has not been found in pubic, parianal, and lumbar areas.[11]

The physiologic transient hypercortisolism of pregnancy, as well as increased ovarian and placental androgen secretion, may contribute to hirsutism.[9] Two cases of generalized hypertrichosis, which developed in pregnancy and resolved postpartum, were attributed to an excess of corticosteroids.[12] If hirsutism occurs to a greater extent than one would expect in pregnancy and/or in an abnormal distribution, polycystic ovary disease, androgen-secreting tumors of the ovary, luteomas, and lutein cysts should be excluded.[13-15] These conditions are characterized by androgen excess and may be associated with a masculinized female fetus.[16] Hirsutism commonly regresses within

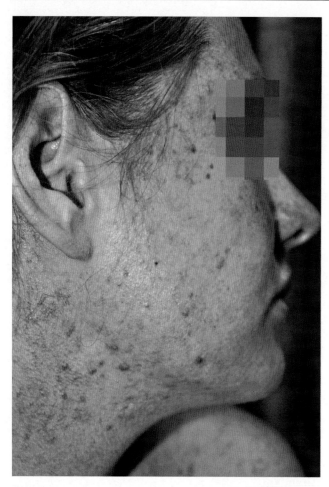

Figure 6.1. Hirsutism is shown at 33 weeks' gestation: excess terminal hairs on the lower cheeks, jaws and neck, and concomitant acne.

6 months' postpartum and occasionally prior to delivery, and often recurs in subsequent pregnancies. Although most of the excess fine hairs resolve, coarse and bristle terminal hairs usually remain (see Fig. 6.2B).[9]

Telogen Effluvium (Telogen Gravidarum)

Hair shedding (telogen effluvium [TE]) develops postpartum, with a latent period of 1 to 16 weeks; 88.7% of cases start between 8 and 16 weeks after delivery.[17] A rapid, synchronous conversion of anagen to telogen hairs, which occurs immediately after delivery (telogen hairs >35% of scalp hairs), following hormonal withdrawal, accounts for this transient hair loss. A similar type of hair loss has been reported after the cessation of oral contraceptive therapy.[18] Lynfield showed that the percentage of anagen hairs fell from 94% in the third trimester to 76% at 6 weeks' postpartum.[8] Other authors reported even higher postpartum telogen counts, such as 65% at 2 months' postpartum.[18] The surgical and emotional stress of delivery, concomitant fever or blood loss, and other hormonal factors, such as prolactin secretion with nursing, can contribute to TE. Behrman suggested that an inhibiting effect on the gonadotrophic activity of the pituitary gland by the high steroid

levels during pregnancy may result in a transient "estrogen deficiency" in the immediate postpartum period, which accounts for TE.[19] The severity of TE varies significantly. The hair loss is not usually noticed until 25% of the hair is lost and becomes more noticeable when more than 40% to 50% of hairs are affected.[20] There appears to be no association between the time of onset and the amount, duration, or final outcome of the shedding.[21]

In a study of 89 patients, the anterior scalp was involved in 59.1%, the entire scalp in 20.4%, and the frontal scalp alone in 11.2% of cases.[17] Prominent temporal thinning is common (Figs. 6.3 and 6.4). Patients with diffuse hair shedding usually have equal part widths over the entire scalp unless they have coexistent pattern hair loss. A pull hair test is positive from several areas of the scalp. A forcible hair pluck shows a percentage of telogen hairs, typically exceeding 20%. Histopathologic diagnosis relies on an increase in the percentage of terminal telogen follicles in horizontal sections of punch biopsy scalp material (Fig. 6.5). Although 20% or more of telogen hairs is typical, lower percentages can be consistent with the diagnosis depending on the baseline telogen count of the patient. There is a slight decrease in the total number of follicles and a normal terminal to vellus follicle ratio.

The duration of shedding is usually less than 6 months but may exceptionally last up to 15 months; two-thirds of patients experience complete regrowth by 6 months' postpartum.[17] The hair, however, may not be as thick as it was prior to pregnancy.[9] Scalp hair density may not return to prepregnancy levels if the patient has a superimposed process, such as female pattern hair loss (Fig. 6.6).[5,17] As indicated by Millikan, a pattern alopecia of female type (Ludwig classification) or male type (Norwood–Hamilton classification) may sometimes become more apparent postpartum because of the change in the number of scalp hairs.[16]

Uncommon Patterns of Hair Loss

A mild **frontoparietal recession** reminiscent of male pattern alopecia toward the end of pregnancy is rare (Fig. 6.7).[22,23] This may be more common in women with a genetic predisposition for pattern hair loss. The frontoparietal recession may resolve spontaneously postpartum,[23] but other authors disagree.[5] **Diffuse hair loss** during the later months of pregnancy has been infrequently reported.[9] It has been attributed to the inhibition of anagen hairs,[24] possibly as a result of decreased gonadotrophic activity secondary to high steroid levels[25]; however, the etiology remains unclear.

Management

Treatment of hirsutism in pregnancy is not recommended because it is expected to improve or resolve postpartum. Patients are advised to wait at least 6 months' postpartum before seeking treatment because fine hairs regress (Table 6.1).

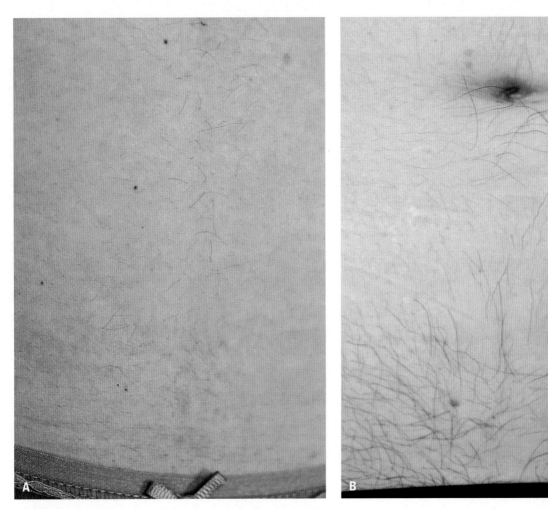

Figure 6.2. Hirsutism is common in the suprapubic area. (**A**) Mild overgrowth of fine hair, expected to resolve postpartum. (**B**) Coarse terminal hairs may persist postpartum.

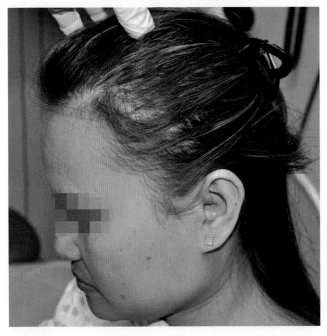

Figure 6.3. Telogen effluvium shown at 11 months' postpartum. Hair regrowth was slow in this patient.

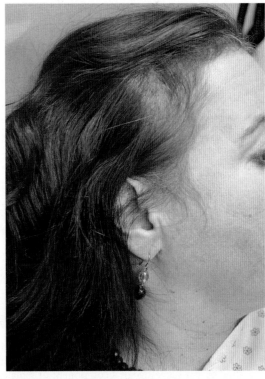

Figure 6.4. Telogen effluvium shown at 6 months' postpartum. Hair regrowth was never complete in this patient.

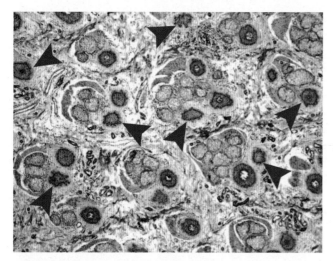

Figure 6.5. A scalp biopsy specimen horizontally sectioned at the level of the infundibulum from a patient with postpartum telogen effluvium. A high proportion of hairs (approximately 30%) are in the telogen phase (*arrows* show some of the telogen hairs). (Courtesy of Dr. Lisa M. Cohen.)

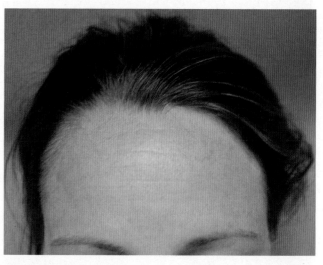

Figure 6.7. Mild frontoparietal recession (shown at 5 months' postpartum), reminiscent of a male pattern alopecia, developed in late pregnancy and persisted postpartum.

Lasers and electrolysis are effective treatment options for terminal hairs that persist. Management of TE involves education, reassurance, and the alleviation of emotional stress as well as good scalp and hair care. Patients with TE should be advised that complete recovery should occur, but it may take up to 15 months. Patients with a superimposed process, such as female pattern alopecia, should be counseled that hair regrowth may not be complete, and treatment of the superimposed process can be initiated postpartum. Topical minoxidil may be utilized postpartum in these cases.[16]

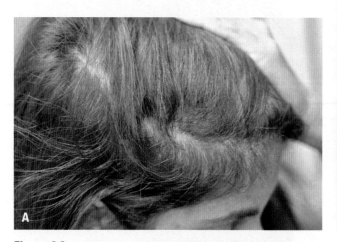

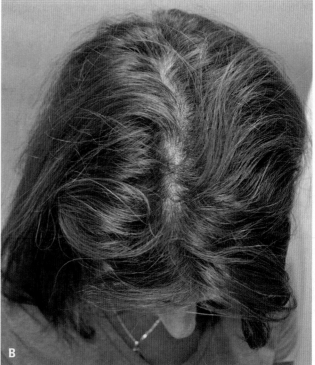

Figure 6.6. Postpartum telogen effluvium with concomitant early pattern hair loss that was proven by scalp biopsy. (**A**) Temporal thinning, as shown by a widened part, consistent with telogen effluvium. (**B**) A widened midline part is suggestive of a component of female-type hair loss. The frontal accentuation of hair loss (a "Christmas tree" pattern) is a clue to differentiating pattern hair loss from telogen effluvium in women. Patients with combined features, such as those shown, do not typically experience complete hair regrowth.

TABLE 6.1	Summary of Management Options
Condition	**Management Options**
Hirsutism	■ Counsel about the transient nature and postpartum improvement/resolution ■ Search for other etiologies, such as polycystic ovary syndrome, androgen-secreting tumors, luteomas, and lutein cysts in cases of severe hirsutism ■ Delay postpartum treatment for 6 months because fine hair is expected to resolve spontaneously ■ Consider hair removal postpartum for persistent terminal hairs
Telogen effluvium	■ Counsel about the transient nature and postpartum improvement/resolution ■ Consider postpartum treatment, such as topical minoxidil, in patients with concomitant pattern hair loss
Nail changes	■ Counsel about the transient nature and postpartum improvement/resolution ■ Rule out other etiologies in case of color change, brittleness, or onycholysis ■ Reduce the use of drying, solvent-based nail products and external sensitizers such as nail polish and nail polish remover ■ Keep nails short if brittle or show onycholysis; use of a moisturizer may be helpful

NAIL CHANGES

Nail changes can be observed as early as the sixth week of gestation.[9] These changes include faster growth (Fig. 6.8), softening, transverse grooving, brittleness (Fig. 6.9), distal onycholysis (separation of nail plate from nail bed) (Fig. 6.10), and subungual hyperkeratosis. Brittleness was the most common change in a study of 2,000 pregnant women.[1] These nail changes typically resolve in 6 to 12 months' postpartum. Beau lines are transverse grooves on the nail plate; these may develop postpartum.[25] The etiology of most of these changes remains unclear. Some authors have noted similarities between pregnancy-associated onycholysis and onycholysis secondary to thyrotoxicosis.[26]

Ponnapula and Boberg reported an increased toenail growth in 89% and a rough toenail texture in 60% of pregnant patients.[27] The faster toenail growth is supported by a faster fingernail growth in earlier studies.[28] Increased peripheral blood flow, as indicated also by capillaroscopy studies, can be triggered by high estrogen levels[29] and may lead to faster nail growth in pregnancy.[27] However, the intake of multivitamin supplements may contribute to increased nail growth because many patients on these supplements report faster growing, soft nails. The study by Ponnapula and Boberg also showed some degree of toenail curvature in pregnancy, in accordance to a previous study,[30] and a similar report in fingernails.[31] The pathogenesis of toenail incurvation may be related to mechanical pressure from excessive pedal edema in restrictive shoe gear.[27] Ingrown toenails were reported in 10% of patients,[27] which is likely associated with the increased curvature.

Two cases of longitudinal melanonychia (LM) affecting multiple nails with the onset in pregnancy have been reported.[32,33] Both patients were of skin type III. There was spontaneous resolution within 3 to 6 months' postpartum. Other authors mentioned two additional cases of transient LM with the involvement of multiple nails.[34] A case of one-nail LM is shown in Figure 6.11A; the epiluminescence microscopy (Fig. 6.11B) showed no features suspicious for an atypical melanocytic process. Signs suggestive of melanocytic atypia, such as band width >5 mm, and multiple streaks of different hues have not been reported; a positive Hutchinson sign in one case[32] was not associated with concerning features of the periungual pigmentation, such as polychromia and asymmetry. Melanocyte activation by high estrogen levels seems to be the most likely mechanism in LM because more than one finger can be affected; however, some authors suggested the formation of lentigines in the nail matrix during gestation but did not provide biopsy confirmation.[32] Cases of leukonychia have been reported,[2,35] including a case of true transverse leukonychia with spontaneous resolution that developed with the onset of menses, and reappeared during and following each pregnancy.[35] Tumors, such as pyogenic granuloma of pregnancy (*granuloma gravidarum*), can develop on the nail bed or periungual areas during gestation (Fig. 6.12) and can be associated with tenderness and hemorrhage.

Management

Nail changes improve postpartum and, therefore, no specific treatment is required. Patients should be counseled about the benign, transient nature of nail changes. When brittleness and/or distal onycholysis is present, other causes such as lichen planus, psoriasis, and onychomycosis should be ruled out, as should infections if there is yellow or green nail discoloration. The benign features of pregnancy-associated LM should be recognized, which helps minimize patient anxiety and avoid invasive procedures, such as a nail matrix biopsy. The frequency of application of solvent-based nail products, which can be drying, should be reduced, and these products should be

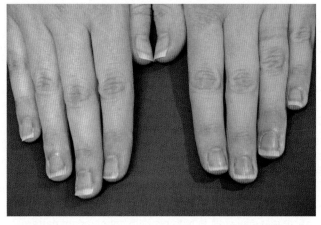

Figure 6.8. Faster growing, soft nails at 16 weeks' gestation.

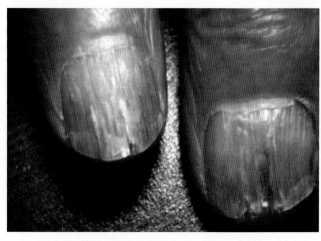

Figure 6.9. Brittle nails may develop in pregnancy.

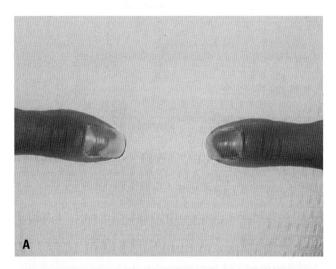

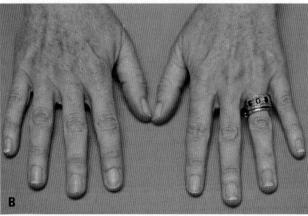

Figure 6.10. Onycholysis in pregnancy. (**A**) Prominent in the thumbnails. (**B**) Affecting most fingernails to varying degrees.

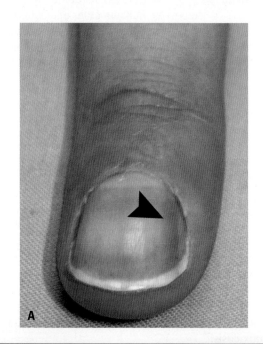

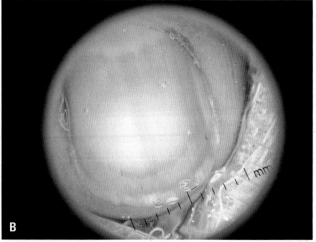

Figure 6.11. (**A**) One-nail longitudinal melanonychia *(arrow)* that developed in pregnancy. (**B**) Dermoscopy of the lesion shows a uniform pigmented band <2 mm wide, comprised of regular, thin, longitudinal gray lines. Signs concerning for atypical melanocytic proliferation such as dark brown or black color, multiple streaks of different hues, and a Hutchinson sign are absent. (Courtesy of Dr. Nathaniel Jellinek.)

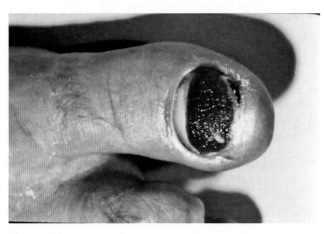

Figure 6.12. A pyogenic granuloma on the nail bed in pregnancy.

used with caution. An effort should be made to reduce the use of external sensitizers, such as nail polish, nail polish removers, and acrylic nails. Aggressive nail techniques should be avoided. It is recommended that nails be kept short, especially if they are brittle or show onycholysis; the use of a moisturizer on nails and cuticles may be helpful.

KEY POINTS

- Hair cycle changes include an increase in anagen and thick hairs of the scalp, the former possibly related to prolongation of the anagen phase.

- Changes in hair growth during pregnancy have been reported in 2.6% to 12.8% of patients, with many women noticing vigorous growth and thickening of scalp hair; however, diffuse hair thinning and a male pattern–like hair loss (frontoparietal recession) in the later months of pregnancy have been reported.

- Mild hirsutism is observed in the majority of pregnant patients and is expected to improve or resolve within 6 months' postpartum; if hirsutism is severe and/or in an abnormal distribution, polycystic ovary disease, androgen-secreting tumors of the ovary, luteomas, and lutein cysts should be ruled out.

- Telogen effluvium occurs as a significant percentage of anagen hairs convert to telogen at or immediately after delivery and usually resolves spontaneously within 15 months' postpartum; hair regrowth may not be complete, especially in cases with concomitant pattern hair loss.

- Nail changes are noticed in 0.66% to 2.1% of patients and resolve postpartum; they include faster growth, softening, transverse grooving, brittleness, distal onycholysis, and subungual hyperkeratosis; longitudinal melanonychia with onset in gestation has been reported.

REFERENCES

1. Rathore SP, Gupta S, Gupta V. Pattern and prevalence of physiological cutaneous changes in pregnancy: a study of 2,000 antenatal women. *Indian J Dermatol Venereol Leprol.* 2011;77(3):402.
2. Muzaffar F, Hussain I, Haroon TS. Physiologic skin changes during pregnancy: a study of 140 cases. *Int J Dermatol.* 1998;37:429–431.
3. Kumari R, Jaisankar TJ, Thappa DM. A clinical study of skin changes in pregnancy. *Indian J Dermatol Venereol Leprol.* 2007;73:141.
4. Pecoraro V, Astore I, Barman JM. The normal trichogram of pregnant women. *Adv Biol Skin.* 1967;9:203–210.
5. Wade TR, Wade SL, Jones HE. Skin changes and diseases associated with pregnancy. *Obstet Gynecol.* 1978;52:233–242.
6. Mohn MP. The effects of different hormonal states on the growth of hair in rats. In: Montagna W, Ellis RA, eds. *Biology of Hair Growth.* New York, NY: Academic Press; 1958:336–393.
7. Nissimov J, Elchalal U. Scalp hair diameter increases during pregnancy. *Clin Exp Dermatol.* 2003;28:525–530.
8. Lynfield YL. Effect of pregnancy on the human hair cycle. *J Invest Dermatol.* 1960;35:323–327.
9. Wong RC, Ellis CN. Physiologic skin changes in pregnancy. *J Am Acad Dermatol.* 1984;10:929–940.
10. Cohen LM, Kroumpouzos G. Pregnancy. In: Callen JP, Jorizzo J, eds. *Dermatological Signs of Internal Disease.* 4th ed. Philadelphia, PA: Elsevier Saunders; 2009:339–348.
11. Trotter M. Activity of hair follicles with reference to pregnancy. *Surg Gynec Obst.* 1935;60:1092–1095.
12. Stoddard F. Hirsutism in pregnancy. *Am J Obstet Gynecol.* 1945;49:417–422.
13. Judd HL, Benirschke K, De Vane G, et al. Maternal virilization developing during a twin pregnancy demonstration of excess ovarian androgen production associated with theca lutein cysts. *N Engl J Med.* 1973;288:118–122.
14. Fayez JA, Bunch TR, Miller GL. Virilization in pregnancy associated with an ovarian cystadenoma. *Am J Obstet Gynecol.* 1974;120:341–346.
15. Fayez JA, Bunch TR, Miller GL. Virilization in pregnancy associated with polycystic ovary disease. *Obstet Gynecol.* 1974;44:511–521.
16. Millikan L. Hirsutism, postpartum telogen effluvium, and male pattern alopecia. *J Cosmet Dermatol.* 2006;5:81–86.
17. Schiff BL, Pawtucket RI, Kern AB. Study of postpartum alopecia. *Arch Dermatol.* 1963;87:609–611.
18. Dawber RP, Connor BL. Pregnancy, hair loss, and the pill. *Br Med J.* 1971;4:234.
19. Behrman H. *The Scalp in Health and Disease.* St Louis, MO: Mosby; 1952.
20. Rapini RP. The skin and pregnancy. In: Creasy RK, Resnik R, eds. *Maternal-Fetal Medicine.* 6th ed. Philadelphia, PA: WB Saunders-Elsevier; 2008:1123–1134.
21. Skelton JB. Postpartum alopecia. *Am J Obstet Gynecol.* 1966;94:125–129.
22. Hellreich PD. The skin changes of pregnancy. *Cutis.* 1974;13:82–86.
23. McKenzie AW. Skin disorders in pregnancy. *Obstet Gynecol.* 1978;52:233–242.
24. Rook A. Endocrine influences on hair growth. *Br Med J.* 1965;1:609–614.
25. Martin AG, Leal-Khouri S. Physiologic skin changes associated with pregnancy. *Int J Dermatol.* 1992;31:375–378.
26. Graham-Brown RAC. Physiologic skin changes related to pregnancy. In: Champion RH, Burton JL, Burns DA, et al., eds. *Rook/*

Wilkinson/Ebling Textbook of Dermatology. 6th ed. London, England: Blackwell Science; 1998:3269–3270.

27. Ponnapula D, Boberg JS. Lower extremity changes experienced during pregnancy. *J Foot Ankle Surg.* 2010;49:452–458.

28. Hewitt D, Hillman RW. Relation between rate of nail growth in pregnant women and estimated previous general growth rate. *Am J Clin Nutr.* 1966;19:436–439.

29. Volterrani M, Rosano G, Coats A, et al. Estrogen acutely increases peripheral blood flow in postmenopausal women. *Am J Med.* 1995;99:119–122.

30. Block RA, Hess LA, Timpano EV, et al. Physiologic changes in the foot during pregnancy. *J Am Podiatr Med Assoc.* 1985;75:297–299.

31. Warraich QA, Cumming GP. Nail deformity in pregnancy. *J Obstet Gynaecol.* 2004;24:822–823.

32. Fryer JM, Werth VP. Pregnancy-associated hyperpigmentation: longitudinal melanonychia. *J Am Acad Dermatol.* 1992;26(3, pt 2): 493–494.

33. Monteagudo B, Suárez O, Rodríguez I, et al. Longitudinal melanonychia in pregnancy [in Spanish]. *Actas Dermosifiliogr.* 2005;96:550.

34. Muallem MM, Rubeiz NG. Physiological and biological skin changes in pregnancy. *Clin Dermatol.* 2006;24:80–83.

35. Chaudhry SI, Black MM. True transverse leukonychia with spontaneous resolution during pregnancy. *Br J Dermatol.* 2006; 154:1199–1219.

CHAPTER 7

Glandular Changes

Elie B. Lowenstein ■ Eve J. Lowenstein

INTRODUCTION

Pregnancy modifies many physiologic functions, including those of the eccrine, apocrine, and sebaceous glands. Glandular changes were noted in up to 36% of pregnant patients in recent studies.[1,2] While many glandular disorders such as acne vulgaris, hidradenitis suppurativa, and Fox–Fordyce disease are thought to be hormonally modulated, surprisingly, their response to pregnancy can be unpredictable. This chapter reviews the physiologic glandular changes of pregnancy, the effects of pregnancy on glandular-related pathologic states, and their management.

PHYSIOLOGIC CHANGES

Activity of the eccrine, apocrine, and sebaceous glands are all affected during pregnancy. Toward the end of pregnancy, eccrine sweating increases, which has been attributed to increased thyroid gland activity or increased weight.[3,4] Nevertheless, palmar sweating may decrease, which is thought to be secondary to increased adrenocortical activity.[5] In addition, apocrine gland activity decreases in pregnancy.[6] Sebaceous gland activity may increase during the third trimester,[4] but several authors believe that there is no consistent change,[3] as also evidenced by the unpredictable course of acne vulgaris in pregnancy.

Breast Changes

Breast changes during pregnancy include enlargement, tenderness, nipple erection, secondary areolae (see Ch. 3, Fig. 3.12), and hypertrophy of the areolar sebaceous glands (Fig. 7.1).[3] The latter, termed Montgomery glands or tubercles, can be seen in up to 36% of pregnant women,[1] are regarded as a reliable early sign of pregnancy, and involute postpartum. Hormonally induced melanocyte stimulation, sebaceous gland hyperactivity, and fluid and sodium retention secondary to the hormonal milieu of pregnancy are postulated to cause these changes.[3]

ACNE VULGARIS

Acne vulgaris, a prevalent disorder of the pilosebaceous unit, shows a diverse clinical picture, ranging from mild comedonal lesions to extensive inflammatory nodules and cysts or fulminant systemic disease. Acne vulgaris is clearly modulated by hormonal influences, as evidenced by typical onset in early puberty and associations with hyperandrogenism, exogenous androgens, and corticosteroids. Acne runs a variable course in pregnancy. Increase in sebaceous gland activity (Fig. 7.2), particularly in the third trimester, is associated with complaints of greasy skin and often coincides with a flare of acne (Fig. 7.3).[3,7] In one study, pregnancy affected acne in approximately 70% of women, with 41% reporting improvement and 29% reporting worsening in pregnancy.[8] An older study had shown improvement of acne in 58% of patients in pregnancy.[9]

Although the course of acne in pregnancy is unpredictable, it is clear that some women will develop acne during pregnancy for the first time or will experience exacerbations during pregnancy, which will subsequently improve after delivery (Fig. 7.4).[3,10] Acne may also develop for the first time in the postpartum period (postgestational acne).[11] Acne conglobata, a severe form of acne vulgaris, has been reported to develop postpartum.[12] Truncal acne may flare (Fig. 7.5), occasionally without concomitant facial involvement. Postinflammatory pigment alteration secondary to acne may develop or worsen during pregnancy and is more prominent in dark skinned patients (see Fig. 7.5). Infants with either parent having a history of severe nodulocystic acne or whose mother has hyperandrogenism are at increased risk of neonatal acne.[13]

Management

Treatment depends on the type and severity of acne, with oral antibiotics reserved for cases with moderate or severe inflammation, including those with extensive truncal involvement (Table 7.1). Topical antibiotics, such as clindamycin and erythromycin, are helpful only in mild cases. Topical azelaic acid is also a safe option (pregnancy category B).[14] Benzoyl peroxide is considered relatively safe to use during pregnancy (pregnancy category C) because of its negligible systemic absorption despite a lack of studies on long-term use in pregnant women. Topical dapsone is pregnancy category C and may be used after weighing benefits and risks; the risks of neonatal kernicterus and methemoglobinemia that have been reported with the oral form are highly unlikely with the topical form. Oral erythromycin base or ethylsuccinate and

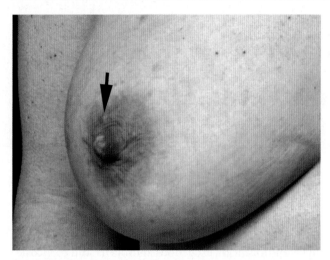

Figure 7.1. Montgomery glands or tubercles are hypertrophic areolar sebaceous glands (shown with *arrow*). They can be seen in up to 36% of pregnant women and typically resolve postpartum. (Courtesy of Dr. George Kroumpouzos.)

penicillins are safe antibiotics to use for moderate-to-severe acne during pregnancy and lactation (pregnancy category B).[14] Nevertheless, their efficacy in the treatment of moderate-to-severe acne is limited. Tetracyclines, retinoids, and the application of salicylic acid over large surface areas should be avoided in pregnant patients (see Chs. 22 and 23).[14,15]

Individual comedo extraction represents a physical modality that can also be utilized during pregnancy. Mild, superficial α-hydroxy acid peels, such as glycolic acid or 2% lactic acid, represent another option for moderate-to-severe acne during pregnancy; although no true safety data exist, most authors consider them safe because of negligible dermal penetration. Microdermabrasion has been used with no reported adverse effects. Peels containing β-hydroxy acid, such as salicylic acid, are an option

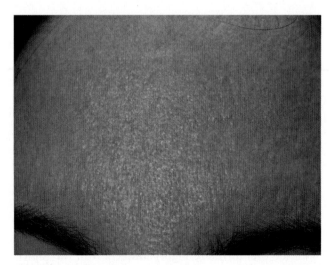

Figure 7.2. Increased sebaceous gland activity during pregnancy.

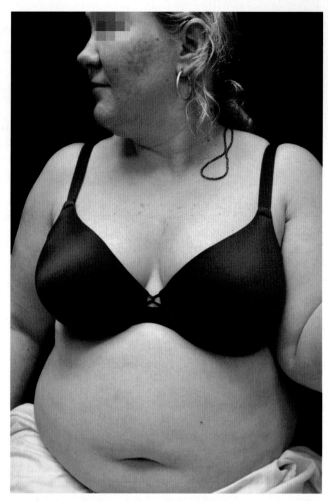

Figure 7.3. Increased acne severity during pregnancy. (Courtesy of Dr. George Kroumpouzos.)

postpartum but should be used with caution because many of the intrapartum medication restrictions remain in effect while lactating. A case of severe acne was treated in pregnancy with narrow band ultraviolet light B (UVB).[16] However, as both broad and narrowband UVB therapies have been associated with photodegradation of folate,[17,18] and low folate levels have been linked to neural tube defects, it is advisable to provide folate supplementation to patients undergoing UVB therapy during pregnancy. No restrictions apply to receiving light therapy for acne postpartum. Laser modalities have been anecdotally used under standard precautions with no adverse effects; however, safety data are lacking.

ACNE ROSACEA

Rosacea is a chronic inflammatory disease that primarily affects pilosebaceous units and blood vessels of the face. It presents with signs of vasodilation, such as flushing, blushing, telangiectasia (erythematotelangiectatic rosacea), and often, papulopustules (papulopustular

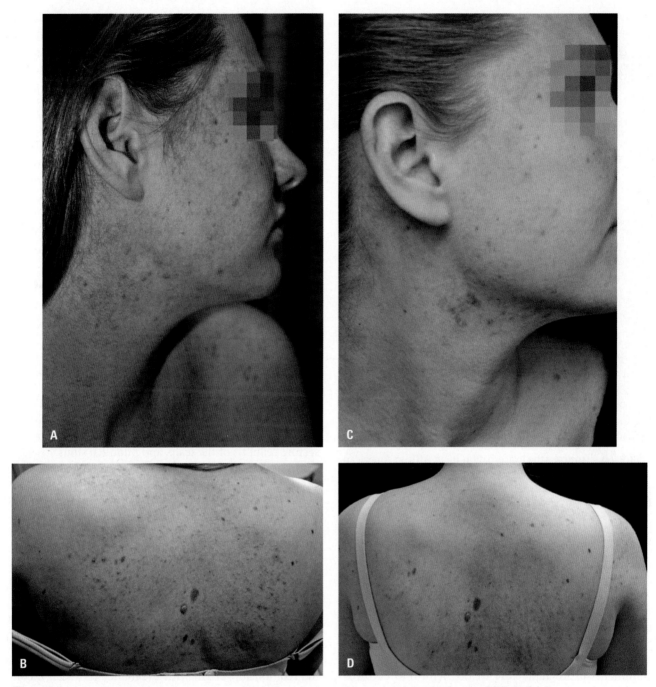

Figure 7.4. A moderate inflammatory acne vulgaris flare during pregnancy. (**A**) On the face, and (**B**) the back. Spontaneous postpartum improvement shown on (**C**) the face and (**D**) the back. (Courtesy of Dr. George Kroumpouzos.)

rosacea) in a centrofacial distribution (Fig. 7.6A). Other presentations include phymatous and ocular rosacea.[19] The etiopathogenesis of rosacea is multifactorial, partly related to vascular hyperactivity, and there is evidence that hormonal factors are involved.[20] The course of rosacea in pregnancy is not predictable and has not been adequately studied. Case studies indicate that certain subtypes of rosacea worsen with pregnancy. Rosacea fulminans, a rarer and more severe subtype of rosacea, has been noted to present during pregnancy or in women taking

oral contraceptives. There have been four reports of rosacea fulminans in pregnancy,[20,21] with dismal obstetric outcomes in two patients.[21]

Management

Patients should be counseled to avoid their unique individual triggers such as sun exposure, spicy foods, emotional stress, and particular cosmetic products. Topical therapy is effective at managing mild papulopustular

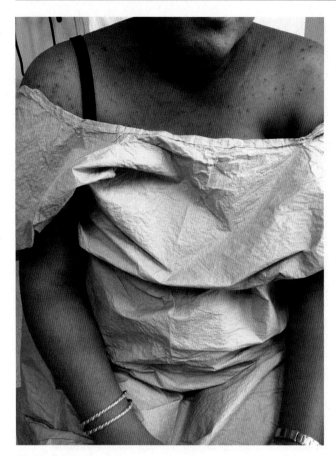

Figure 7.5. Truncal acne exacerbation in an African American woman during the second trimester associated with extensive postinflammatory hyperpigmentation. (Courtesy of Dr. Mital Patel.)

rosacea.[22] Azelaic acid is deemed safe and can be effective (see Fig. 7.6). Topical antibiotics, including metronidazole, clindamycin, and erythromycin, have been effective for the treatment of papulopustular rosacea. Topical and systemic retinoids should be avoided in pregnancy. Systemic antibiotics that are safe for acne (see previous) may also be used for rosacea in pregnancy. Flares of rosacea fulminans in pregnancy are treated with oral erythromycin and oral corticosteroids.[23] Laser or intense pulse light therapy, following standard safety precautions, can be used to treat erythematotelangiectatic rosacea,[19] but such a procedure is usually delayed until the postpartum period because rosacea frequently improves postpartum. The management of ocular rosacea includes ocular hygiene, erythromycin ophthalmic ointment, and sulfa eye drops.[19]

PERIORAL DERMATITIS

Perioral dermatitis is a common dermatosis that primarily affects women of childbearing age.[24] Typical features are shown in Figure 7.7A. The condition is thought to

be pathogenetically related to rosacea because these entities have a similar histopathology and respond to similar therapy. Common trigger factors include topical steroid use and cosmetic products. Little has been published on the prevalence or severity of perioral dermatitis in pregnancy. Perioral dermatitis flares during pregnancy have been noted by the authors (see Fig. 7.7B) and others, but they are not a consistent finding. Perioral dermatitis may be treated in pregnancy with oral and topical antibiotics similar to those discussed for AV and rosacea. Topical metronidazole should be used preferentially over topical calcineurin inhibitors (tacrolimus, pimecrolimus); the latter are pregnancy category C, but their systemic absorption from perioral application should be considered negligible.

HIDRADENITIS SUPPURATIVA

Hidradenitis suppurativa (HS) is a chronic, relapsing, inflammatory skin disease that affects intertriginous areas, especially the axillary and anogenital regions.[25] HS is caused by occlusion and rupture of follicular units, with inflammation of the apocrine glands occurring as a secondary phenomenon.[25,26] HS is also referred to as "acne inversa," reflecting its inclusion in the follicular occlusion tetrad of diseases that also includes acne conglobata, dissecting cellulitis of the scalp, and pilonidal sinus. The disease manifests as painful inflammatory nodules and sterile abscesses. Characteristic lesions include double comedones and deep sinus tracts. Over time, draining sinuses (Fig. 7.8) and progressive scarring develop. Various bacteria have been recovered from HS lesions, but it remains unclear whether they are secondary colonizers or etiologic agents.[27]

HS develops after puberty and tends to resolve with menopause. It appears to be more common among females. HS has been associated with hyperandrogenism, manifesting with elevated androgen levels, acne, hirsutism, and irregular menses.[26] Nevertheless, high levels of androgens were not found in other HS studies.[28] Like acne, the relationship of HS with pregnancy has been inconsistent, with some patients experiencing improvement[6] (Fig. 7.9) and others worsening in pregnancy.[28] Another study showed no consistent relationship between HS and pregnancy.[28] There are no fetal/neonatal risks inherent to the disease; however, a bacterial neonatal infection can develop if there is persistent suppuration at the time of delivery.[29] Although a cesarean delivery would be an option in this case, a neonatal infection can be prevented with maternal antibiotic intake.

Management

Management includes weight loss and smoking cessation because obesity and smoking have been linked to HS. Patients should also be advised to wear loose clothing

TABLE 7.1	Summary of Management Options
Condition	**Management Options**
Acne vulgaris	■ General measures: Mild liquid cleanser ■ Topical medications such as erythromycin, clindamycin, azelaic acid, dapsone, and benzoyl peroxide[14] ■ Oral antibiotics (penicillins, cephalosporins, erythromycin base or ethylsuccinate, clindamycin) for moderate-to-severe acne[14,15] ■ α-Hydroxy acid peels, microdermabrasion, narrowband UVB (safety data limited)[16]
Acne rosacea	■ General measures: As previous; avoid triggers ■ Topical metronidazole, azelaic acid[22] ■ Systemic antibiotics (as previous) for moderate-to-severe disease ■ Ocular hygiene, erythromycin ophthalmic ointment, sulfa eye drops for ocular rosacea[19] ■ Oral erythromycin and oral corticosteroids for flares of rosacea fulminans[23] ■ Laser or intense pulsed light therapy[19]
Perioral dermatitis	■ General measures: As previous; avoid triggers ■ Topical metronidazole, clindamycin, or erythromycin[14,24] ■ Azelaic acid or calcineurin inhibitors[24] ■ Systemic antibiotics (as previous) for moderate-to-severe disease
Hidradenitis suppurativa	■ General measures: Smoking cessation, wear loose clothes ■ Topical antibiotics (erythromycin, clindamycin)[27] ■ Intralesional steroids[27] ■ Oral antibiotics (as previous) ■ TNF-α inhibitors for severe disease (safety data limited)[30] ■ Surgical modalities for severe disease unresponsive to drug therapy[33]
Fox–Fordyce disease	■ Topical antibiotics, such as clindamycin[35] ■ Topical/intralesional steroids[35] ■ UVB therapy, dermabrasion, electrocautery, or excision for severe involvement[35]
Hyperhidrosis	■ General measures: Wear light clothes, shower frequently ■ Topical aluminum chloride[35]
Miliaria	■ General measures: Avoid triggers, wear light clothes, shower frequently, cool with fan ■ Low potency topical steroids for pruritus relief[35]

TNF, tumor necrosis factor; UVB, ultraviolet light B.

so as not to aggravate their lesions and to keep the affected areas clean. HS can result in psychological disability, and emotional support is indicated.[27] Intralesional steroid injections are relatively safe and helpful in pregnancy. The aforementioned oral antibiotics for acne, as well as clindamycin, are safe options for HS in pregnancy and can help suppress inflammation. Antiandrogens and other hormonal therapies, in addition to oral retinoids, are used for patients with moderate-to-severe HS[26] but are contraindicated in pregnancy (see Ch. 22). For severe HS, tumor necrosis factor (TNF)-α inhibitors such as infliximab and adalimumab have been successful as a presurgical treatment.[30] Although TNF-α inhibitors are pregnancy category B, available human

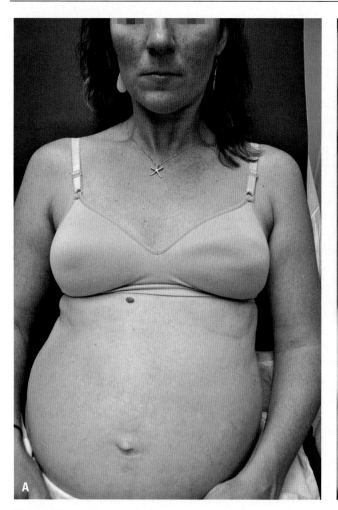 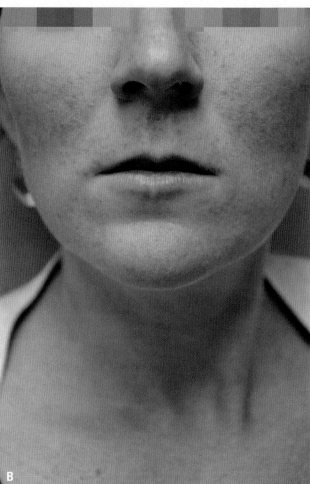

Figure 7.6. (**A**) Rosacea flare (erythematotelangiectatic and papulopustular lesions) during late pregnancy. (**B**) Same patient after 1-month treatment with topical 5% azelaic acid gel. (Courtesy of Dr. George Kroumpouzos.)

exposure data in pregnancy are sparse, and their effects on the fetus are unknown. Some authors recommend discontinuing these agents early on in pregnancy out of fetal anomaly concerns, whereas others recommend discontinuing them during the third trimester in order to minimize the immunosuppressive effects on the neonate.[31,32] In severe cases, the benefits of these agents may outweigh the risks. Surgical procedures, including incision and drainage, exteriorization of sinus tracts, laser evaporation, and local or wide excision, are useful in the most severe forms of HS that do not respond well to drug therapy, or where drug options are limited.[33]

FOX–FORDYCE DISEASE

Fox–Fordyce disease (FFD), also known as apocrine miliaria, is a rare, often intensely pruritic disorder that develops as a result of plugging of the follicular infundibulum,

which obstructs the entrance of the apocrine gland. It occurs primarily in women 15 to 35 years of age (female to male ratio, 9:1) and runs a prolonged course with spontaneous remission after menopause. The condition presents as perifollicular papules primarily in the hair-bearing axillae and in the anogenital and periareolar skin (Fig. 7.10). Hormonal factors appear to play a significant role in the pathogenesis. Apocrine gland activity decreases during pregnancy but may rebound postpartum.[6] FFD reflects this decrease in apocrine activity in pregnancy with improvement during pregnancy, particularly in the last trimester.

Treatment in pregnancy is limited because contraceptives and antiandrogens, which are effective, are contraindicated.[34] Topical antibiotics and mild topical steroids[35] may be used during pregnancy, and topical retinoids may be used postpartum. UVB therapy, dermabrasion, and surgical excision (liposuction-assisted curettage)[35] may be considered for severe involvement during pregnancy; however, each has its associated risks to consider. As

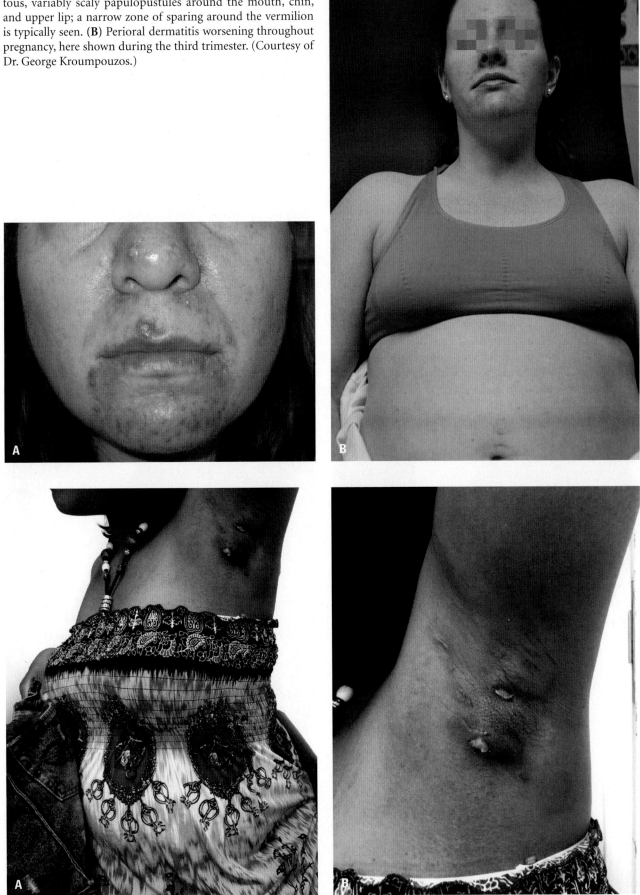

Figure 7.7. (**A**) Perioral dermatitis presenting with erythematous, variably scaly papulopustules around the mouth, chin, and upper lip; a narrow zone of sparing around the vermilion is typically seen. (**B**) Perioral dermatitis worsening throughout pregnancy, here shown during the third trimester. (Courtesy of Dr. George Kroumpouzos.)

Figure 7.8. Draining abscesses in axillary hidradenitis suppurativa in the third trimester. (**A**) A distant view. (**B**) A close-up view. (Courtesy of Dr. Mital Patel.)

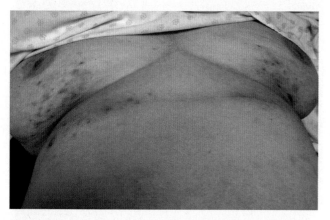

Figure 7.9. Quiescent hidradenitis in the beginning of the second trimester. There is scarring and extensive postinflammatory hyperpigmentation but minimal inflammation. (Courtesy of Dr. George Kroumpouzos.)

mentioned previously, providing folate supplementation to patients undergoing UVB therapy during pregnancy is recommended.[17,18] Dermabrasion and surgical interventions each have risks from anesthesia and other complications to consider.

HYPERHIDROSIS AND MILIARIA

Eccrine sweating tends to increase in the last trimester, which may lead to an increased incidence of hyperhidrosis, miliaria, and dyshidrosis. Hyperhidrosis can be controlled with topical 20% aluminum chloride hexahydrate in ethyl alcohol (pregnancy category C). The manufacturers of iontophoresis units advise against the use of this procedure during pregnancy.[32] Injectable botulinum toxin is pregnancy category C and is generally deferred during pregnancy and lactation.[36] Oral drugs such as clonidine or glycopyrrolate (pregnancy category C) are best deferred until after pregnancy and lactation.

Miliaria is a relatively common skin eruption that is due to a blockage of the eccrine sweat ducts and is usually seen in humid conditions or during overheating.[35] If the blockage occurs at the level of the stratum corneum, the name miliaria crystallina (sudamina) is given. This appears as fine clear noninflammatory, superficial vesicles (Fig. 7.11). If the obstruction occurs deeper in the (intraepidermal portion of the) duct, the terms miliaria rubra (prickly heat) and profunda (the deepest form) are used. Miliaria rubra manifests with minute, nonfollicular erythematous macules and papules with superimposed punctate vesicle; lesions are usually pruritic, and can become pustular. Creating a

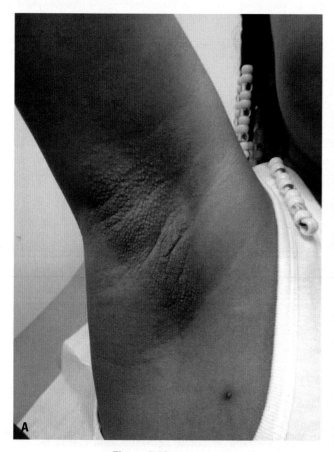

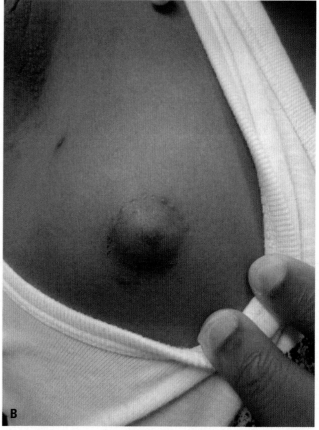

Figure 7.10. Fox–Fordyce disease. **(A)** Axillary involvement. **(B)** Periareolar involvement.

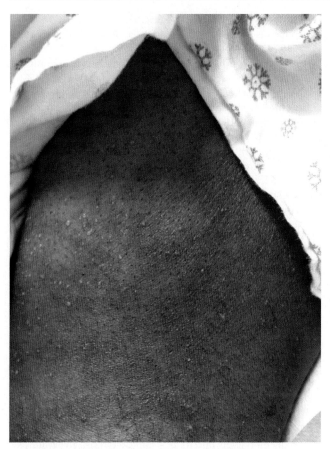

Figure 7.11. Miliaria crystallina presenting with fine superficial vesicles in a febrile hospitalized woman. (Courtesy of Dr. Katy Burris.)

cool environment with the use of fans, wearing lightweight, nonocclusive clothing, and taking frequent showers help resolve the eruption within days. Other triggering factors, such as the use of occlusive ointments, should be avoided.

Acknowledgment: We would like to thank Eleanor Feldman, student at SUNY HSCB College of Medicine, for her assistance in the preparation of this manuscript.

MATERNAL RISKS

Exacerbation of acne, rosacea, and hidradenitis suppurativa
Risks related to bacterial superinfection of hidradenitis lesions
Heat intolerance in third trimester
Risks from pharmacologic treatment

FETAL RISKS

Case reports of stillbirth and intrauterine death in rosacea fulminans
Neonatal infection from severe superinfected hidradenitis
Risks from pharmacologic treatment

- Hormonally induced breast changes in pregnancy include enlargement, tenderness, nipple erection, secondary areolae, and hypertrophy of the areolar sebaceous glands.

- Acne vulgaris, acne rosacea, and hidradenitis suppurativa run an unpredictable course in pregnancy; these disorders have not been associated with fetal risks.

- Treatment of severe acne, acne rosacea, and hidradenitis suppurativa in pregnancy can be challenging because safe antibiotic options in pregnancy show only mild efficacy in these diseases; rosacea fulminans requires an oral antibiotic, such as erythromycin, and oral corticosteroids.

- Apocrine gland activity decreases in pregnancy, which can result in an improvement of Fox–Fordyce disease.

- Eccrine sweating tends to increase, particularly in the last trimester of pregnancy, which can result in an increased incidence of hyperhidrosis and miliaria.

REFERENCES

1. Kumari R, Jaisankar TJ, Thappa DM. A clinical study of skin changes in pregnancy. *Indian J Dermatol Venereol Leprol.* 2007; 73:141.
2. Rathore SP, Gupta S, Gupta V. Pattern and prevalence of physiological cutaneous changes in pregnancy: a study of 2000 antenatal women. *Indian J Dermatol Venereol Leprol.* 2011;77: 402.
3. Wong RC, Ellis CN. Physiologic skin changes in pregnancy. *J Am Acad Dermatol.* 1984;10:929–940.
4. Winton GB, Lewis CW. Dermatoses of pregnancy. *J Am Acad Dermatol.* 1982;6:977–998.
5. MacKinnon PCB, MacKinnon IL. Palmar sweating in pregnancy. *J Obstet Gynecol Br Emp.* 1955;62:298–299.
6. Cornbleet T. Pregnancy and apocrine diseases: hidradenitis, Fox-Fordyce disease. *Arch Dermatol Syph.* 1952;65:12–19.
7. Geraghty LN, Pomeranz MK. Physiologic changes and dermatoses of pregnancy. *Int J Dermatol.* 2011;50:771–782.
8. Shaw JC, White LE. Persistent acne in adult women. *Arch Dermatol.* 2001;137:1252–1253.
9. Ratzer MA. The influence of marriage, pregnancy and childbirth on acne vulgaris. *Br J Dermatol.* 1964;76:165–168.
10. Kroumpouzos G, Cohen LM. Dermatoses of pregnancy. *J Am Acad Dermatol.* 2001;45:1–19.
11. Aman W. Development of acne following pregnancy (postgestational acne) [in German]. *Hautarzt.* 1979;30:319–320.
12. Van Pelt HP, Juhlin L. Acne conglobata after pregnancy. *Acta Derm Venereol.* 1999;79:169.
13. Bekaert C, Song M, Delvigne A. Acne neonatorum and familial hyperandrogenism. *Dermatology.* 1998;196:453–454.

14. Akhavan A, Bershad S. Topical acne drugs: review of clinical properties, systemic exposure, and safety. *Am J Clin Dermatol.* 2003;4:473–492.

15. Mylonas I. Antibiotic chemotherapy during pregnancy and lactation period: aspects for consideration. *Arch Gynecol Obstet.* 2011;283:7–18.

16. Zeichner JA. Narrowband UV-B phototherapy for the treatment of acne vulgaris during pregnancy. *Arch Dermatol.* 2011;147: 537–539.

17. Park KK, Murase JE. Narrowband UV-B phototherapy during pregnancy and folic acid depletion. *Arch Dermatol.* 2012;148: 132–133.

18. Juzeniene A, Stokke KT, Thune P, et al. Pilot study of folate status in healthy volunteers and in patients with psoriasis before and after UV exposure. *J Photochem Photobiol B.* 2010;101:111–116.

19. Culp B, Scheinfeld N. Rosacea: a review. *P T.* 2009;34:38–45.

20. Ferahbas A, Utas S, Mistik S, et al. Rosacea fulminans in pregnancy: case report and review of the literature. *Am J Clin Dermatol.* 2006;7:141–144.

21. Jarrett R, Gonsalves R, Anstey AV. Differing obstetric outcomes of rosacea fulminans in pregnancy: report of three cases with review of pathogenesis and management. *Clin Exp Dermatol.* 2010;35:888–891.

22. Goldgar C, Keahey DJ, Houchins J. Treatment options for acne rosacea. *Am Fam Physician.* 2009;80:461–468.

23. Jansen T, Plewig G, Kligman AM. Diagnosis and treatment of rosacea fulminans. *Dermatology.* 1994;188:251–254.

24. Hafeez ZS. Perioral dermatitis: an update. *Int J Dermatol.* 2003; 42:514–517.

25. Yu CC, Cook MG. Hidradenitis suppurativa: a disease of follicular epithelium, rather than apocrine glands. *Br J Dermatol.* 1990;122:763–769.

26. Mortimer PS, Dawber RP, Gales MA, et al. Mediation of hidradenitis suppurativa by androgens. *Br Med J (Clin Res Ed).* 1986;292:245–248.

27. Alikhan A, Lynch PJ, Eisen DB. Hidradenitis suppurativa: a comprehensive review. *J Am Acad Dermatol.* 2009;60:539–561.

28. Barth JH, Layton AM, Cunliffe WJ. Endocrine factors in pre- and postmenopausal women with hidradenitis suppurativa. *Br J Dermatol.* 1996;134:1057–1059.

29. Revuz J. Hidradenitis suppurativa - patients' frequently asked questions. In: Jemec GBE, Revuz J, Leyden JJ eds. *Hidradenitis Suppurativa.* Heidelberg, Germany: Springer Verlag; 2006: 187–192.

30. Haslund P, Lee RA, Jemec GB. Treatment of hidradenitis suppurativa with tumour necrosis factor-alpha inhibitors. *Acta Derm Venereol.* 2009;89:595–600.

31. Chambers CD, Johnson DL. Emerging data on the use of anti-tumor necrosis factor-alpha medications in pregnancy. *Birth Defects Res A Clin Mol Teratol.* 2012;94:607–611.

32. Ali YM, Kuriya B, Orozco C, et al. Can tumor necrosis factor inhibitors be safely used in pregnancy? *J Rheumatol.* 2010;37:9–17.

33. Yazdanyar S, Jemec GB. Hidradenitis suppurativa: a review of cause and treatment. *Curr Opin Infect Dis.* 2011;24:118–123.

34. Kronthal HL, Pomeranz JR, Sitomer G. Fox-Fordyce disease: treatment with an oral contraceptive. *Arch Dermatol.* 1965;91: 243–245.

35. Miller JL, Hurley HJ. Diseases of the eccrine and apocrine sweat glands. In: Bolognia JL, Jorizzo JL, Rapini RP, eds. *Dermatology.* 2nd ed. Philadelphia, PA: Mosby Elsevier; 2008:531–548.

36. Botulinum toxin. *Consens Statement.* 1990;8:1–20.

37. Frequently asked questions – Iontophoresis. Hyperhidrosis Support Group Web site. http://www.hyperhidrosisuk.org/faq/iontophoresis.html. Accessed October 17, 2012.

CHAPTER 8

Autoimmune Progesterone Dermatitis

Jennifer Jenkins ■ Leslie Robinson-Bostom ■ Giampiero Girolomoni ■ George Kroumpouzos

INTRODUCTION

Autoimmune progesterone dermatitis (AIPD) is a rare hypersensitivity to progesterone. AIPD clinically presents as a cyclic mucocutaneous eruption, which occurs during the luteal phase of the menstrual cycle when progesterone levels are elevated. The concept of allergy to endogenous sex hormones was first proposed by Géber in 1921, who documented a cyclic urticarial eruption that was reproduced upon investigational provocation with premenstrual serum.[1] In addition, desensitization with systematic injections of autologous premenstrual serum was successful at alleviating symptomatology.[1,2] In 1964, Shelley, Preucel, and Spoont demonstrated a partial response to estrogen therapy, documented a cure by oophorectomy, and termed this distinct entity AIPD.[3] Pregnancy has variable effects on the clinical course of AIPD. This chapter reviews AIPD and also autoimmune estrogen dermatitis, a less common cyclic hormone allergy that must be considered in the clinical differential diagnosis of AIPD.

EPIDEMIOLOGY

AIPD is a rare entity. Since the first description by Géber, approximately 60 cases have been reported.[4]

ETIOLOGY

The variable clinical presentations of AIPD are united by an underlying hypersensitivity to endogenous progesterone. Although the sequence of events that leads to the development of hypersensitivity to progesterone has not been adequately clarified, exposure to exogenous progesterone may be involved in the sensitization.

CLINICAL FEATURES

AIPD manifests with variable clinical presentations (Table 8.1). Symptoms present or worsen significantly during the luteal phase of the menstrual cycle. Historical evidence of a cyclical eruption is bolstered by the use of a diary, noting flares of symptoms in the days prior to menses. The clinical presentations include, among others, urticaria[5,6] (Fig. 8.1), erythema multiforme[7,8] (Fig. 8.2), eczematous dermatitis[9,10] (Fig. 8.3), fixed drug eruption[11,12] (Fig. 8.4), stomatitis,[12] purpura and petechiae,[13] vesiculobullous eruptions,[14] deep type of erythema annulare centrifugum,[15] angioedema,[16] and exceptionally, anaphylaxis.[16–18] Cutaneous symptoms begin to flare during the second half of the menstrual cycle and peak 3 to 10 days before menses (Fig. 8.5). Symptoms typically resolve or significantly abate within 1 to 2 days following menstruation. Approximately two-thirds of patients have a known exposure to exogenous progesterone, typically in the form of oral contraceptive therapy.[2] There is a subset of patients without known exogenous progesterone exposure.[19] The pathophysiology in these cases remains unclear, although steroid cross-sensitivity has been proposed as a mechanism.[20] The natural course of AIPD is chronic until menopause. In several reports, AIPD resolved spontaneously after a period of multiple years.

Presentation in Pregnancy

Pregnancy has variable effects on the course of AIPD because both exacerbations and remissions have been reported. AIPD may first occur during pregnancy or in the postpartum period with or without subsequent premenstrual recurrences.[21,22] Pregnancy may also exacerbate the course of preexisting AIPD, and spontaneous abortion has been reported in two cases.[22,23] Recurrences of urticaria and angioedema may occur in pregnancy. Intraoperative angioedema and extensive urticaria have been reported during cesarean sections with concurrent oophorectomy; spinal anesthesia was chosen in order to avoid airway manipulation.[24] Conversely, the pregnant state may improve the course of AIPD during gestation.[25] As an explanation, the gradual rise in hormone levels during pregnancy may desensitize affected patients. Alternatively, elevated maternal cortisol levels may dampen the immunologic response during pregnancy.[18] Maternal and fetal risks of AIPD in pregnancy are summarized in the box.

PATHOLOGY

The histologic findings are dependent on the morphology of the clinical presentation. A subacute spongiotic dermatitis with eosinophils has been demonstrated in

TABLE 8.1	**Clinical Presentation of Autoimmune Progesterone Dermatitis**[a]

Urticaria

Erythema multiforme

Eczematous dermatitis

Vesiculobullous eruption

Stomatitis

Nonspecific papular erythema

Dermatitis herpetiformis–like eruption

Fixed drug eruption

Acneiform eruption

Purpura/petechiae

Erythema annulare centrifugum

Angioedema

Anaphylaxis

[a] Frequency of presentations are presented in descending order.

LABORATORY TESTS

Serologic testing may show an elevated eosinophil count. The underlying hypersensitivity to progesterone is supported by a positive intradermal skin test to progesterone, oral, or intramuscular progesterone challenge or the detection of circulating antibodies to progesterone, particularly in cases with an urticarial or angioedema presentation.

Intradermal Skin Testing

Intradermal skin testing with aqueous progesterone is recommended to confirm progesterone hypersensitivity. Intradermal skin testing should be performed under physician supervision, especially in cases with an urticarial presentation. Skin testing should not be attempted in patients presenting with angioedema or anaphylaxis. Using a tuberculin syringe, diluted aqueous synthetic progesterone (typically 0.01%, 0.1%, and 1%) is injected into the dermis of the anterior forearm, forming a superficial bleb. A normal saline control should also be placed. Readings are performed every 10 minutes for the first 4 hours and then at 24, 48, and, if needed, 96 hours. Positive reactions include an immediate urticarial reaction and a delayed hypersensitivity reaction at the site (a persistent wheal and flare reaction between 24 and 48 hours) (Fig. 8.8). A cautious interpretation must be rendered to avoid false-positive readings due to irritant reaction to diluents.[2,26]

Provocative Challenge

Challenges from the intramuscular or oral administration of progesterone are less preferable given the risk of systemic reactions; rare reports describe severe exacerbation of urticaria with angioedema. Provocative testing may, however, prove diagnostic in those patients with negative

eczematous lesions mimicking allergic contact dermatitis both clinically and histopathologically[9] (Fig. 8.6). Erythema multiforme–like presentations show histopathologic features of vacuolar interface dermatitis, with necrotic basal keratinocytes overlying a superficial perivascular infiltrate of lymphocytes, neutrophils, and some eosinophils.[8] A cutaneous and mucosal fixed drug eruption demonstrated a superficial perivascular mononuclear cell infiltrate with spongiosis and pigment incontinence.[11,12] Other eczematous presentations show histopathologic features of a hypersensitivity reaction (Fig. 8.7).

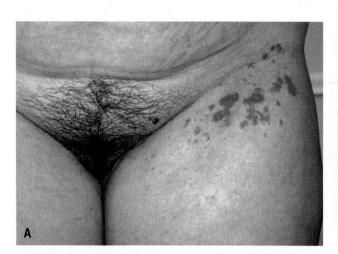
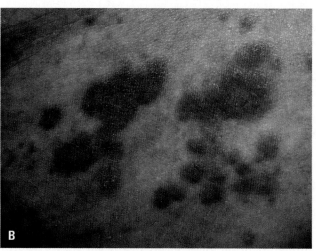

Figure 8.1. A clinical presentation with urticarial lesions in a 33-year-old female. (**A**) A distant view and (**B**) a close view. Lesions appeared 4 to 5 days before menses and resolved with residual hyperpigmentation a few days after menses.

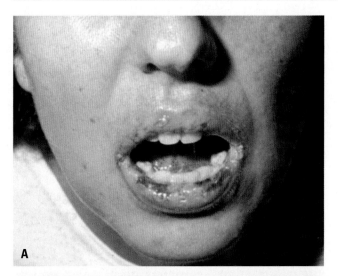

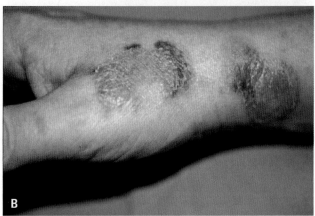

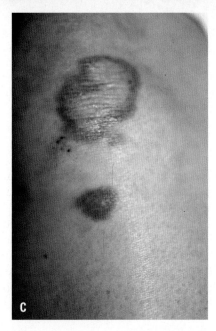

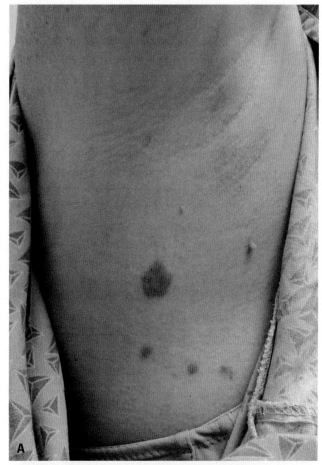

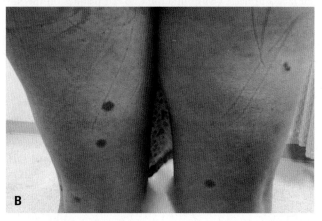

Figure 8.3. Clinical features of eczematous dermatitis. **(A)** Round, pink to red scaly plaques located on the axilla. **(B)** Round, pink scaly plaques located on the posterior upper legs. This patient, with a known history of autoimmune progesterone dermatitis, was undergoing in vitro fertilization and was managed with topical corticosteroids.

Figure 8.2. The clinical features of erythema multiforme. **(A)** Eroded and crusted lesions on the oral mucosa and lips. Similar lesions were present on the vulva and perineal area. **(B)** Targetoid erythematous plaques with central bulla formation on the forearm and wrist. **(C)** A similar targetoid lesion on the knee.

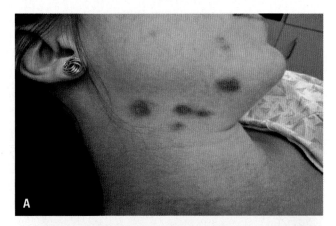

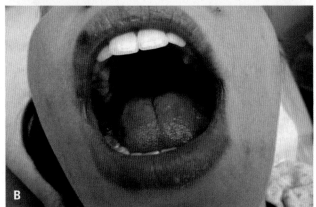

Figure 8.4. Clinical features of a fixed drug eruption. (**A**) Round, 1- to 2-cm, pink to red erythematous plaques with scale located on face and neck. (**B**) Round, pink to red plaques on the lips and cheek. These lesions faded between menstrual cycles, leaving a dark purple discoloration, and recurred in the same location each month. (Courtesy of Dr. Mariana Castells.)

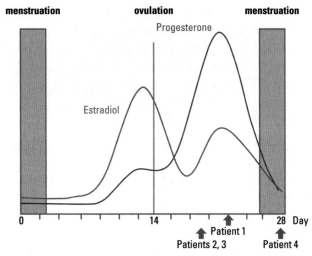

Figure 8.5. Estradiol and progesterone levels in the menstrual cycle. *Arrows* show the day of the cycle when symptoms started in each of the four patients presented in Figures 8.1 to 8.4. (Figure modified from Prieto-Garcia A, Sloane DE, Gargiulo AR, et al. Autoimmune progesterone dermatitis: clinical presentation and management with progesterone desensitization for successful in vitro fertilization. *Fertil Steril.* 2011;3:e9–e13.)

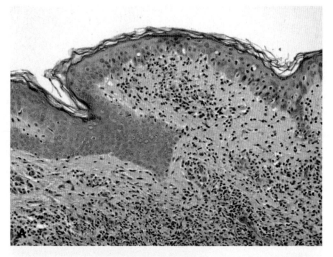

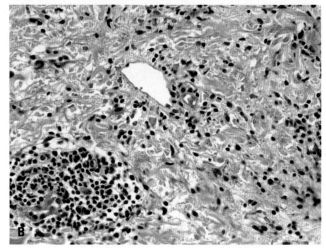

Figure 8.6. Histopathology of vacuolar interface dermatitis. (**A**) The vacuolar interface change at the dermoepidermal junction overlying a superficial dermal lymphohistiocytic infiltrate (hematoxylin-eosin, ×20). (**B**) Superficial to mid-dermal perivascular and interstitial lymphohistiocytic infiltrate with few eosinophils (hematoxylin-eosin, ×40).

skin testing. Aqueous progesterone is strongly preferred as an intramuscular progesterone formulation so as to avoid irritant reactions to the vehicle. Provocative testing should be performed during the first half of the menstrual cycle when endogenous progesterone levels are low. An oral challenge with synthetic progesterone may not reliably reproduce symptoms. Intravaginal progesterone provocation has demonstrated utility when an aqueous solution is not available for intradermal testing.[21,27]

DIAGNOSIS

Diagnostic criteria for AIPD include (1) cyclic cutaneous or mucosal lesions related to the menstrual cycle, (2) positive progesterone sensitivity, and (3) symptomatic improvement upon ovulation suppression.[28]

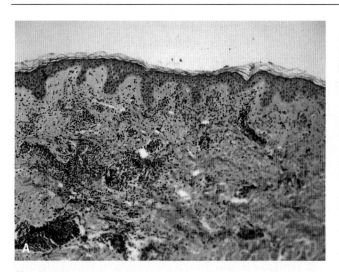
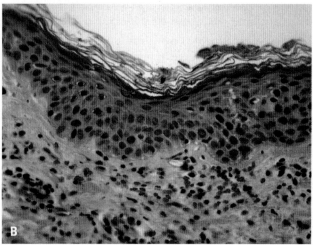

Figure 8.7. Histopathology of hypersensitivity reaction. (**A**) Superficial to mid-dermal perivascular and predominantly lymphohistiocytic infiltrate with few eosinophils (hematoxylin-eosin, ×10). (**B**) Mild epidermal spongiosis with focal parakeratosis. Papillary dermis with focal erythrocyte extravasation and a superficial perivascular lymphocytic infiltrate (hematoxylin-eosin, ×40). (Courtesy of Dr. Lisa M. Cohen.)

DIFFERENTIAL DIAGNOSIS

The differential diagnosis is dependent on the morphologic features of AIPD. When acneiform features are present, AIPD should be differentiated from perimenstrual flares of acne, which are often encountered in the spectrum of premenstrual syndrome. AIPD with eczematous features should be differentiated from atopic and contact dermatitis, whereas AIPD with targetoid or bullous lesions should be differentiated from erythema multiforme and bullous diseases. Other diseases that show premenstrual flares, such as psoriasis, lupus erythematosus, lichen planus, dermatitis herpetiformis, and urticaria, may need to be included in the differential diagnosis. A history of flares during the luteal phase of the menstrual cycle favors the diagnosis of AIPD, but a final confirmation of diagnosis requires a positive progesterone testing.

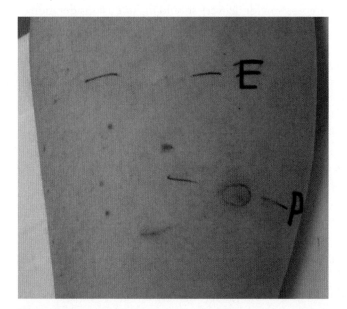

Figure 8.8. Intradermal testing with progesterone (0.1 ml of an aqueous suspension at 1 mg/ml), resulted in a >1-cm area of erythema and edema (*P site*) 8 hours after the injection. Intradermal testing with estrogen benzoates (0.1 ml of an aqueous suspension at 1 mg/ml) was negative (*E site*) as was the control intradermal testing with distilled water on the contralateral forearm. (Testing performed by Dr. Girolomoni.)

PATHOGENESIS

It has been postulated that an allergy to endogenous progesterone occurs after sensitization from an exogenous exposure. Indeed, most reported cases have a history of exogenous progesterone exposure, often in the form of oral contraceptive therapy. The uptake of exogenous progesterone by antigen-presenting cells and the presentation of T-helper cells may result in sensitization.[29] However, not all cases of AIPD have been associated with a prior exposure to exogenous progesterone and, in some cases, similar steroids were suggested.[30] One case report describes familial AIPD in three sisters.[31] Several mechanisms may be involved. The dermatologic findings range from eczematous eruptions to anaphylactic reactions, representing either a type IV or type I hypersensitivity reaction, respectively. A type III hypersensitivity reaction has also been proposed in those cases with circulating immunoglobulin (Ig)G antibodies against progesterone.[32] In patients with anaphylaxis and negative skin tests, progesterone may have a direct histamine-releasing effect on mast cells[33] because human mast cells express progesterone receptors.[29]

MANAGEMENT

The goal of treatment is ovulation suppression to eliminate the luteal phase surge of progesterone. Symptomatic treatment with oral H_1 and H_2 antihistamines and topical or oral corticosteroids (prednisolone) has been effective in mild cases and may be tried when ovulation suppression is contraindicated (Table 8.2).[10,25] Oral contraceptive therapy has demonstrated some effectiveness because spikes of progesterone are inhibited under the ovarian suppression that is induced by oral contraception.[31] Nevertheless, oral contraceptives can cause exacerbation in some cases.[4] Gonadotropin-releasing hormone (GnRH) analog therapy has been used successfully in the perimenopausal period[9,18,27] but is less preferable for the majority of patients because it induces premature menopause. Estrogen supplementation and bone density monitoring are required. Danazol has been used with variable success.[34] Progesterone desensitization is uncommonly performed,[29] and therapy with conjugated estrogens alone[32] is associated with an increased risk of endometrial cancer. Tamoxifen is a less favorable long-term treatment option due to its increased risk for uterine and breast malignancy, thromboembolism, and negative effects on bone metabolism.[12,25,35] Intermittent perimenstrual use of tamoxifen is an option. Definitive therapy is achieved with a hysterectomy and bilateral salpingo-oopherectomy but should be reserved for severe and recalcitrant cases.[36,37]

Treatment of Progesterone-Induced Anaphylaxis

Treatment rests on oral antihistamines, systemic corticosteroids, epinephrine, and bronchodilators as needed. Patients with a known anaphylactic response or angioedema should be equipped with epinephrine autoinjectors. Anovulatory treatment options are similar as listed previously. In more severe cases, definitive treatment is surgical oophorectomy. Before the consideration of an oophorectomy, a trial of chemical oophorectomy with a GnRH analogue is recommended. Hormonal confirmation of anovulation should be followed by a positive progesterone challenge. Once these criteria are met, thereby confirming both sensitivity to progesterone and the effectiveness of an oophorectomy, surgical oophorectomy may be offered as a definitive therapy.[18]

Preconception Management

The management of AIPD for patients trying to conceive rests on symptomatic treatment with antihistamines, topical corticosteroids, and, if needed, oral corticosteroids. A unique therapeutic challenge arises in afflicted patients who must undergo in vitro fertilization. Effective treatment options in this clinical scenario include progesterone desensitization and topical corticosteroids.[10,29]

Management in Pregnancy and Delivery

During pregnancy, treatment options are limited. In cases with a mild clinical presentation, topical corticosteroids are a good treatment option. Cases with a history of urticaria or angioedema/anaphylaxis may need repeated courses of systemic corticosteroids, epinephrine (administered subcutaneously or intravenously), and oral antihistamines (see Table 8.2). Management recommendations for delivery are dependent on the clinical presentation (Table 8.3). In cases presenting with urticaria or angioedema, the preparation for delivery should include a consideration of premedication with corticosteroids, antihistamines, and

TABLE 8.2	Summary of Management Options	

Treatment	Comment
Pregnant/Lactating Patient	
Symptomatic treatment (dependent on clinical presentation)	Oral antihistamines, topical corticosteroids, oral corticosteroids, subcutaneous epinephrine when indicated[10,25]
Additional Options Postpartum in Nonlactating Patient	
Oral contraceptive therapy	Safe option[31]
GnRH analog	Leuprolide and buserelin used effectively in case reports; appealing option in the perimenopausal period[4,9,18]
Danazol	200 mg twice daily starting 1–2 days prior to expected menses and continued for 3 days upon onset[34]
Progesterone desensitization	Uncommonly performed; effective option if patient plans to undergo in vitro fertilization[29]
Conjugated estrogens	Increased risk of endometrial cancer[32]
Tamoxifen	20–30 mg/d, less favorable long-term option because of its safety profile; intermittent perimenstrual use is an option[25,35]

GnRH, gonadotropin-releasing hormone.

TABLE 8.3	Obstetric Management

If there is a history of papulosquamous or vesiculobullous presentation,

■ Provide routine obstetric management

If there is a history of urticaria, angioedema, or anaphylaxis,

■ Provide prepartum planning with consideration of anesthesia options, if needed
■ Consider regional anesthesia to avoid airway manipulation if cesarean section
■ Consider prophylaxis with systemic corticosteroids, antihistamines, and intravenous fluids
■ Provide periodic monitoring for signs and symptoms of eruption
■ Provide standard anaphylaxis treatment for symptomatic cases

intravenous fluids. If a cesarean section is performed, further consideration should be made for regional anesthesia to avoid airway manipulation.[24] Severe acute reactions in the immediate postpartum period have been described and should be treated as standard anaphylaxis.

AUTOIMMUNE PROGESTERONE DERMATITIS OF PREGNANCY

Some authors distinguish AIPD from autoimmune progesterone dermatitis of pregnancy, with the latter being more closely associated with pregnancy. AIPD of pregnancy has been reported only once in the English literature.[22] This report described a 25-year-old woman with a nonpruritic, acneiform eruption and polyarthritis, which manifested only in pregnancy and resolved postpartum. Recurrent skin and joint symptoms occurred within the first weeks of gestation in three pregnancies. Each pregnancy was complicated by a spontaneous abortion. Despite the absence of premenstrual flares between pregnancies, the patient demonstrated a positive oral challenge to contraceptive and positive intradermal skin testing to progesterone. The histopathology demonstrated a pandermal perivascular infiltrate with lymphocytes and eosinophils, eosinophilic lobular panniculitis, and intraepidermal eosinophilic abscess formation. This patient was treated only in the nonpregnant state with antiovulation therapy (1.25 mg conjugated equine estrogen for 21 days per month).

AUTOIMMUNE ESTROGEN DERMATITIS

Sensitivity to endogenous estrogen manifests with a cyclic eruption called autoimmune estrogen dermatitis (AED). As in AIPD, the clinical presentation is variable and a diagnosis relies on the identification of the cyclical premenstrual flare. Cutaneous manifestations include eczema, urticaria, papulovesicular eruptions, hand eruptions, and generalized or localized (vulvar, perianal) pruritus. Some cases have demonstrated localization of the lesions to the head, neck, upper trunk, and arms, possibly because estrogen receptor density is the highest in this region. Intradermal skin testing to estrogen is required to confirm the diagnosis. Shelley, Shelley, and Talanin used a subepidermal injection of a sterile aqueous suspension of pure estrone (0.1 ml in a 1:1,000 dilution).[38] Positive test results are the persistence of a papule for more than 24 hours or, in cases of urticaria, an immediate urticarial wheal that fades in hours. Reactivation of the test area during premenstrual periods is a convincing proof of the diagnosis.[38] An oral challenge can be performed with ethinyl estradiol. A positive oral challenge confirms an estrogen-aggravated dermatosis; however, positive intradermal skin testing is required for a diagnosis. Intradermal progesterone testing is routinely performed to rule out AIPD.

AED has been reported in a patient presenting with urticaria in early gestation[39]; no fetal complications were noted. Treatment with tamoxifen 10 mg one to three times daily for 10 to 14 days before menses has been effective.[38] However, the safety profile of tamoxifen limits its use, and intermittent, brief administration is recommended. Progesterone-only therapy in oral or intramuscular form is an option, but it carries the risk of metrorrhagia. Mild symptoms may be treated with topical corticosteroids, oral antihistamines, or short courses of oral corticosteroids. Like AIPD, AED runs a chronic course with remission at menopause, although spontaneous remission after several years has been reported.[2,38]

MATERNAL RISKS

Depending on presentation:
Eczematous or vesiculobullous eruption: Secondary infection
Erythema multiforme–like eruption or stomatitis: Difficulty eating, malaise, pain, loss of appetite
Urticaria: Respiratory difficulty
Angioedema/anaphylaxis: Respiratory compromise, hemodynamic instability
Risks from pharmacologic treatment

FETAL RISKS

Spontaneous abortion (two cases)
Risks from pharmacologic treatment

KEY POINTS

■ Autoimmune progesterone dermatitis is a hypersensitivity reaction to endogenous progesterone that manifests as a mucocutaneous eruption during the luteal phase of the menstrual cycle.

- Skin manifestations vary, which makes diagnosis challenging; the most common are urticaria, erythema multiforme, and eczematous dermatitis.

- Additional diagnostic criteria are a provocative test, such as intradermal skin testing, and symptomatic improvement upon ovulation suppression.

- Autoimmune progesterone dermatitis may start, worsen, or improve in pregnancy; a case developed only in pregnancy (autoimmune progesterone dermatitis of pregnancy).

- Treatment in pregnancy includes oral antihistamines, topical and/or systemic corticosteroids, and epinephrine in cases of angioedema/anaphylaxis.

- The preparation for delivery in cases with history of urticaria or angioedema should include premedication with corticosteroids, antihistamines, and intravenous fluids; regional anesthesia should be considered if a cesarean section is performed.

- Sensitivity to endogenous estrogen (autoimmune estrogen dermatitis) causes a clinical syndrome similar to autoimmune progesterone dermatitis, which presents with a cyclical premenstrual flare.

REFERENCES

1. Géber H. Einige Daten zur Pathologie der Urticaria menstruationalis. *Dermatol Z.* 1921;32:143–150.
2. Black M, Stephens C. Perimenstrual skin eruptions, autoimmune progesterone dermatitis, autoimmune estrogen dermatitis. In: Black MM, Ambros-Rudolph C, Edwards L, et al., eds. *Obstetric and Gynecologic Dermatology.* 3rd ed. London, England: Mosby Elsevier; 2008:13–22.
3. Shelley W, Preucel R, Spoont S. Autoimmune progesterone dermatitis. Cure by oophorectomy. *JAMA.* 1964;190:35–38.
4. Toms-White LM, John LH, Griffiths DJ, et al. Autoimmune progesterone dermatitis: a diagnosis easily missed. *Clin Exp Dermatol.* 2010;36:378–380.
5. Vasconcelos C, Xavier P, Vieira AP, et al. Autoimmune progesterone urticaria. *Gynecol Endocrinol.* 2000;14:245–247.
6. Walling HW, Scupham RK. Autoimmune progesterone dermatitis. Case report with histologic overlap of erythema multiforme and urticaria. *Int J Dermatol.* 2008;47:380–382.
7. Nasabzadeh T, Stefanato C, Doole J, et al. Recurrent erythema multiforme triggered by progesterone sensitivity. *J Cutan Pathol.* 2010;37:1164–1167.
8. Cocuroccia B, Gisondi P, Gubinelli E, et al. Autoimmune progesterone dermatitis. *Gynecol Endocrinol.* 2006;22:54–56.
9. Lee MK, Lee WY, Yong SJ, et al. A case of autoimmune progesterone dermatitis misdiagnosed as allergic contact dermatitis. *Allergy Asthma Immunol Res.* 2011;2:141–144.
10. Jenkins J, Geng A, Robinson-Bostom L. Autoimmune progesterone dermatitis associated with infertility treatment. *J Am Acad Dermatol.* 2008;58:353–355.
11. Asai J, Katoh N, Nakano M, et al. Case of autoimmune progesterone dermatitis presenting as fixed drug eruption. *J Dermatol.* 2009;36:643–645.
12. Moghadam BK, Hersini S, Barker BF. Autoimmune progesterone dermatitis and stomatitis. *Oral Surg Oral Med Oral Pathol Oral Radiol Endod.* 1998;85:537–541.
13. Wintzen M, Goor-van Egmond MB, Noz KC. Autoimmune progesterone dermatitis presenting with purpura and petechiae. *Clin Exp Dermatol.* 2004;29:316.
14. Leitao EA, Bernhard JD. Perimenstrual nonvesicular dermatitis herpetiformis. *J Am Acad Dermatol.* 1990;22:331–334.
15. Halevy S, Cohen AD, Lunenfeld E, et al. Autoimmune progesterone dermatitis manifested as erythema annulare centrifugum: confirmation of progesterone sensitivity by in vitro interferon-gamma release. *J Am Acad Dermatol.* 2002;47:311–313.
16. Bernstein IL, Bernstein DI, Lummus ZL, et al. A case of progesterone-induced anaphylaxis, cyclic urticaria/angioedema, and autoimmune dermatitis. *J Womens Health.* 2011;4:643–648.
17. Bemanian MH, Gharagozlou M, Farashahi MH, et al. Autoimmune progesterone anaphylaxis. *Iran J Allergy Asthma Immunol.* 2007;6:97–99.
18. Snyder JL, Krishnaswamy G. Autoimmune progesterone dermatitis and its manifestation as anaphylaxis: a case report and literature review. *Ann Allergy Asthma Immunol.* 2003;90:469–477.
19. Kakarla N, Zurawin RK. A case of autoimmune progesterone dermatitis in an adolescent female. *J Pediatr Adolesc Gynecol.* 2006;19:125–129.
20. Moody BR, Schatten S. Autoimmune progesterone dermatitis: onset in a woman without previous exogenous progesterone exposure. *South Med J.* 1997;90:845–846.
21. Le K, Wood G. A case of autoimmune progesterone dermatitis diagnosed by progesterone pessary. *Australas J Dermatol.* 2011;52:139–141.
22. Bierman SM. Autoimmune progesterone dermatitis of pregnancy. *Arch Dermatol.* 1973;107:896–901.
23. Wojnarowska E, Greaves MW, Peachey RD. Progesterone-induced erythema multiforme. *J R Soc Med.* 1985;78:407–408.
24. O'Rourke J, Khawaja N, Loughrey, et al. Autoimmune progesterone dermatitis in a parturient for emergency caesarean section. *Int J Obstetric Anesthesia.* 2004;13:275–279.
25. Stephens CJ, Wojnarowska FT, Wilkinson JD. Autoimmune progesterone dermatitis responding to Tamoxifen. *Br J Dermatol.* 1989;121:135–137.
26. Stranahan D, Rausch D, Deng A, et al. The role of intradermal skin testing and patch testing in the diagnosis of autoimmune progesterone dermatitis. *Dermatitis.* 2006;17:39–42.
27. Németh H, Kovács E, Gödény S, et al. Autoimmune progesterone dermatitis diagnosed by intravaginal progesterone provocation in a hysterectomised woman. *Gynecol Endocrinol.* 2009;25:410–412.
28. Warin AP. Case 2. Diagnosis: erythema multiforme as a presentation of autoimmune progesterone dermatitis. *Clin Exp Dermatol.* 2001;26:107–108.
29. Prieto-Garcia A, Sloane DE, Gargiulo AR, et al. Autoimmune progesterone dermatitis: clinical presentation and management with progesterone desensitization for successful in vitro fertilization. *Fertil Steril.* 2011;3:e9–e13.
30. Dedecker F, Graesslin O, Quereux C, et al. Autoimmune progesterone dermatitis: a rare pathology. *Eur J Obstet Gynecol Reprod Biol.* 2005;123:120–121.
31. Chawla SV, Quirk C, Sondheimer SJ, et al. Autoimmune progesterone dermatitis. *Arch Dermatol.* 2009;145:341–342.

32. Hart R. Autoimmune progesterone dermatitis. *Arch Dermatol.* 1977;113:426–430.

33. Slater JE, Kaliner M. Effects of sex hormones on basophil histamine release in recurrent idiopathic anaphylaxis. *J Allergy Clin Immunol.* 1987;80:285–290.

34. Shahar E, Bergman R, Pollack S. Autoimmune progesterone dermatitis: effective prophylactic treatment with danazol. *Int J Dermatol.* 1997;36:708–711.

35. Nabai H, Rahbari H. Autoimmune progesterone dermatitis treated with tamoxifen. *Cutis.* 1994;54:181–182.

36. Medeiros S, Rodrigues-Alves R, Costa M, et al. Autoimmune progesterone dermatitis: treatment with oophorectomy. *Clin Exp Dermatol.* 2010;35:e12–3.

37. Ródenas JM, Herranz MT, Tercedor J. Autoimmune progesterone dermatitis: treatment with oophorectomy. *Br J Dermatol.* 1998;139:508–511.

38. Shelley WB, Shelley ED, Talanin NY, et al. Estrogen dermatitis. *J Am Acad Dermatol.* 1995;32:25–31.

39. Lee AY, Lee KH, Lim YG. Oestrogen urticaria associated with pregnancy. *Br J Dermatol.* 1999;141:774.

CHAPTER 9

Inflammatory Skin Disease

George Kroumpouzos ■ Annalisa Patrizi

INTRODUCTION

Inflammatory skin disease can worsen or, less often, improve during gestation.[1] Diseases that may develop and/or often worsen in gestation include atopic dermatitis (AD), urticarias, and erythema annulare centrifugum (EAC).[1–3] Chronic plaque psoriasis may improve in pregnancy, whereas generalized pustular psoriasis (impetigo herpetiformis) can be triggered by pregnancy (see Ch. 10).[1] This chapter highlights the clinical features, the pathogenesis, and the management of inflammatory skin disease in pregnancy.

ATOPIC DERMATITIS

Epidemiology

A large prospective study did not show an increased prevalence,[4] but two subsequent studies indicated a high prevalence of AD, including "new AD" (AD developing for the first time in gestation), which comprises up to 80% of all AD cases in pregnancy.[5,6] AD was the most common pregnancy dermatosis in these two studies. Two other studies confirm deterioration of AD in 52% to 61% of patients.[7,8] There is a personal history of atopy and/or infantile AD in 27% of pregnant females with AD, a family history of atopy in 50% of cases, and infantile AD in 19% of the offspring.[5]

Clinical Features

Most pregnant patients with AD present with lesions on typical atopic sites, such as the flexural aspects of the extremities (Fig. 9.1), face, neck (Fig. 9.2), and décolleté (Fig. 9.3),[5] although hand and/or foot (Fig. 9.4) and truncal involvement (Figs. 9.5A and 9.5B) are also common.[6] Lesions often become generalized (see Fig. 9.5). Less common presentations are follicular and nummular eczema (Fig. 9.6), and eczema of the nipple and/or areola (Fig. 9.7). As indicated in a peer review,[2] the prevalence of several important (xerosis) or associated features (keratosis pilaris, atypical vascular responses, ocular/periorbital changes, hyperlinear palms, ichthyosis, perifollicular accentuation, lichenification) of AD[9] in gestation has not been reported in recent studies.[5–7] In the authors' experience, xerosis, worsening of keratosis pilaris (Fig. 9.8), and lichenification (Fig. 9.1B) are common features, especially in patients with AD prior to gestation.

AD can develop bacterial (typically from Staphylococcus aureus) (see Figs. 9.2, 9.7, and 9.9) or, less often, herpetic superinfection (eczema herpeticum) in pregnancy,[10,11] although there are no epidemiologic data on this.[2]

Cases of recurring AD in pregnancy due to sensitization caused by contact allergens, such as ultrasound gel, have been reported.[12] Figure 9.10 shows a sensitization to the rubber in a pump used for breastfeeding in an atopic patient, which resulted in a widespread eczematous eruption. Worsening of hand eczema is seen intrapartum and commonly postpartum; often, the latter shows a component of irritant dermatitis secondary to the use of wipes and other irritants during direct infant care (Fig. 9.11).[1] Up to 2% of breastfeeding mothers develop eczema of the areola and/or nipple, and approximately half of these have AD.[10] Nipple eczema may show painful fissures that can become secondarily infected with S. aureus, and thus develop impetiginization and crusting, which can be severe (Fig. 9.12). The prevalence of dyshidrosis during pregnancy has not been studied. In the series of the authors, dyshidrotic dermatitis was more likely to flare than remit during pregnancy, especially in patients with AD (Fig. 9.13).

A clinical overlap among gestational AD, prurigo of pregnancy (PP), and pruritic folliculitis of pregnancy (PFP) was suggested.[6] These entities were grouped together under a new disease complex (atopic eruption of pregnancy [AEP]) in a reclassification of specific dermatoses (see Ch. 21).[6] The study found that AEP starts earlier in gestation (first or second trimester in 75% of patients) than specific dermatoses of pregnancy, such as polymorphic eruption and pemphigoid gestationis, which may help differentiate it from them. AEP includes both patients with typical eczematous features (E-type AEP; 67% of AEP) (see Ch. 21, Fig. 21.15) and prurigo/papular lesions (P-type AEP; 33% of AEP) (see Figs. 9.5 and Ch. 21, Fig. 21.16), although a combination of features is also common (see Ch. 21, Fig. 21.17). Of the AEP patients in the study, 80% never had AD, but were characterized as atopic based on personal and/or family history of atopy and/or elevated serum immunoglobulin E (IgE) levels (uncontrolled). However, the association between PP and atopy was not corroborated in a prospective study,[4] and other authors suggested that AEP be restricted to the widespread types of AD in pregnancy and that cases with distribution on extensor extremities be classified under PP.[13] The recurrence of AEP in subsequent pregnancies can be observed in one-third of patients[6]; however, the postpartum prognosis of AEP has not been studied in the nonpregnant state.

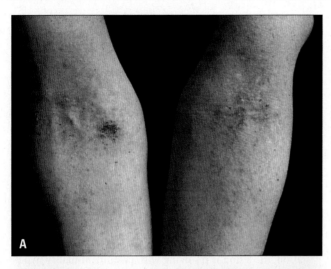

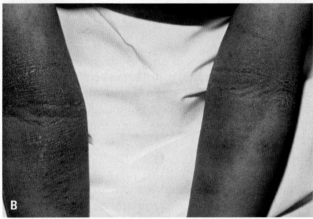

Figure 9.1. The typical presentation of atopic dermatitis in a flexural distribution (antecubital fossae and forearms). (**A**) Mild lichenification and pruritic papules. (**B**) Prominent lichenification in a patient with long-standing atopic dermatitis.

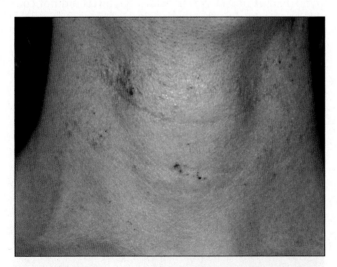

Figure 9.2. Pruritic, scaly papules and erythema on the neck in a 24-year-old pregnant patient. The lesions were infected with *Staphylococcus aureus*. (Courtesy of Dr. Iria Neri.)

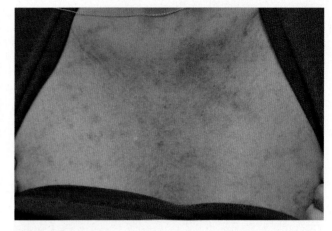

Figure 9.3. Pruritic eczematous papules and plaques as well as erythematous areas are shown on the chest in the first trimester.

Diagnosis

AD is a clinical diagnosis because the histopathologic features depend on the stage and type of lesions and do not always allow for a differentiation between AD and other dermatoses. Two studies on AD in pregnancy[7,8] used Hanifin's and Rajka's criteria,[14] and another two studies[5,6] used the U.K. Working Party criteria[15] (Table 9.1). However, including uncontrolled IgE elevations as an additional criterium in the studies that used the U.K. Working Party criteria[5,6] has been challenged, because IgE regulation in pregnancy has not been adequately studied. Of note, IgE is not included in the U.K. Working Party criteria, and only a high IgE level was included in the atopy criteria by Hanifin and Rajka.[14]

Differential Diagnosis

The differential diagnosis of AD in gestation is shown in Chapter 21, Table 21.1. The differentiation of AD from specific dermatoses, such as polymorphic eruption, PP,

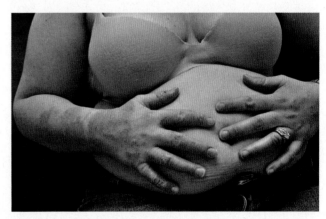

Figure 9.4. Atopic hand dermatitis is shown in the first trimester in a 41-year-old patient with a history of atopic dermatitis. Note the fissures on the fingers of the right hand and the eczematous lesions on the right forearm.

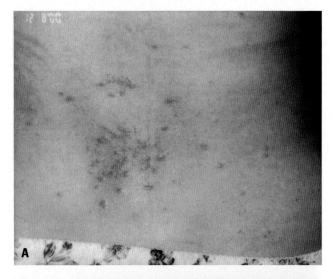

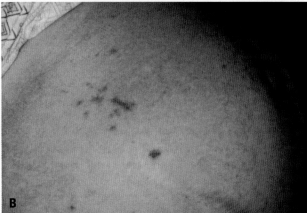

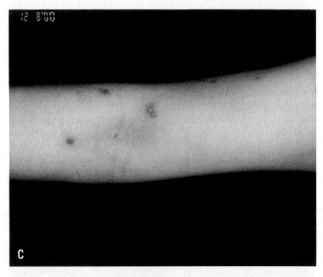

Figure 9.5. Generalized pruritic papules and prurigo-like lesions are shown on the trunk (**A and B**) and the upper extremities (**C**) in the third trimester. The morphology of the lesions is consistent with the P-type of atopic eruption of pregnancy.

and PFP, can be challenging, especially when these specific dermatoses present with eczematous clinical features in early gestation.[2] Also, the criteria[14,15] that were used in recent studies[5–8] do not allow for an easy differentiation between AEP and other specific dermatoses, such as

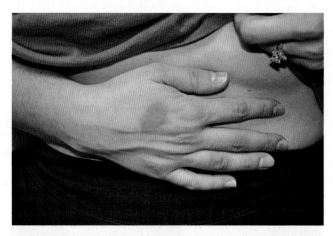

Figure 9.6. Nummular eczematous plaque shown at 14 weeks' gestation; the lesion is resolving with postinflammatory hyperpigmentation.

polymorphic eruption, in cases in which AEP presents in an atypical (nonflexural) distribution because the AEP diagnosis in these cases would rely solely on historical data (history of atopy and/or eruption in a flexural distribution) (see Table 9.1).[2]

Pathogenesis

Pregnancy is characterized by decreased maternal cell-mediated immunity (Th1 response) but intact humoral immunity (Th2 response), which helps prevent fetal rejection. This Th2 deviation seems to be associated with deterioration of mainly Th2-driven diseases, such as AD, and improvement of Th1-driven diseases, such as psoriasis. The placenta produces interleukin-4 (IL-4), a Th2 cytokine that may be critical to the induction of IgE and pathogenesis of AD. Nevertheless, IgE levels did not correlate with the deterioration of disease in a recent study,[7] which may indicate that it is the intrinsic AD (non–IgE-associated subtype of AD[16]) that is mostly affected by

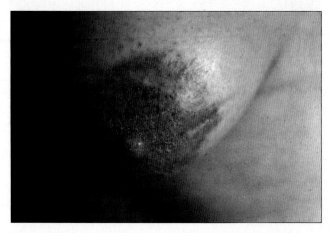

Figure 9.7. Eczema of the nipple and areola in the same patient as in Figure 9.2. Lesions were infected with *Staphylococcus aureus*. (Courtesy of Dr. Iria Neri.)

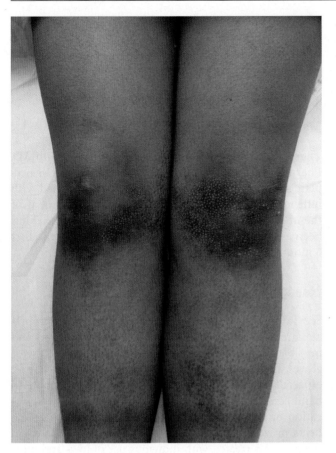

Figure 9.8. Severe keratosis pilaris with accentuation in gestation is shown in a Brazilian pregnant patient with atopic dermatitis. (Courtesy of Dr. Tania Cestari.)

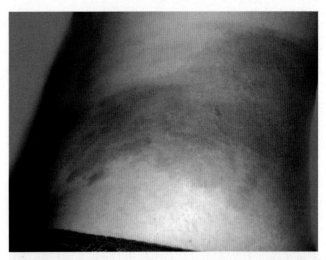

Figure 9.9. Cellulitis that resulted from a staphylococcal superinfection of truncal eczema is shown in the first trimester. The affected area was tender and warm. The lesions responded to a 2-week course of oral cephalexin.

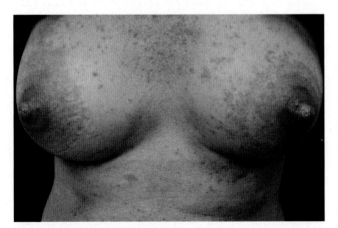

Figure 9.10. Contact dermatitis was caused 3 days after delivery by a rubber pump that the patient used for nursing; the erythema on the periareolar areas follows the contour of the pump. The patient was an atopic individual, and sensitization by rubber caused a generalized eczematous dermatitis on the chest and abdomen.

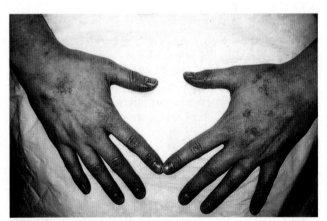

Figure 9.11. Postpartum hand eczema is shown. It was aggravated by the use of irritants during infant care. Patients with atopic dermatitis are prone to develop irritant dermatitis on the dorsal aspects of the hands.

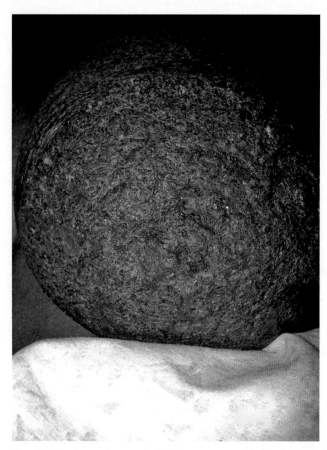

Figure 9.12. Severe impetiginization of the nipple and areola is shown. The patient was seen in the clinic a month before delivery and treated with hydrocortisone, which did not help. She developed impetigo that required a systemic antibiotic during labor and delivery. The mother decided not to nurse. (Courtesy of Dr. Eve Lowenstein.)

pregnancy. Along the same lines, a study indicated that total IgE levels were increased during early pregnancy in sensitized women with allergic symptoms but not in the nonsensitized women without allergic symptoms.[17] Experimental studies show that estrogen and progesterone

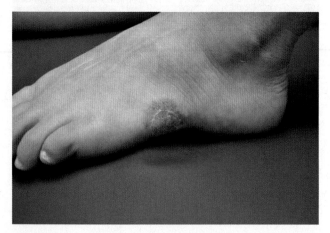

Figure 9.13. A cluster of minute itchy vesicles, a presentation of dyshidrosis on the feet, is shown in the second trimester.

enhance IgE induction but have opposite effects on histamine release (induced by estrogen).[2] It needs to be investigated whether other factors, such as maternal stress and epidermal barrier disruption, can play a role in gestational AD.[2]

Maternal and Fetal Risks

There are no maternal or fetal risks associated with AD. Pharmacologic risks and risks related to bacterial or herpetic superinfection of the lesions can be managed with judicious use of medications and prompt treatment of the infection, respectively. A maternal history of AD has been associated with an increased risk of AD in the first 6 months of life.[18]

Management

See Table 9.2. Counseling includes reviewing appropriate care and emphasizing the avoidance of sensitizers and possible allergens. Hand protection, including the use of gloves, is important in those cases involving the hands, especially because external sensitizers may contribute to hand eczema, which is common postpartum. The application of a mild emollient on the nipple and/or areola helps prevent lesions in the postpartum period. AD in pregnancy is treated with judicious use of low- and mid-potency topical corticosteroids, along with an H_1 antihistamine, which is safe in pregnancy (diphenhydramine, chlorpheniramine, loratadine).[2] A short taper of oral corticosteroid, such as prednisolone, may be used in the second or third trimester for severe or recalcitrant AD.[2] Ultraviolet light B (UVB) is a safe second-line treatment[10] and especially useful in the first trimester, a time during which oral steroids should be avoided. UVB has been associated with an increased risk of recurrent herpes simplex infections[19] and degradation of folate,[20] and, because low serum folate levels have been linked to neural tube defects, folate supplementation should be provided to patients undergoing UVB phototherapy during pregnancy. The use of topical calcineurin inhibitors (tacrolimus, pimecrolimus; pregnancy category C) can be considered in UVB-unresponsive cases after an appropriate discussion with the patient; their use should be restricted to localized areas, such as the face and intertriginous areas.[10]

Cyclosporine is the safest systemic medication and can be used as a third-line option; it should be used for a short period of time (typically effective in <2 months) in order to minimize maternal and fetal risks.[10] The use of azathioprine as a third-line option remains controversial because its safety profile is not superior to that of cyclosporine. Systemic antibiotics, such as penicillins, cephalosporins, and erythromycin base or ethylsuccinate, are safe during gestation and can be administered in superinfected AD.[2] Prompt intravenous acyclovir treatment is warranted if there is clinical suspicion of herpetic superinfection[11] (Table 9.2).

TABLE 9.1	Sets of Diagnostic Criteria That Have Been Used in Studies on Atopic Dermatitis in Pregnancy[5–8]		
AD Diagnostic Criteria		**H&R[14]**	**U.K. WP[15]**
Mandatory+++			1+++
Major++		≥3/4++	
Minor+		≥3/25+	≥3/5+
Itchy skin condition (>12 months)			+++
Pruritus		++	
Typical morphology and distribution of skin lesions		++	+
Chronic/relapsing course[a]		++	
Personal or family h/o atopy		++	+
H/o dry skin		+	+
H/o flexural involvement			+
Rash younger than age 2 years[a]			+
29 other minor criteria (include ↑ serum IgE)		+	
Validation of criteria		Twice (hospital setting)	Extensive (hospital and population settings)

[a] Criteria that cannot be easily applied in gestation to "new AD."

AD, atopic dermatitis; H/o, history of; H&R, Hanifin and Rajka criteria; IgE, immunoglobulin E; UK WP, U.K. Working Party criteria; ↑, elevated.

(Modified from Koutroulis I, Papoutsis J, Kroumpouzos G. Atopic dermatitis in pregnancy: current status and challenges. *Obstet Gynecol Surv.* 2011;66:654–663.)

TABLE 9.2	Summary of Management Options
Atopic dermatitis	■ Dry skin care, emollients, avoidance of trigger factors, prevention of hand dermatitis and nipple eczema postpartum ■ Low- to mid-potency topical corticosteroids, oral H_1 antihistamines[2] ■ A short taper of oral corticosteroid for severe cases[2] ■ UVB phototherapy as second-line option[10] ■ Pimecrolimus, tacrolimus on small skin areas (third-line option)[10] ■ Cyclosporine as third-line option[10] ■ Penicillins/cephalosporins for bacterial superinfection[2] ■ Intravenous acyclovir for *eczema herpeticum*[11]
Psoriasis	■ Counseling on lifestyle modification, control of comorbidities ■ Mid-potency topical corticosteroids[21] ■ Calcipotriene, topical tacrolimus, anthralin[21] ■ UVB therapy as second-line option[31]; first-line for generalized disease ■ Cyclosporine as third-line option[31]; second-line for generalized disease ■ Continuation of biologics in pregnancy not recommended but can be considered only after appropriate discussion with patient
Urticaria	■ Oral H_1 antihistamines (loratadine, chlorpheniramine)[39] ■ A short taper of oral corticosteroid for very symptomatic cases[39] ■ Aminocaproic acid may be beneficial in severe cases associated with angioedema[34] ■ Epinephrine in cases with concomitant angioedema affecting the upper airway[39]
Erythema annulare centrifugum	■ Search for underlying etiology if trigger factors other than pregnancy are suspected

UVB, ultraviolet light B.

PSORIASIS

Epidemiology

Chronic plaque psoriasis is the most common type of psoriasis to develop or exacerbate during pregnancy.[21] It is more likely to improve (55% to 63%) than worsen (13% to 26%)

during gestation,[21–23] especially in the first two trimesters[22] (Fig. 9.14). Psoriasis flares within 4 months of delivery in 65% to 87% of patients.[21,22] The response to subsequent pregnancies is likely to be the same.[19] Pustular psoriasis is less affected by pregnancy,[19] although generalized pustular psoriasis can be exceptionally triggered by gestation (*impetigo herpetiformis*) (see Ch. 10).[24] Breastfeeding does not seem to affect psoriasis.[19] Psoriatic arthritis improves or remits in up to 80% of pregnancies and flares within 3 months' postpartum in 70% of pregnancies[25]; the onset of psoriatic arthritis within 3 months' postpartum has been reported in 30% of mothers with psoriasis.[26]

Clinical Features

The manifestations of chronic plaque psoriasis do not differ from those of the nonpregnant patient. The extensor surfaces of the extremities (Fig. 9.15), especially elbows, knees, and the dorsa of hands and feet, buttocks, and scalp are commonly affected; however, other areas of the trunk, face, and intertriginous and genital areas may be involved. Severe, erythrodermic psoriasis can be exceptionally seen

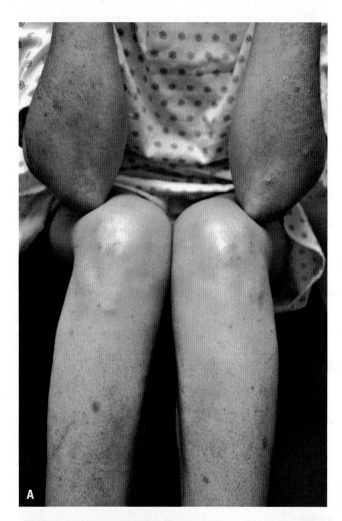
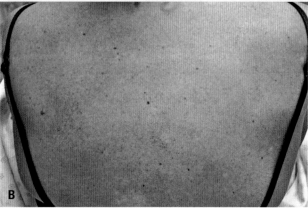

Figure 9.14. The remission of severe generalized psoriasis in gestation is shown. The patient had large generalized psoriatic plaques prior to gestation, and most lesions cleared spontaneously in the first two trimesters. Only small thin lesions (**A**) on the knees, legs, elbows and (**B**) back remained during gestation, and most lesions resolved with hypopigmentation.

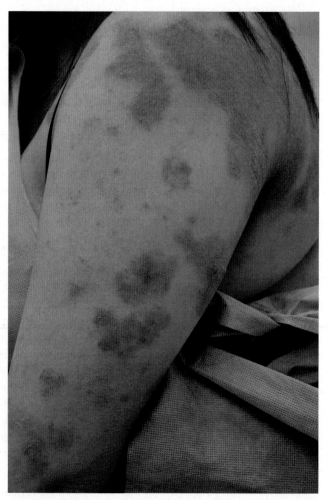

Figure 9.15. Chronic plaque psoriasis remained unchanged during gestation in this Asian primigravida patient. Typical large, scaly, erythematous plaques on the extensor surfaces of the upper extremities and back are shown in the third trimester.

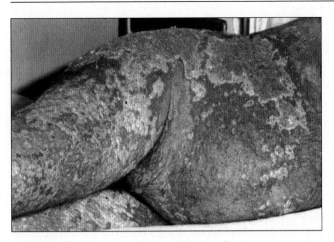

Figure 9.16. Severe, erythrodermic psoriasis is shown in pregnancy.

in pregnancy (Fig. 9.16). Lesions of guttate psoriasis are smaller (drop-like), thinner, and typically generalized (Fig. 9.17). Generalized pustular psoriasis of pregnancy (*impetigo herpetiformis*) (see Ch. 10, Figs. 10.1 to 10.4) is discussed in Chapter 10.[24]

Diagnosis

Psoriasis in pregnancy can be diagnosed by the characteristic morphology and distribution of lesions, with a personal/family history usually suggestive of the diagnosis. A biopsy is not usually required.

Differential Diagnosis

The differentiation from other psoriasiform dermatoses and eczematous processes is based on typical clinical features, often in the presence of a personal and/or family history of psoriasis.

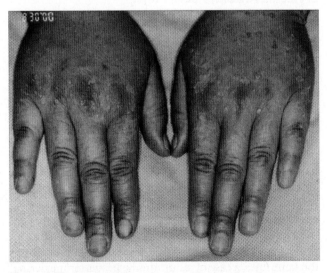

Figure 9.17. Thin, mildly scaly, drop-like papules of guttate psoriasis in a pregnant Hispanic patient. The patient had a history of chronic plaque psoriasis.

Pathogenesis

Improvement of psoriasis in pregnancy has been attributed to the high levels of IL-10 in gestation,[27] a cytokine that has a beneficial effect on psoriasis. Boyd, Morris, and Phillips postulated that the improvement of psoriasis is secondary to hormone-induced downregulation of the immune system, with progesterone playing the greatest role.[21] They also suggested that hormones affect keratinocytes directly because these cells metabolize sex hormones. Fetal suppression of the immune system may provide an alternative explanation, with hormones such as human placental lactogen and human chorionic gonadotropin being involved.[21]

Maternal and Fetal Risks

A recent study showed that women with severe psoriasis have an increased risk for low–birth-weight infants,[28] and another study showed higher odds of poor pregnancy outcome, including preterm birth and low birth weight, in women with psoriasis.[29] A recent study showed that moderate-to-severe psoriasis is associated with spontaneous and induced abortions, pregnancy-induced hypertension, premature rupture of membranes, large-for-gestational age newborns, and macrosomia.[30] Other authors attribute these findings to comorbidities or other health behaviors associated with the disease.[31]

Management

First, the extent (localized versus generalized) and severity of disease should be determined; severe disease involves >10% of body surface area. Because psoriasis has been associated with certain comorbidities, which, as aforementioned, may be associated with poor pregnancy outcomes, management includes advice on lifestyle modification that should be optimally started prior to pregnancy. Topical medications such as mid-potency corticosteroids, calcipotriene, tacrolimus, and anthralin (all pregnancy category C) appear to be safe first-line treatment options for localized psoriasis in pregnancy.[19] Coal tars should be avoided and very potent topical steroids should be used on small areas in order to minimize systemic absorption. Topical tazarotene should be discontinued in cases of known or suspected pregnancy, particularly in the first trimester.[19]

UVB is the safest second-line treatment for localized psoriasis that has not responded to topical medications[32] or when using topical medications is impractical[19]; however, it is the first-line treatment option for generalized disease. Psoralen (methoxsalen is pregnancy category C) with UVA (PUVA) therapy should be avoided because of a risk of mutagenicity; PUVA should be discontinued when pregnancy is confirmed or suspected. Topical PUVA provides a safer option, especially for psoriasis of the palms and soles, because levels of 8-methoxypsoralen are undetectable after topical application of psoralen.[19]

A short course of cyclosporine is a second-line option for severe and/or generalized disease.[32] Systemic medications such as methotrexate and retinoids (pregnancy category X) should be avoided, and a minimum drug-free interval of 3 months (for men and women) and 2 years (for women only), respectively, before conception is recommended.[32] Manufacturers of biologics such as etanercept, infliximab, adalimumab, and ustekinumab (all pregnancy category B) advise avoidance during pregnancy because the long-term effects on the newborn are unknown. Nevertheless, registry studies do not indicate fetal harm, and no toxicity or teratogenicity has been reported in animal studies.[33] Some authors recommend limiting infliximab use to the first 30 weeks of pregnancy because transplacental transport of IgG is poor until the late second trimester.[33] Biologics can be found at low levels in breast milk, and they are probably safe during breastfeeding because the oral bioavailability of monoclonal antibody drugs is very poor.[33]

OTHER INFLAMMATORY SKIN DISEASE

Urticarias

Sex hormones are known to have an effect on chronic urticaria,[34] and flares of chronic urticaria during the premenstrual phase of the menstrual cycle have been documented. The onset of urticaria in pregnancy is shown in Figures 9.18 and 9.19. Exacerbation of chronic urticaria in pregnancy has been reported,[1] but its course in gestation is inconsistent. In some cases, recurrent urticaria flares during pregnancy showed common features with hereditary angioedema[35] (Fig. 9.19C); however, the C1 esterase inhibitor levels and complement components were consistently normal. In these cases, attacks of urticaria were also caused by oral contraceptives or occurred before menses. Pressure urticaria may occur or become aggravated by pregnancy and appears on the abdomen in the second or, more often, the third trimester.[36] Precipitating factors include heat, constrictive clothing, or even the distention of the abdominal wall.[36] Urticarial lesions can develop in autoimmune progesterone dermatitis.[37] Autoimmune estrogen dermatitis has been reported in a patient presenting with urticaria in early pregnancy.[38]

Urticaria should be differentiated from specific dermatoses of pregnancy such as polymorphic eruption and pemphigoid gestationis, drug eruptions, papular urticaria (arthropod bites), and urticaria vasculitis. Polymorphic eruption typically presents in the third trimester in the primigravida with skin lesions along the abdominal striae that show periumbilical sparing. When the diagnosis of prebullous, pemphigoid gestationis is a consideration (see Fig. 9.19), a skin biopsy should be taken for immunofluorescence (positive in pemphigoid gestationis). Urticaria vasculitis can be triggered by pregnancy[39]; however, it often shows a purpuric component, is associated with systemic symptoms, and demonstrates features of vasculitis in histopathology and immunofluorescence studies.

Treatment of urticaria in pregnancy includes a newer generation, nonsedating oral H_1 antihistamine that is safe during gestation, such as loratadine; chlorpheniramine is a safe alternative (both are pregnancy category B).[40] Using the lowest possible dose is recommended[40]; however, the dose often needs to be increased to achieve satisfactory response, and adding another antihistamine may be required. A short taper of oral corticosteroid can provide symptomatic relief in cases not responding to antihistamines. Aminocaproic acid (pregnancy category C) may be helpful in cases associated with angioedema[35] but should be used only after safer options have been exhausted. Epinephrine is required in rare cases, presenting with features of angioedema involving the upper airway (i.e., throat swelling, respiratory difficulties).[40] Second-generation antihistamines, such as loratadine and cetirizine, appear at very low levels in breast milk and can be safely used in breastfeeding mothers.

Erythema Annulare Centrifugum

Erythema annulare centrifugum (EAC), the most common type of figurate erythemas, has been reported to start in pregnancy in a handful of cases.[3,41–43] Lesions started as early as the 12th[41] and as late as the 33rd week[42] and showed typical clinical features of EAC (i.e., centrifugal expansion with central clearing, desquamation at the inner margin [trailing scale] of an annular erythematous border) (Fig. 9.20). The onset in pregnancy and spontaneous resolution by delivery[43] or within 1 month postpartum[3] were suggestive of pregnancy-triggered EAC. The authors suggested that the hormonal changes of gestation can trigger EAC because high progesterone levels can aggravate inflammation at the tissue level, and, in one case, the onset of EAC coincided with the peak of human chorionic gonadotropin[41] in the 12th week of gestation. Along the same lines, a case of autoimmune progesterone dermatitis showed EAC features,[44] and EAC has been associated with the menstrual cycle or estrogenic compounds.[42]

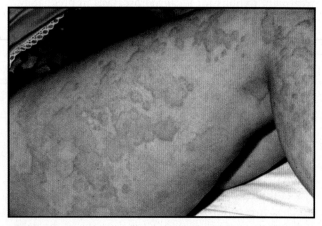

Figure 9.18. Urticaria, which developed in a 32-year-old pregnant female.

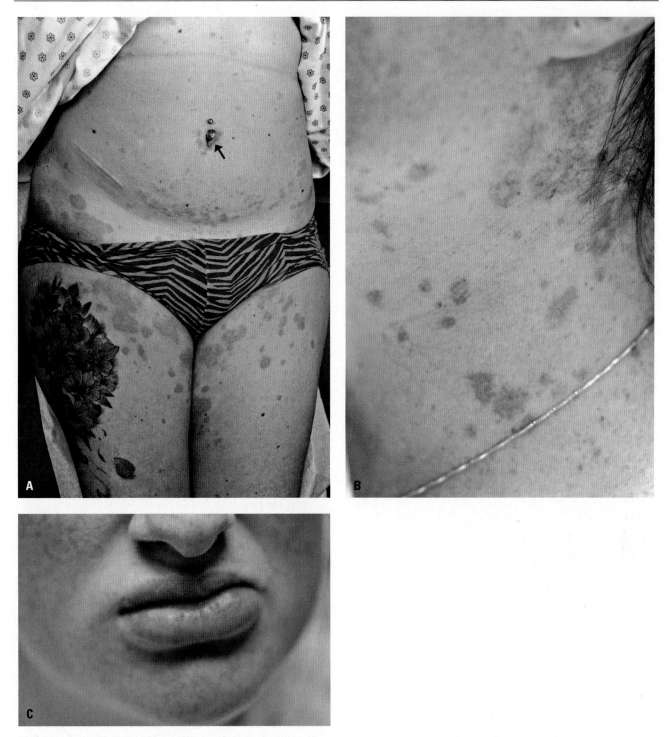

Figure 9.19. Acute severe urticaria is shown at the 6th week of pregnancy. Generalized urticarial lesions are shown (**A**) on the abdomen, lower extremities, (**B**) face, and neck. There were some features of angioedema (i.e., tender swelling of the lips [especially the lower lip, shown in (**C**)], chin, hands, and feet). The presentation, including the involvement of the umbilicus (shown with *arrow* in [**A**]), was suggestive of pemphigoid gestationis. Direct immunofluorescence helped rule out pemphigoid gestationis, and normal C4, C1q, and functional C1 inhibitor levels ruled out hereditary and acquired C1 inhibitor deficiency.

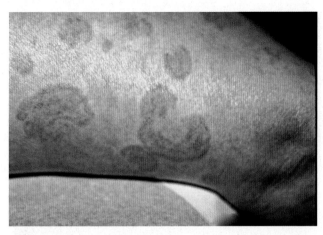

Figure 9.20. The typical features of erythema annulare centrifugum are shown: lesions expanding centrifugally with central clearing and desquamation at the inner margin (trailing scale) of the erythematous border. Annular and polycyclic configurations result.

MATERNAL RISKS

Atopic dermatitis: Risks related to bacterial and herpetic superinfection; risks from pharmacologic treatment
Psoriasis: Risks from pharmacologic treatment; risks from severe, erythrodermic psoriasis (rare)
Urticaria: Risks (throat swelling, respiratory distress) in cases with concomitant features of angioedema (rare)
Erythema annulare centrifugum: None

FETAL RISKS

Atopic dermatitis: Risks from pharmacologic treatment
Psoriasis: Low birth weight (two studies), prematurity (one study); association with abortion, pregnancy-induced hypertension, premature rupture of membranes, large-for-gestational age infants (one study)
Urticaria: Risks from pharmacologic treatment
Erythema annulare centrifugum: None

KEY POINTS

- Two recent studies showed that atopic dermatitis is the most common pregnancy dermatosis, manifesting in the first two trimesters in 75% of cases; in these studies, new onset during pregnancy was more common than exacerbation of preexisting atopic dermatitis.
- Treatment of atopic dermatitis includes emollients, low- and mid-potency topical corticosteroids, short courses of an oral corticosteroid, and oral H_1 antihistamines; UVB is a safe second-line option and cyclosporine is a third-line option; a superinfection requires prompt treatment.

- Chronic plaque psoriasis may improve in pregnancy in 55% to 63% of patients and flares postpartum in 65% to 87% of cases; psoriatic arthritis may improve or remit in pregnancy and start or flare postpartum.
- Chronic plaque psoriasis has been associated with adverse pregnancy outcomes that are possibly related to its comorbidities; treatment includes mid-potency topical corticosteroids, calcipotriene, topical tacrolimus, and anthralin; UVB is a safe second-line option, and a short course of cyclosporine is a third-line option for moderate to severe psoriasis.
- The course of chronic idiopathic urticaria in pregnancy is inconsistent, and some cases have shown concomitant features of angioedema; physical urticaria can be aggravated by pregnancy.
- Erythema annulare centrifugum has been associated with pregnancy and may be triggered by the hormonal changes of gestation; there have been no maternal or fetal risks.

REFERENCES

1. Kroumpouzos G, Cohen LM. Dermatoses of pregnancy. *J Am Acad Dermatol.* 2001;45:1–19.
2. Koutroulis I, Papoutsis J, Kroumpouzos G. Atopic dermatitis in pregnancy: current status and challenges. *Obstet Gynecol Surv.* 2011;66:654–663.
3. Rosina P, D'Onghia FS, Barba A. Erythema annulare centrifugum and pregnancy. *Int J Dermatol.* 2002;41:516–517.
4. Roger D, Vaillant L, Fignon A, et al. Specific pruritic dermatoses of pregnancy: a prospective study of 3192 women. *Arch Dermatol.* 1994;130:734–739.
5. Vaughan Jones SA, Hern S, Nelson-Piercy C, et al. A prospective study of 200 women with dermatoses of pregnancy correlating the clinical findings with hormonal and immunopathological profiles. *Br J Dermatol.* 1999;141:71–81.
6. Ambros-Rudolph CM, Müllegger RR, Vaughan-Jones SA, et al. The specific dermatoses of pregnancy revisited and reclassified: results of a retrospective two-center study on 505 pregnant patients. *J Am Acad Dermatol.* 2006;54:395–404.
7. Cho S, Kim HJ, Oh SH, et al. The influence of pregnancy and menstruation on the deterioration of atopic dermatitis symptoms. *Ann Dematol.* 2010:22180–22185.
8. Kemmett D, Tidman MJ. The influence of menstrual cycle and pregnancy on atopic dermatitis. *Br J Dermatol.* 1991;125:59–61.
9. Eichenfield LF, Hanifin JM, Luger TA, et al. Consensus conference on pediatric atopic dermatitis. *J Am Acad Dermatol.* 2003;49:1088–1095.
10. Weatherhead S, Robson SC, Reynolds NJ. Eczema in pregnancy. *BMJ.* 2007;335:152–154.
11. Latta RA, Baker DA. Treatment of recurrent eczema herpeticum in pregnancy with acyclovir. *Infect Dis Obstet Gynecol.* 1996;4:239–242.
12. Moreno E, Macías E, Dávila I, et al. Recurring eczema during pregnancy and after delivery due to sensitization caused by an ultrasound gel. *Ultrasound Obstet Gynecol.* 2009;34:120–121.
13. Ingber A. Atopic eruption of pregnancy. *J Eur Acad Dermatol Venereol.* 2010;24:984.

14. Hanifin JM, Rajka G. Diagnostic features of atopic eczema. *Acta Derm Venereol*. 1980;92:s44–s47.

15. Williams HC, Burney PGJ, Hay RJ, et al. The U.K. Working Party's diagnostic criteria for atopic dermatitis. I: derivation of a minimum set of discriminators for atopic dermatitis. *Br J Dermatol*. 1994;131:383–396.

16. Wuthrich B, Schmid-Grendelmeier P. The atopic eczema/dermatitis syndrome. Epidemiology, natural course, and immunology of the IgE-associated ("extrinsic") and the nonallergic ("intrinsic") AEDS. *J Investig Allergol Clin Immunol*. 2003;13:1–5.

17. Sandberg M, Frykman A, Jonsson Y, et al. Total and allergen-specific IgE levels during and after pregnancy in relation to maternal allergy. *J Reprod Immunol*. 2009;81:82–88.

18. Moore MM, Rifas-Shiman SL, Rich-Edwards JW, et al. Perinatal predictors of atopic dermatitis occurring in the first six months of life. *Pediatr*. 2004;113:468–474.

19. Tauscher AE, Fleischer AB Jr, Phelps KC, et al. Psoriasis and pregnancy. *J Cutan Med Surg*. 2002;6:561–570.

20. Park KK, Murase JE. Narrowband UV-B phototherapy during pregnancy and folic acid depletion. *Arch Dermatol*. 2012;148:132–133.

21. Boyd AS, Morris LF, Phillips CM, et al. Psoriasis and pregnancy: hormone and immune system interaction. *Int J Dermatol*. 1996;35:169–172.

22. Murase JE, Chan K, Garite TJ, et al. Hormonal effect on psoriasis in pregnancy and post partum. *Arch Dermatol*. 2005;141:601–606.

23. Raychaudhuri SP, Navare T, Gross J, et al. Clinical course of psoriasis during pregnancy. *Int J Dermatol*. 2003;42:518–520.

24. Vaidya DC, Kroumpouzos G, Bercovitch L. Recurrent postpartum impetigo herpetiformis presenting after a "skip" pregnancy. *Acta Dermatol Venereol*. 2013;93:102–103.

25. Ostensen M. The effect of pregnancy on ankylosing spondylitis, psoriatic arthritis, and juvenile rheumatoid arthritis. *Am J Reprod Immunol*. 1992;28:235–237.

26. McHugh NJ, Laurent MR. The effect of pregnancy on the onset of psoriatic arthritis. *Br J Rheumatol*. 1989;28:50–52.

27. Trautman MS, Collmer D, Edwin SS, et al. Expression of interleukin-10 in human gestational tissues. *J Soc Gynecol Invest*. 1997;1:247–253.

28. Yang YW, Chen CS, Chen YH, et al. Psoriasis and pregnancy outcomes: a nationwide population-based study. *J Am Acad Dermatol*. 2011;64:71–77.

29. Lima XT, Janakiraman V, Hughes MD, et al. The impact of psoriasis on pregnancy outcomes. *J Invest Dermatol*. 2012;132:85–91.

30. Cohen-Barak E, Nachum Z, Rozenman D, et al. Pregnancy outcomes in women with moderate-to-severe psoriasis. *J Eur Acad Dermatol Venereol*. 2011;25:1041–1047.

31. Bandoli G, Johnson DL, Jones KL, et al. Potentially modifiable risk factors for adverse pregnancy outcomes in women with psoriasis. *Br J Dermatol*. 2010;163:334–339.

32. Weatherhead S, Robson SC, Reynolds NJ. Management of psoriasis in pregnancy. *BMJ*. 2007;334:1218–1220.

33. Puig L, Barco D, Alomar A. Treatment of psoriasis with anti-TNF drugs during pregnancy: case report and review of the literature. *Dermatology*. 2010;220:71–76.

34. Kasperska-Zajac A, Brzoza Z, Rogala B. Sex hormones and urticaria. *J Dermatol Sci*. 2008;52:79–86.

35. Warin RP, Cunliffe WJ, Greaves MW, et al. Recurrent angioedema: familial and oestrogen-induced. *Br J Dermatol*. 1986;115:731–734.

36. Oumeish OY, Al-Fouzan AS. Miscellaneous diseases affected by pregnancy. *Clin Dermatol*. 2006;24:113–117.

37. Vasconcelos C, Xavier P, Vieira AP, et al. Autoimmune progesterone urticaria. *Gynecol Endocrinol*. 2000;14:245–247.

38. Lee AY, Lee KH, Lim YG. Oestrogen urticaria associated with pregnancy. *Br J Dermatol*. 1999;141:774.

39. Nürnberg W. [Urticaria-vasculitis-syndrome]. In: Czarnetzki BM, Grabbe J, eds. *Urtikaria: Klinik, Diagnostik, Therapie*. 1st ed. Heidelberg, Germany: Springer-Verlag; 1993:159–167.

40. Powell RJ, Du Toit GL, Siddique N, et al. BSACI guidelines for the management of chronic urticaria and angio-oedema. *Clin Exp Allergy*. 2007;37:631–650.

41. Dogan G. Pregnancy as a possible etiologic factor in erythema annulare centrifugum. *Am J Clin Dermatol*. 2009;10:33–35.

42. Choonhakarn C, Seramethakun P. Erythema annulare centrifugum associated with pregnancy. *Acta Derm Venereol*. 1998;78:237–238.

43. Senel E, Gulec AT. Erythema annulare centrifugum in pregnancy. *Indian J Dermatol*. 2010;55:120–121.

44. Halevy S, Coen AD, Lunenfeld E, et al. Autoimmune progesterone dermatitis manifested as erythema annulare centrifugum: confirmation of progesterone sensitivity by in vitro interferon-gamma release. *J Am Acad Dermatol*. 2002;47:311–313.

CHAPTER 10

Impetigo Herpetiformis

Darshan C. Vaidya ■ Aleksandr Itkin ■ George Kroumpouzos

INTRODUCTION

Impetigo herpetiformis (IH) (generalized pustular psoriasis of pregnancy)[1] is a potentially life threatening, pustular dermatosis that typically occurs in the third trimester and demonstrates a progressive course with eventual rapid resolution upon delivery. The term IH was originally coined by Hebra in 1872.[2] Although familial cases and occurrence in twins have been reported, patients do not typically have a personal or family history of psoriasis and are not likely to subsequently develop chronic plaque psoriasis.[3] Patients are mostly disease free between pregnancies, but the disease has a tendency to recur in subsequent pregnancies with an earlier onset and greater morbidity.[4,5] Nevertheless, a skip pregnancy has been reported, with the disease starting later in gestation than in prior pregnancies.[6]

EPIDEMIOLOGY

The disease is rare, with approximately 150 cases reported in the English literature.

ETIOLOGY

The pathogenesis of IH is elusive. Possible triggers of IH include hypocalcemia,[3,7] occasionally secondary to hypoparathyroidism,[8] hypovitaminosis D,[9] stress,[5] and bacterial infections.[10] Whether hypocalcemia is a primary or secondary phenomenon has yet to be elucidated. Nevertheless, there have been cases of IH associated with hypoparathyroidism and/or hypocalcemia in nonpregnant women, which may indicate a primary role of hypocalcemia in the disease process.[7,8] Furthermore, normalization of serum calcium levels in patients with hypoparathyroidism and IH has resulted in dramatic improvement of the skin disease.[2,8,11] In contrast, it has been hypothesized that hypocalcemia may be secondary to the exudative inflammatory skin lesions of IH that lead to hypoproteinemia with a subsequent loss of free and protein-bound serum calcium.[7] As a result, compensatory secondary hyperparathyroidism may ensue.[9] Patients with impaired compensatory mechanisms, such

as postsurgical parathyroidectomy or thyroidectomy, may be at risk for developing a more severe course of IH.[9] Some authors suggest that hypocalcemia secondary to hypoalbuminemia (resulting mostly in a decrease of the nonionized fraction), along with decrease of vitamin D during pregnancy and puerperium, plays a role in IH development during these states.[3] The genetic background of patients has not been elucidated. Two patients showed expression of human leukocyte antigen (HLA)-Cw6,[9,12] similar to that reported in generalized pustular psoriasis. One group reported two sisters with IH, neither with a prior history of psoriasis, who shared common HLA antigens (A11, AW24, BW44, BW54, and DR6Y).[13] The authors suggested that alterations in a patient's metabolic milieu may uncover an underlying genetic predisposition.

The role of high estrogen or progesterone levels as a trigger for IH has been stressed by several authors. It is known that generalized pustular psoriasis can be precipitated or exacerbated by pregnancy, miscarriage, menstruation, or systemic progesterone intake. IH can similarly manifest as a response to the triggers listed previously, but lesions generally resolve after the triggers are removed. Interestingly, a patient with recurrent menstrual exacerbations of IH for 7 years postpartum has been reported.[14] Finally, some authors have claimed a common pathway between IH and pustular psoriasis, namely a decrease in skin-derived antileucoproteinase/elafin, leading to an imbalance between human leukocyte elastase and its inhibitor.[15]

CLINICAL FEATURES

IH begins typically in the third trimester but has been reported as early as the first trimester and also in puerperium.[2,3,6] It follows a progressive course with rapid postpartum resolution. The disease has also been reported in men,[16] postmenopausal women,[17] and nonpregnant women taking oral contraceptives.[4] IH has been associated with cholestasis[17] or RhE isoimmunization.[18]

IH manifests distinctively as an eruption of tiny pustules on erythematous patches in a symmetric, flexural distribution, typically in the inguinal region.[19] The lesions have a tendency to spread centrifugally onto the trunk,

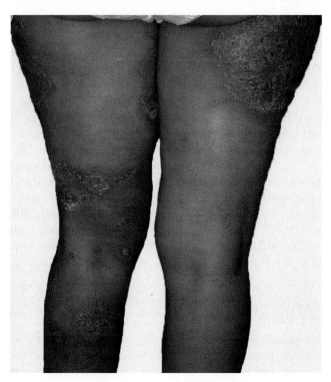

Figure 10.1. Erythematous plaques with central crust and pustules along the peripheral, active edge are distributed on the lower extremities.

around the umbilicus and proximal extremities, and eventually cover the entire body, forming large polycyclic erythematous patches and plaques studded with pustules along their periphery (Figs. 10.1 to 10.3). The pustules are sterile but can become secondarily infected. The central portion of the lesions may become crusted and impetiginized, or even vegetative. Lesions can become confluent, and may occasionally take on a pseudoverrucous appearance (Fig. 10.4). Facial edema has been exceptionally reported when lesions involved the face (Fig. 10.5), but

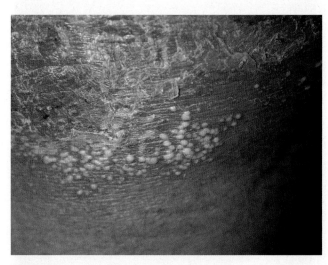

Figure 10.2. Pustules are characteristically seen at the active edge of the lesions.

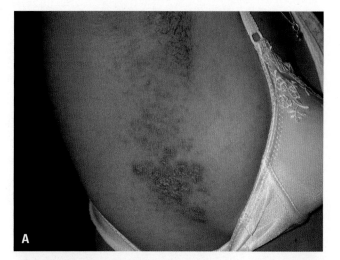

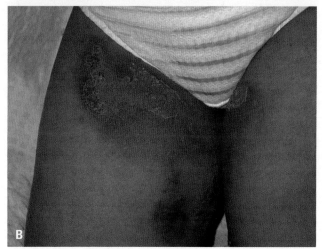

Figure 10.3. Erythematous crusted plaques involving (**A**) the axilla and (**B**) the groin and inner thighs.

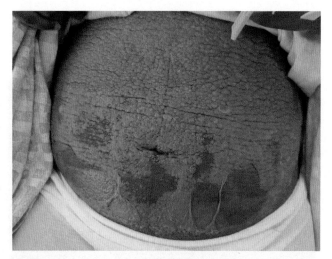

Figure 10.4. Confluent, vesicopustular lesions on the abdomen, associated with extensive erosions and pseudoverrucous features. (Reprinted with permission from Acta Dermato-Venereologica 2013.[6])

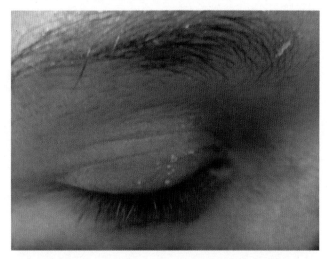

Figure 10.5. Edema and erythema are demonstrated on the eyelid and eyebrow. Minute pustules, healing with desquamation, are seen on the upper eyelid.

edema can also occur elsewhere, often in the setting of hypoalbuminemia.[6,20] Pustular involvement of acral sites may also be seen.[6,20]

In severe cases or flares occurring during the tapering of treatment, erythroderma may result (Fig. 10.6). In con-

trast to entities such as acute generalized exanthematous pustulosis (AGEP), IH is a nonpruritic eruption. In the initial response to treatment, the center of the lesion clears first (Fig. 10.7A), whereas the margins may still show activity (Fig. 10.7B). Lesions often heal with erosions (see Fig. 10.4) and/or crusting with desquamation (Fig. 10.8). Postinflammatory hyperpigmentation commonly develops upon resolution of the lesions (Fig. 10.9). Unusual cases may show erosive or circinate mucous membrane lesions.[21] Figure 10.10 shows pustules on the tongue and buccal mucosa. Nail changes, such as uplifting, distal onycholysis, and/or subungual pustules may be exceptionally noticed (Fig. 10.11).[19] A case showed bullae distributed in an annular configuration and associated with unilateral lower limb edema that mimicked deep vein thrombosis.[22]

PATHOLOGY

Histopathologic features are those of pustular psoriasis, including spongiform pustules (spongiform pustules of Kogoj), which are formed by the aggregation of neutrophils and degenerated keratinocytes beneath the stratum corneum and in the upper Malpighian layer, and a superficial perivascular infiltrate of lymphocytes and neutrophils

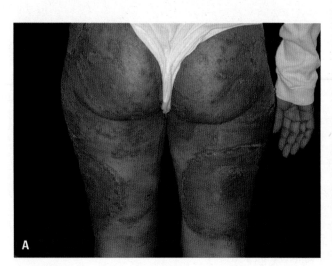

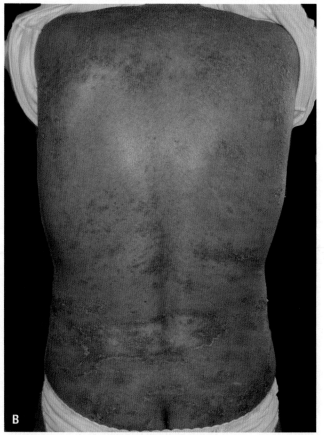

Figure 10.6. An erythrodermic flare after patient ran out of cyclosporine. Lesions are shown on (**A**) the buttocks and lower extremities and (**B**) the back.

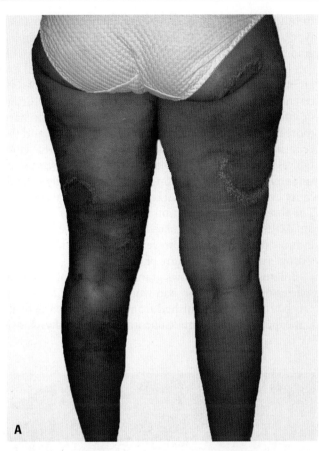
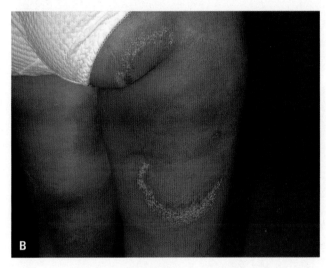

Figure 10.7. (**A**) The initial response to treatment with oral prednisone and topical steroids; compare to Figure 10.1. (**B**) Note the central clearing and pustules at the active edge.

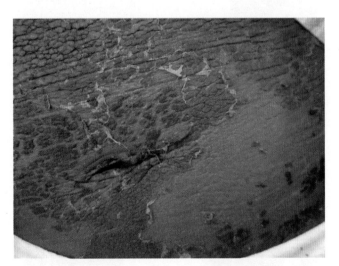

Figure 10.8. Extensive lesions on the abdomen healing with crusting and desquamation following successful treatment with oral corticosteroid; compare with Figure 10.4, which shows the lesions prior to corticosteroid treatment.

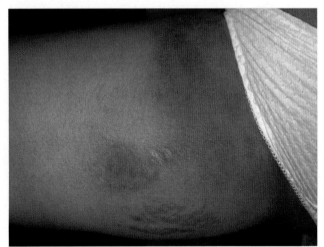

Figure 10.9. The resolution of lesions with postinflammatory hyperpigmentation following oral prednisone treatment (compare to Fig. 10.3B).

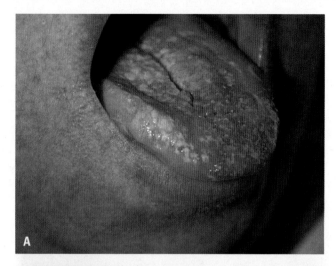

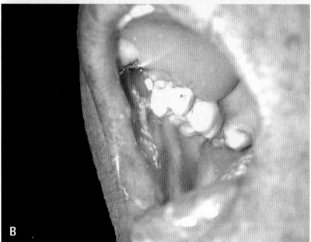

Figure 10.10. Pustules on (**A**) the tongue, and (**B**) buccal and labial mucosa.

(Fig. 10.12). The neutrophils within the spongiform pustule eventually migrate into the stratum corneum (Fig. 10.13), resembling a large Munro abscess. At the edges of the abscess, spongiform degeneration and a shell of thin epidermal cells can be noticed (Fig. 10.14). Psoriasiform hyperplasia and parakeratosis may not be seen in early lesions (Fig. 10.15).[6,19] An absence of eosinophils helps differentiate IH from AGEP.

DIAGNOSIS

The diagnosis of IH can be made based on distinct clinical features and can be confirmed by pathology of pustular psoriasis.

DIFFERENTIAL DIAGNOSIS

The differential diagnosis includes AGEP, pustular drug eruption, bacterial infection (e.g., bullous impetigo), *id*-reaction, subcorneal pustular dermatosis,

immunoglobulin (Ig)A pemphigus (subcorneal pustular type), and specific pregnancy dermatoses such as pemphigoid gestationis (see Ch. 19). Differentiation from AGEP can be challenging and is based on history, physical examination, and histopathologic features. AGEP may represent a variant of pustular psoriasis triggered by drugs or infection.[23] Clinically, patients with AGEP tend to have more facial involvement, accompanied by edema, and the eruption tends to be pruritic. Histologically, AGEP lacks typical psoriasiform hyperplasia and shows numerous eosinophils along with eosinophil exocytosis, single-cell keratinocyte necrosis, and marked papillary dermal edema.[23] The absence of an association with medications helps rule out AGEP and other pustular drug eruptions, such as that induced by ritodrine[24]; however, the final confirmation of a drug eruption may require patch testing.

Bullous impetigo shows gram-positive staphylococcal species on a Gram stain and wound culture. *Id*-reaction can be readily distinguished from IH on the basis of its clinicopathologic features. Subcorneal pustular dermatosis

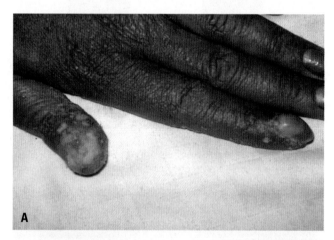

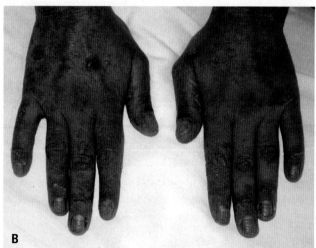

Figure 10.11. (**A**) The extension of lesions onto the proximal nail fold, subungual pustules, and distal onycholysis. The entire nail plate of the index finger is uplifted and yellow. (**B**) Significant improvement after oral corticosteroid treatment. (Courtesy of Dr. Maria Magdalena Roth.)

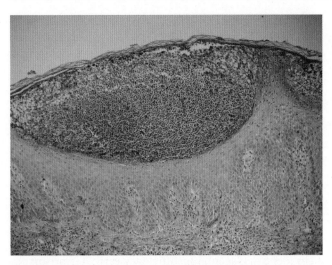

Figure 10.12. Psoriasiform hyperplasia with a large subcorneal pustule containing numerous neutrophils and a superficial perivascular infiltrate of lymphocytes and neutrophils (hematoxylin-eosin, ×10).

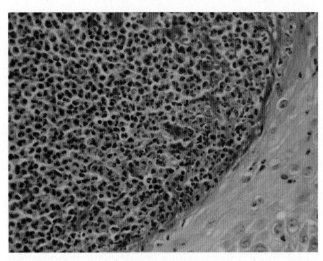

Figure 10.14. A shell of thin epidermal cells and spongiform degeneration can be noticed at the edges of the macropustule (hematoxylin-eosin, ×40).

(Sneddon-Wilkinson disease) is characterized by sterile pustules within flexural annular plaques but is associated with IgA paraproteinemia and responds to dapsone. IgA pemphigus can be clinically indistinguishable from IH and subcorneal pustular dermatosis, but lesions are generally pruritic and direct immunofluorescence shows IgA deposition on the cell surfaces of upper epidermal keratinocytes.

MATERNAL AND FETAL RISKS

Maternal risks include symptomatic aggravation (malaise, fever, hypothermia, chills, nausea, vomiting, severe dehydration, diarrhea), risks associated with hypocalcemia (tetany, seizures, paresthesias, delirium), sepsis secondary to superinfection of exudative skin lesions, and, rarely, death secondary to cardiac or renal failure.[1,3,25] These historically reported maternal risks are currently uncommon because most cases are treated promptly.[19] An association with gestational hypertension[26,27] needs to be clarified. Laboratory abnormalities may be seen, including leukocytosis, hypocalcemia, hypoalbuminemia, hypophosphatemia, iron deficiency anemia, and fluid/electrolyte abnormalities.[1,19] Fetal risks include low birth weight, intrauterine growth restriction, premature rupture of membranes, stillbirth, and neonatal death, which are thought to be secondary to placental insufficiency and/or fluid/electrolyte imbalance.[3]

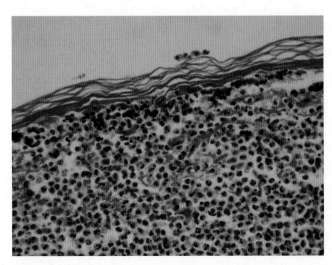

Figure 10.13. Neutrophils migrating to the stratum corneum (hematoxylin-eosin, ×20).

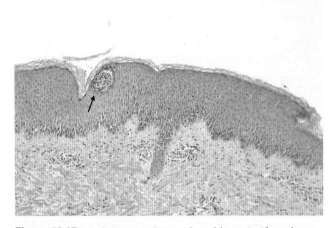

Figure 10.15. Early lesions show only mild psoriasiform hyperplasia and acanthosis as well as a sparse dermal infiltrate with scattered neutrophils. A small subcorneal spongiform pustule *(arrow)* is seen (hematoxylin-eosin, ×10).

Fetal risks may occasionally be unavoidable even with successful control of the skin disease.[4,9,19]

MANAGEMENT

Due to the rarity of IH, treatment recommendations arise from case reports and series. Important factors to consider when deciding on a treatment regimen include the extent of the disease, the impact on overall maternal and fetal well-being, pregnancy status, lactation status, and relevant past medical history. Prompt treatment is imperative given the increased maternal and fetal morbidity and the risk of fetal demise. Table 10.1 highlights management options. Systemic corticosteroids remain the cornerstone of treatment, often resulting in a dramatic response (see Figs. 10.7A and 10.9).[4,9,19] Nevertheless, relapses are common with tapering (Fig. 10.16) or with the discontinuation of steroid treatment. In these cases as well as in cases refractory to oral steroids or when oral steroids are contraindicated, oral cyclosporine is an effective second-line treatment (Fig. 10.17), which can provide complete remission of the disease (Fig. 10.18).[20,28,29] A gradual tapered dose is recommended because relapses are common with abrupt discontinuation of cyclosporine (see Fig. 10.6). Although fetal growth restriction and prematurity may occur with cyclosporine treatment, infants who experience these adverse effects recover rapidly after birth with no long-term sequelae.[28] Methotrexate can be used successfully in nonlactating mothers.[3,11,21,22,30] As shown in Figure 10.19, low-dose acitretin can maintain the remission postpartum,[31] but its use is restricted to nonlactating mothers.

The obstetric management is outlined in Table 10.2. Early diagnosis and treatment are of utmost importance in the prevention of maternal and fetal risks. Careful fetal monitoring is imperative, and placental function tests can help identify placental insufficiency early.[26] If pregnancy is near term, labor may be induced, and the method used for labor induction depends on the state of the cervix.[27] Although there are no restrictions for epidural or spinal anesthesia, general anesthesia may need to be conducted when the lesions occupy sites of puncture.[32]

TABLE 10.1	Summary of Management Options
Treatment	**Comment**
Pregnant/Lactating Patient	
Correction of metabolic/electrolyte abnormalities	Has resulted in resolution[2,8,11,20,25]
High-potency topical corticosteroids	Administered in combination with systemic steroids[9,19]
Systemic corticosteroids	First-line Rx[4,9,19]; prednisone dose typically up to 60–80 mg/d
Cyclosporine	Effective second-line Rx (3–10 mg/kg/d) with[28,29] or without systemic steroids[20]
Narrowband UVB	Safe adjunctive Rx,[33] typically in conjunction with topical or systemic steroids
Tumor necrosis factor-α inhibitors	Infliximab (one case)[34]
Clofazimine	200 mg/d in combination with oral steroids (one case)[35]
Broad-spectrum systemic antibiotics	For superinfection or cases triggered by infection[10]
Termination of pregnancy	Has resulted in resolution[4,9,22,25]
Additional Options Postpartum in Nonlactating Patient	
Methotrexate	7.5–20 mg weekly as monotherapy, or in combination with systemic steroids, with slow taper[3,11,21,22,30]
Acitretin	Dose up to 30 mg/d[31] (see Fig. 10.19)
Etretinate	Dose up to 1 mg/kg/d, often combined with systemic steroids[12,36]
Isotretinoin	Combination with PUVA[1]
Phototherapy	PUVA as monotherapy or in combination with systemic steroids or retinoids[1,3] or clofazimine[37]; narrowband UVB Rx in combination with systemic steroids[38]
Hormonal treatment	Ethynodiol/mestranol (one case)[39]

PUVA, psoralen plus ultraviolet light A; Rx, treatment; UVB, ultraviolet light B.

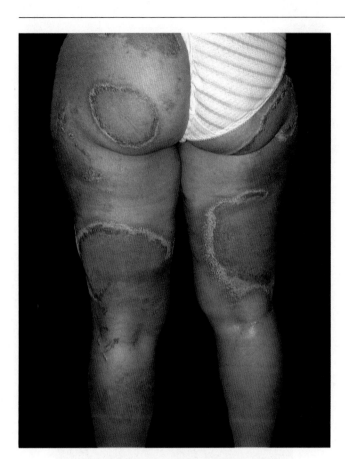

Figure 10.16. In the same patient (compare to Fig. 10.7A), a quick relapse with prednisone tapering prior to starting oral cyclosporine.

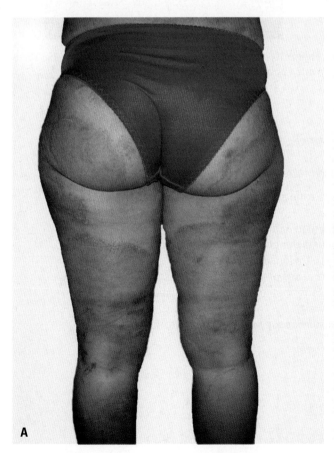

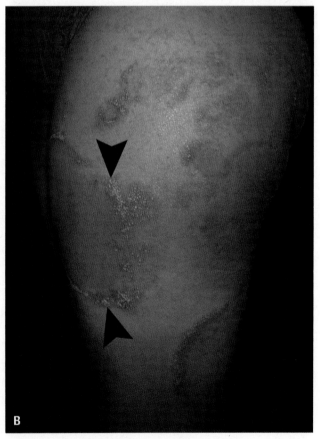

Figures 10.17. The initial response to oral cyclosporine; (**A**) compare to Figure 10.16. (**B**) Note that the edges of the lesions are still active (*arrows* show pustules).

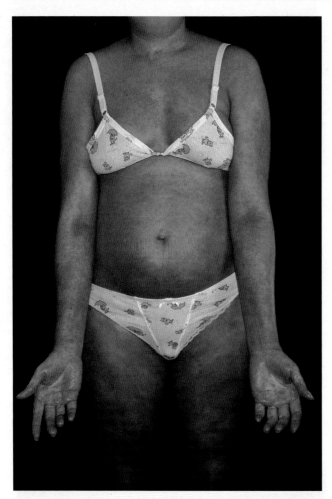

Figure 10.18. The resolution of lesions with oral cyclosporine (5 mg/kg/d) shortly before delivery. Note that the edge of the lesions is inactive (i.e., no pustules are seen).

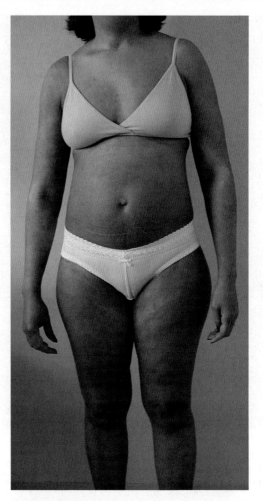

Figure 10.19. Durable remission in the same patient (Fig. 10.18) with a postpartum course of acitretin (25 mg/d).

TABLE 10.2	**Obstetric Management**

- Replace fluid and electrolytes; administer systemic steroids early, especially because they also promote fetal lung maturity
- Monitor fetus carefully (ultrasonography and regular nonstress testing)
- Monitor for placental insufficiency with placental function tests (serum biochemistry, placental morphology, uterine artery Doppler ultrasound)
- Consider terminating pregnancy in intractable cases or when fetal status is uncertain
- Consider inducing labor if pregnancy is near term; method used for labor induction depends on the state of cervix
- Avoid epidural or spinal anesthesia when lesions occupy sites of puncture; no other restrictions as to the type of anesthesia

MATERNAL RISKS

Malaise
High fever
Hypothermia
Nausea, vomiting, diarrhea, dehydration
Iron deficiency anemia
Tetany, seizures, delirium
Sepsis
Renal failure
Heart failure
Risks from pharmacologic treatment

FETAL RISKS

Intrauterine growth restriction
Premature rupture of membranes
Low–birth-weight infant
Stillbirth
Neonatal death
Risks from pharmacologic treatment

KEY POINTS

■ Impetigo herpetiformis occurs predominantly in the third trimester and can recur in subsequent pregnancies with earlier onset and greater morbidity; possible triggers include hypocalcemia, hypoparathyroidism, hypovitaminosis D, stress, and bacterial infections.

■ The eruption starts with sterile pustules at the margins of erythematous patches in intertriginous areas and can generalize; histopathologic features are those of pustular psoriasis.

■ Maternal risks include symptomatic aggravation, risks associated with hypocalcemia, sepsis, and, rarely, death from renal or heart failure; fetal risks include growth restriction, premature rupture of membranes, low birth weight, stillbirth, and neonatal death.

■ Close maternal and fetal monitoring and prompt treatment are required; oral corticosteroids remain the cornerstone of treatment, and cyclosporine is an effective second-line treatment option.

■ Postpartum treatment options in nonlactating patients include those listed previously as well as methotrexate, oral retinoids, and phototherapy.

REFERENCES

1. Breier-Maly J, Ortel B, Breier F, et al. Generalized pustular psoriasis of pregnancy (impetigo herpetiformis). *Dermatology.* 1999;198:61–64.

2. Fouda UM, Fouda RM, Ammar HM, et al. Impetigo herpetiformis during the puerperium triggered by secondary hypoparathyroidism: a case report. *Cases J.* 2009;2:9338.

3. Katsambas A, Stavropoulos PG, Katsiboulas V, et al. Impetigo herpetiformis during the puerperium. *Dermatology.* 1999;198: 400–402.

4. Oumeish OY, Farraj SE, Bataineh AS. Some aspects of impetigo herpetiformis. *Arch Dermatol.* 1982;118:103–105.

5. Sahin HG, Sahin HA, Metin A, et al. Recurrent impetigo herpetiformis in a pregnant adolescent: case report. *Eur J Obstet Gynecol Reprod Biol.* 2002;101:201–203.

6. Vaidya D, Kroumpouzos G, Bercovitch L. Recurrent postpartum impetigo herpetiformis presenting after a "skip" pregnancy. *Acta Derm Venereol.* 2013;93:102–103.

7. Holm AL, Goldsmith LA. Impetigo herpetiformis associated with hypocalcemia of congenital rickets. *Arch Dermatol.* 1991; 127:91–95.

8. Moynihan GD, Ruppe JP Jr. Impetigo herpetiformis and hypoparathyroidism. *Arch Dermatol.* 1985;121:1330–1331.

9. Wolf R, Tartler U, Stege H, et al. Impetigo herpetiformis with hyperparathyroidism. *J Eur Acad Dermatol Venereol.* 2005;19: 743–746.

10. Rackett SC, Baughman RD. Impetigo herpetiformis and *Staphylococcus aureus* lymphadenitis in a pregnant adolescent. *Pediatr Dermatol.* 1997;14:387–390.

11. Sardy M, Preisz K, Berecz M, et al. Methotrexate treatment of recurrent impetigo herpetiformis with hypoparathyroidism. *J Eur Acad Dermatol Venereol.* 2006;20:742–743.

12. Winzer M, Wolff HH. Impetigo herpetiformis. *Hautarzt.* 1998; 39:110–113.

13. Tada J, Fukushiro S, Fujiwara Y, et al. Two sisters with impetigo herpetiformis. *Clin Exp Dermatol.* 1989;14:82–84.

14. Chaidemenos G, Lefaki I, Tsakiri A, et al. Impetigo herpetiformis: menstrual exacerbations for 7 years postpartum. *J Eur Acad Dermatol Venereol.* 2005;19:466–469.

15. Kuijpers AL, Schalkwijk J, Rulo HF, et al. Extremely low levels of epidermal skin-derived antileucoproteinase/elafin in a patient with impetigo herpetiformis. *Br J Dermatol.* 1997;137:123–129.

16. Hanno R, Saleeby E, Krull E. Disorders of pregnancy. In: Demis D, ed. *Clinical Dermatology.* Philadelphia, PA: Lippincott; 1991:1–15.

17. Fan P, Gao T, Li M, et al. A case of impetigo herpetiformis associated with intrahepatic cholestasis of pregnancy. *J Dermatol.* 2006;33:563–566.

18. Trevisan G, Kokelj F. Impetigo herpetiformis and RhE isoimmunization: a case report. *Cutis.* 1996;58:87–89.

19. Roth MM, Feier V, Cristodor P, et al. Impetigo herpetiformis with postpartum flare-up: a case report. *Acta Dermatovenerol Alp Panonica Adriat.* 2009;18:77–82.

20. Lakshmi C, Srinivas CR, Paul S, et al. Recurrent impetigo herpetiformis with diabetes and hypoalbuminemia successfully treated with cyclosporine, albumin, insulin and metformin. *Indian J Dermatol.* 2010;55:181–184.

21. Luewan S, Sirichotiyakul S, Tongsong T. Recurrent impetigo herpetiformis successfully treated with methotrexate: a case report. *J Obstet Gynaecol Res.* 2011;37:661–663.

22. Lim KS, Tang MB, Ng PP. Impetigo herpetiformis—a rare dermatosis of pregnancy associated with prenatal complications. *Ann Acad Med Singapore.* 2005;34:565–568.

23. Halevy S, Kardaun SH, Davidovici B, et al. The spectrum of histopathological features in acute generalized exanthematous pustulosis: a study of 102 cases. *Br J Dermatol.* 2010;163:1245–1252.

24. Kuwabara Y, Sato A, Abe H, et al. Ritodrine-induced pustular eruptions distinctly resembling impetigo herpetiformis. *J Nippon Med Sch.* 2011;78:329–333.

25. Arslanpence I, Dede FS, Gokcu M, et al. Impetigo herpetiformis unresponsive to therapy in a pregnant adolescent. *J Pediatr Adolesc Gynecol.* 2003;16:129–132.

26. Huang YH, Chen YP, Liang CC, et al. Impetigo herpetiformis and gestational hypertension: a case report and literature review. *Dermatology.* 2011;222:221–224.

27. Wolf Y, Groutz A, Walman I, et al. Impetigo herpetiformis during pregnancy: case report and review of the literature. *Acta Obstet Gynecol Scand.* 1995;74:229–232.

28. Finch TM, Tan CY. Pustular psoriasis exacerbated by pregnancy and controlled by cyclosporin A. *Br J Dermatol.* 2000;142:582–584.

29. Imai N, Watanabe R, Fujiwara H, et al. Successful treatment of impetigo herpetiformis with oral cyclosporine during pregnancy. *Arch Dermatol.* 2002;138:128–129.

30. Cravo M, Vieira R, Tellechea O, et al. Recurrent impetigo herpetiformis successfully treated with methotrexate. *J Eur Acad Dermatol Venereol.* 2009;23:336–337.

31. Gao QQ, Xi MR, Yao Q. Impetigo herpetiformis during pregnancy: a case report and literature review. *Dermatology.* 2013; 226:35–40.

32. Samieh-Tucker A, Rupasinghe M. Anaesthesia for caesarean section in a patient with acute generalised pustular psoriasis. *Int J Obstet Anesthesia.* 2007;16:375–378.

33. Vun YY, Jones B, Al-Mudhaffer M, et al. Generalized pustular psoriasis of pregnancy treated with narrowband UVB and topical steroids. *J Am Acad Dermatol.* 2006;54:s28–s30.

34. Sheth N, Greenblatt DT, Acland K, et al. Generalized pustular psoriasis of pregnancy treated with infliximab. *Clin Exp Dermatol.* 2009;34:521–522.

35. Zabel J, Erenski P. [Clofazimine in the treatment of impetigo herpetiformis]. *Przegl Dermatol.* 1984;71:161–163.

36. Gimenez Garcia R, Gimenez Garcia MC, Llorente de la Fuente A. Impetigo herpetiformis: response to steroids and etretinate. *Int J Dermatol.* 1989;28:551–552.

37. Rubisz-Brzezinska J, Zebracka T, Sobczyk M, et al. [Impetigo herpetiformis—a peculiar form of pustular psoriasis. Treatment with clofazimine and PUVA]. *Przegl Dermatol.* 1981;68: 505–509.

38. Bozdag K, Ozturk S, Ermete M. A case of recurrent impetigo herpetiformis treated with systemic corticosteroids and narrowband UVB. *Cutan Ocul Toxicol.* 2012;31:67–69.

39. Gligora M, Kolacio Z. Hormonal treatment of impetigo herpetiformis. *Br J Dermatol.* 1982;107:253.

Galen Foulke ■ Jennie T. Clarke ■ Jeffrey P. Callen

INTRODUCTION

The complex immunologic alterations occurring during gestation can alter the course of rheumatic skin disease, in some cases quelling symptoms and, in others, causing flares. The disease process itself or the medications used to control its course can make planning, achieving, and completing pregnancy a challenge. This chapter will discuss the cutaneous manifestations of the following diseases, as encountered in pregnancy: lupus erythematosus, neonatal lupus, rheumatoid arthritis, scleroderma, dermatomyositis, and the antiphospholipid antibody syndrome.

LUPUS ERYTHEMATOSUS

Lupus erythematosus (LE) has a predilection for women in their childbearing years, with an incidence almost 10 times greater than that of age-matched males.[1] Although a complex dysregulation of the immune system underlies LE, the disease appears to be principally mediated through humoral immunity, which is upregulated in pregnancy. It would logically follow then that pregnancy should induce flares in LE disease activity. However, an impressive body of research has failed to reach a clear consensus,[1–12] and the extent to which pregnancy itself enhances the risk for LE flares remains debatable. In general, it appears as though many patients with systemic LE (SLE) experience a two- to threefold increase in disease severity during pregnancy, and at least 50% of pregnancies in women with SLE are associated with some degree of disease activity.[8,9] Independent risk factors for SLE flare in pregnancy include a flare within the 6 months prior to conception, the discontinuation of hydroxychloroquine (HCQ) therapy prior to conception or during pregnancy, and a history of severe disease or frequent flares.[7–9,11]

Clinical Features

Skin disease may occur as a component of SLE or as the primary manifestation in patients without organ-threatening disease. Primarily cutaneous LE (CLE) is two to three times more common than SLE, but 72% to 85% of SLE patients have some degree of skin involvement.[13,14] CLE is subdivided into lupus-specific skin disease and lupus-nonspecific skin disease.[13–16] Lupus-specific skin disease is characterized by distinct histopathologic changes, whereas lupus-nonspecific skin disease includes an array of dermatologic conditions that have been reported to coincide with either CLE or SLE. Lupus-specific skin disease is classified into three major subtypes: **acute CLE** (ACLE), **subacute CLE** (SCLE), and **chronic** (CCLE) or **discoid LE** (DLE). Most patients with CLE have only one of the three subtypes, but nearly one-third will have two types, and 3% will have all three concurrently.[14]

ACLE presents in localized and generalized forms, which may exist independently or concurrently. Localized ACLE is the classic malar or "butterfly" rash. Pink to red papules, macules, or patches coalesce symmetrically over the bridge of the nose and the malar eminences (Figs. 11.1A and 11.1B). The erythema characteristically spares the nasolabial folds. The rash can be markedly edematous and is often quite pruritic. Photoexposed areas of the forehead, chin, anterior neck, and chest may also be involved. ACLE generally does not result in scarring following resolution. In its generalized form, ACLE presents as an eruption that appears as morbilliform or exanthematous most commonly on the chest, extensor arms, and dorsal hands sparing the knuckles. Less commonly, vesicles and bullae may arise, and exceptionally, full thickness skin necrosis can occur with subsequent sloughing, creating an appearance that is similar to toxic epidermal necrolysis (Fig. 11.1C). Nearly all cases of ACLE occur in patients with active SLE as either a presenting symptom or a herald of an imminent flare of systemic disease. Because ACLE has the highest association with active SLE, the risk for a poor pregnancy outcome is probably highest in this subtype.

SCLE is the least common type of CLE. Of patients with SCLE, 50% will meet diagnostic criteria for SLE[10,13,14]; however, SCLE patients have a much lower risk of severe systemic disease (i.e., cerebritis or nephritis).[12,13,16–18] The average age at onset of SCLE is 40 to 60 years, so most patients are past reproductive years. Clinically, SCLE presents in two forms: pink to red papulosquamous psoriasiform plaques or arcuate, annular, or polycyclic, scaly pink/red plaques (Figs. 11.2A and 11.2B). Bullae and vesicles may exceptionally be seen (Fig. 11.2C). Patients are photosensitive, and lesions are photodistributed on the extensor arms, shoulders, neck, chest, and the back. The majority of patients with SCLE have an elevated titer of the anti-Ro/SSA antibody.[14–18] Maternal anti-Ro/SSA antibodies cross the placenta and can cause neonatal LE.

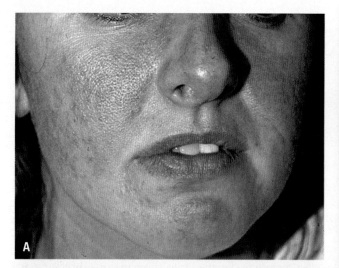

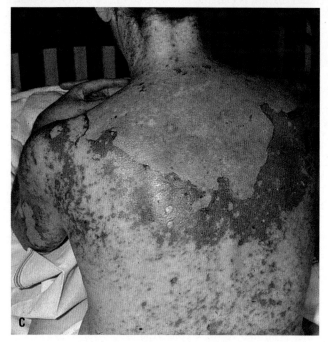

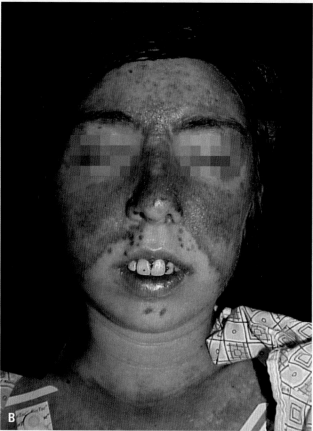

Figure 11.1. Acute cutaneous lupus erythematosus. (**A**) Erythematous macules on the sun-exposed malar cheeks, nose, and chin typify the so-called butterfly rash. (**B**) Red to purple plaques on the malar eminences, forehead, nose, and lower lip in a thrombocytopenic patient during a flare of systemic lupus. (**C**) Severe widespread erosions and full thickness epidermal necrosis resembling toxic epidermal necrolysis.

Pregnant patients known to have this antibody must be closely monitored for fetal cardiac conduction abnormalities (see "Neonatal Lupus Erythematosus," that follows).

DLE is the most common form of CLE. Patients with localized DLE (involving the head and neck only) have an approximately 5% risk of concurrent SLE,[10,13,14,17,18] whereas the risk of SLE in those with the generalized form is probably closer to 20%.[13] Both types have a low risk of developing severe systemic disease, and, therefore, DLE is the CLE subtype associated with the best pregnancy outcomes. Active lesions (Fig. 11.3) are characterized by pink/red plaques with thick, densely adherent, keratotic scales. The plaques develop hyperpigmented borders with an atrophic, hypo- or depigmented center that often contains telangiectases. Lesions result in permanent scarring. Scarring alopecia occurs when hair-baring skin is involved.

Maternal and Fetal Risks

The reported risk of skin disease flares during pregnancy ranges from 21% to 90%[1,7,8]; however, few studies have specifically evaluated the effect of pregnancy on cutaneous manifestations of lupus. Normal skin changes in pregnancy, such as palmar erythema and facial flushing due to vasodilation and postpartum telogen effluvium, can be mistaken for a lupus flare in patients with known SLE at pregnancy onset. The maternal and fetal prognosis is intrinsically tied to the severity of disease.[7–9] Overall, around one in five pregnancies with SLE will result in miscarriage or fetal death, with the highest risk occurring in the second trimester.[8–12] The risks of preterm delivery (~33%), often due to premature rupture of membranes, low birth weight, cesarean delivery (~33%), and preeclampsia (~20%), are increased.[7–9,11,12]

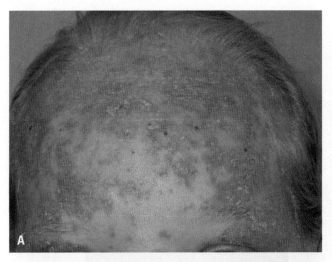

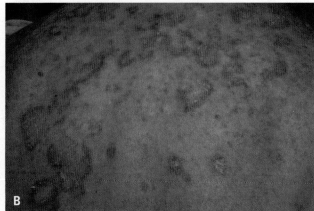

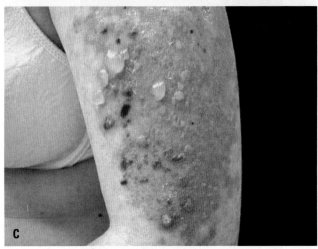

Figure 11.2. Subacute cutaneous lupus erythematosus. **(A)** Photodistributed, pink, scaly patches on the forehead of a young woman with systemic lupus erythematosus flaring 3 months' postpartum. **(B)** Annular, scaly, pink patches on the upper back. **(C)** Scaly, psoriasiform, pink plaque with overlying vesicles and bullae on the extensor surface of the upper arm. Bullous lesions are exceptionally seen in subacute cutaneous lupus.

Management

Management begins prior to conception so that pregnancies in patients with LE can be planned to minimize disease-related maternal and fetal risks as well as those due to drug therapy. Ideally, patients with SLE should be free of disease flares for 6 months prior to conception. If the patient or her partner is taking methotrexate, the drug should be stopped three ovulatory cycles prior to conception and folate supplementation should be initiated at 400 mcg per day. If the patient is on HCQ, it should be continued in pregnancy and breastfeeding because cessation has been demonstrated as a risk factor for lupus flares and increased corticosteroid use. HCQ use has not been associated with adverse pregnancy outcomes.[8,19–21] Nonsteroidal anti-inflammatory drugs (NSAIDs) may be used for arthralgias but have been associated with fetal risks (Table 11.1). For SLE that is not controlled with antimalarial therapy and NSAIDs, the lowest dosage of systemic corticosteroid should be utilized (ideally ≤10 mg per day prednisone). Prednisone, prednisolone, and methylprednisolone are the safest glucocorticoid choices during pregnancy because they cross the placenta at very low concentrations. Stress doses of glucocorticoids are recommended at delivery in patients with prolonged use of ≥20 mg per day of prednisone for >3 weeks in the 6 months prior to delivery. Azathioprine is currently the safest immunosuppressive drug used in organ-threatening SLE, and, if necessary, it can be continued as a steroid-sparing agent for systemic disease control during pregnancy.

Treatment of CLE starts with sun protection (see Table 11.1). Patients should be counseled to avoid sun exposure and employ protective clothing, barrier cosmetics, and broad spectrum sunscreen with SPF ≥30. Topical corticosteroids are the first-line treatment in pregnancy. Topical tacrolimus may be beneficial when atrophy is a concern.[22,23] Intralesional corticosteroids can be very beneficial for DLE. Systemic corticosteroids should be avoided for CLE during pregnancy. HCQ is the first-line systemic agent used for CLE that is refractory to topical therapy.

Laboratory monitoring in pregnancy requires careful interpretation because pregnancy can result in a significant elevation in inflammatory markers such as ESR and CRP, and the hormonal milieu enhances hepatic synthesis of C3 and C4. Anemia and thrombocytopenia secondary to dilution are common as well. Patients should be monitored with urinalyses and routine blood work at least once per trimester and screened for antiphospholipid antibodies (aPL).[11,24]

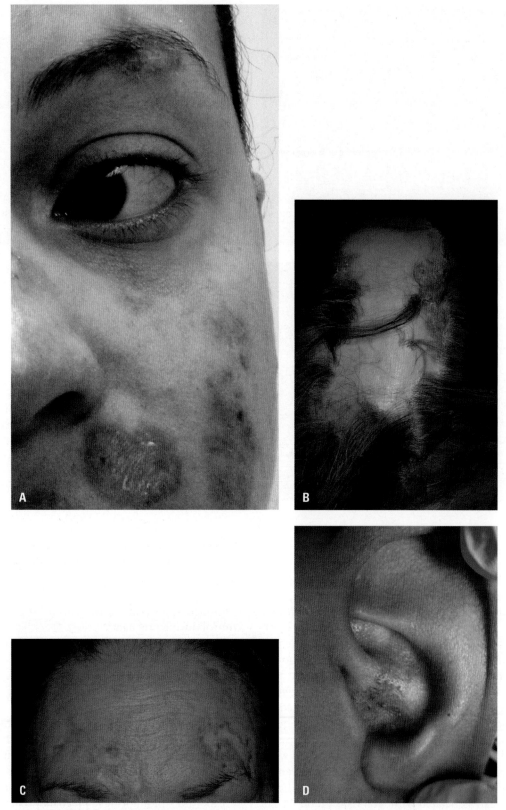

Figure 11.3. Discoid lupus erythematosus. **(A)** Scaly, erythematous, hyperpigmented, atrophic plaques on the face. Erythema and scales are signs of active disease. **(B)** Scarring (permanent) alopecia and red scaly atrophic plaques on the crown of the scalp. **(C)** Depigmented atrophic plaques with hyperpigmented borders are typical of "burnt out" inactive discoid lupus; these changes are permanent. **(D)** Pink, scaly, hyperpigmented patches with follicular plugging. The conchal bowl is a common site of involvement in discoid lupus erythematosus.

TABLE 11.1	Summary of Management Options in the Pregnant/Lactating Patient	

Rheumatic Skin Disease	Management	Comment
Lupus erythematosus	Sun protection	■ Clothing, hats, shade, broad spectrum sunscreen with SPF $\geq$30
	Topical corticosteroids	■ Use lowest effective potency to avoid skin atrophy
	Intralesional corticosteroids	■ Useful for limited areas of cutaneous lupus
	HCQ	■ For SLE/severe CLE; typically 200–400 mg/d[19]
	NSAIDs	■ For arthralgias; avoid during third trimester due to risk of premature closure of ductus arteriosus and inhibition of labor
		■ Ibuprofen may inhibit implantation; hold during conception cycles until after a positive pregnancy test
	Aspirin	■ Low-dose (81 mg/d); may be used throughout pregnancy for patients with antiphospholipid syndrome; safety discussed in Ch. 22
	Systemic corticosteroids	■ For extracutaneous manifestations
		■ Low-moderate doses if NSAIDs/aspirin and HCQ fail; try to limit prednisone to $\leq$10 mg/d
		■ Maternal and fetal risks associated with systemic steroids (see Ch. 22); stress doses of glucocorticoids are recommended perioperatively in patients with prolonged use
	Azathioprine	■ For organ-threatening SLE when benefit of immunosuppression outweighs risk
Neonatal lupus erythematosus	Serial fetal echocardiography	■ Weekly fetal echocardiograms from week 18–26, then every other week through week 32
	Fluorinated corticosteroids (maternal)	■ Betamethasone (3 mg/d)/dexamethasone (4 mg/d) may reverse first- or second-degree fetal heart block if started immediately on detection of the block (observational data)[27]; Rx continued until delivery
		■ If heart block progresses to third degree and persists for 1 week, fluorinated steroids should be discontinued
	HCQ	■ Rx during pregnancy may reduce risk of NLE
	Cardiac pacemaker	■ Often required at birth for congenital heart block
	Photoprotection	■ For infants with NLE-associated skin disease (as previous)
Rheumatoid arthritis	NSAIDs	■ See previous
	Aspirin	■ See previous
	Systemic corticosteroids	■ May be given at low-moderate doses if low-dose NSAIDs/aspirin fail to provide adequate control
		■ Try to limit prednisone to $\leq$10 mg/d; higher doses can be used if required but are associated with maternal and fetal risks (see Ch. 23)
	HCQ	■ Can be used in patients with inadequate response to NSAIDs and prednisone
	Sulfasalazine	■ Can be used in patients with inadequate response to NSAIDs and prednisone
	TNF inhibitors	■ Risk appears to be low, but data are limited; avoid use unless disease is inadequately controlled with other measures

(continued)

TABLE 11.1	Summary of Management Options in the Pregnant/Lactating Patient *(continued)*	

Rheumatic Skin Disease	Management	Comment
Systemic sclerosis	Cimetidine/ranitidine/omeprazole	■ Can be safely used for gastroesophageal reflux not adequately controlled with conservative measures
	ACE inhibitors	■ Benefits in hypertension and renal crises may outweigh risks
Dermatomyositis	Sun protection	■ See previous
	Topical corticosteroids	■ See previous
	HCQ	■ See previous
	Systemic corticosteroids	■ For myopathy or interstitial lung disease
	IVIG (data limited)	■ For severe systemic disease
Antiphospholipid antibody syndrome	Aspirin	■ Begin Rx (81 mg/d) as soon as conception is attempted[44]
		■ Considered in women with aPL who lack h/o thrombosis or obstetric complications
		■ Stop Rx after 36 weeks' gestation
	Heparin/LMWH	■ LMWH is more costly, but advantages include ease of administration; longer bioavailability; no need for laboratory monitoring; and reduced risks of hemorrhage, thrombocytopenia, and osteoporosis
		■ Anticoagulation should begin once intrauterine pregnancy is confirmed and continue until delivery; strongly recommended if h/o thrombotic event
		■ Resume heparin 4–6 hours after vaginal delivery and 12 hours after cesarean delivery to prevent postpartum thrombosis; continue for 6 weeks' postpartum; may switch to warfarin Rx once INR is therapeutic
	Plasmapheresis (data limited)	■ Could be considered in patients for whom aspirin and/or heparin failed to prevent pregnancy loss
	HCQ	■ Observational studies in nonpregnant patients demonstrate reduced risk of thrombosis
	Fetal ultrasonography	■ Early in pregnancy to establish estimated date of delivery
		■ Every 3–4 weeks starting in late second trimester to asses fetal growth and amniotic fluid volume
		■ Umbilical artery Doppler flow analyses if fetal growth restriction detected
	Warfarin	■ Used for 4–6 weeks' postpartum to prevent thromboses

ACE, angiotensin-converting enzyme; aPL, antiphospholipid antibodies; CLE, cutaneous lupus erythematosus; HCQ, hydroxychloroquine; h/o, history of; INR, international normalized ratio; IVIG, intravenous immunoglobulin; LMWH, low–molecular-weight heparin; NLE, neonatal lupus erythematosus; NSAIDs, nonsteroidal anti-inflammatory drugs; Rx, treatment; SLE, systemic lupus erythematosus; SPF, sun protection factor; TNF, tumor necrosis factor.

Neonatal Lupus Erythematosus

Neonatal lupus erythematosus (NLE) is a disease of the fetus/newborn related to transplacental passage of maternal anti-Ro/SSA or, less commonly, anti-La/SSB or anti-U1RNP antibodies to the fetus. Cardiac disease (i.e., congenital heart block [CHB]), the less frequently reported endocardial fibroelastosis, and a transient skin rash resembling SCLE are the most common manifestations of NLE; the less common are hematologic, hepatobiliary, and/or neurologic disease. It is most common for infants with NLE to have only one of these manifestations, although they may occur together in any combination as well. Anti-Ro/SSA antibody is present in ~2% of the population; however, far fewer than 2% of pregnancies result in NLE. The risk for NLE in a patient known to have Ro/SSA antibodies is ~2%.[25] The most reliable predictor of risk for NLE is a history of a prior baby with NLE (~20% to 33% chance in subsequent pregnancies). Although the transplacental transfer of autoantibodies is a crucial factor in the development of NLE, fetal susceptibility and other maternal factors appear to be at play as well.

Clinical Features

The cutaneous manifestations of NLE are clinically and histologically similar to SCLE: with scaly annular, arcuate, or polycyclic plaques (Fig. 11.4). The rash typically appears on the face, especially on the periorbital areas, and the scalp within the first 8 weeks of life (but has also been noted at delivery) and typically resolves by week 22 of life as maternal immunoglobulin (Ig)G clears from the infant's system. Ultraviolet (UV) light exposure may trigger the eruption. Scarring and atrophy are rare, although telangiectases and hypopigmentation may persist. The most common manifestation of NLE is CHB caused by fibrosis of the atrioventricular (AV) node.[24–28] In fact, NLE is the most common cause of CHB.[26] CHB typically develops during the second trimester. Hepatobiliary disease approximately affects 10% of babies with NLE. It can present with liver failure (in utero or shortly after birth) with histologic evidence of excessive iron storage, transient cholestasis with conjugated hyperbilirubinemia and

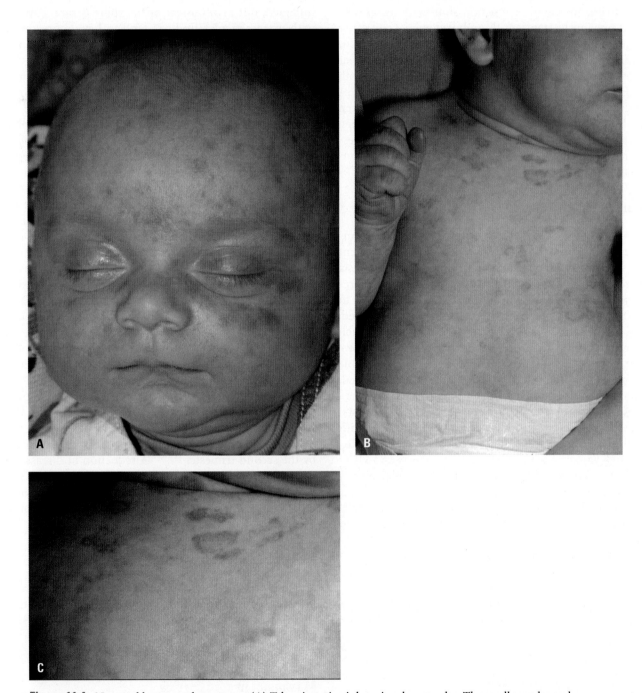

Figure 11.4. Neonatal lupus erythematosus. **(A)** Telangiectatic pink periocular macules. The small papules and pustules, however, are due to neonatal acne. (Courtesy of Dr. Andrea L. Zaenglein.) **(B)** Annular pink patches on the trunk in neonatal lupus. (Courtesy of Dr. Howard Pride.) **(C)** Pink annular patches with minimal scale. (Courtesy of Dr. Howard Pride.)

minimal transaminasemia (several weeks after birth), or transient mild-to-moderate transaminasemia occurring weeks to months after birth.[29] Transient thrombocytopenia is the most common hematologic abnormality (10%), although there are also reports of neutropenia, anemia, and pancytopenia.[25]

Fetal and Neonatal Risks

CHB is associated with a 15% to 30% mortality rate.[26] Two-thirds of patients require a permanent pacemaker.[24–26] Other risks include liver function abnormalities, as outlined previously, transient thrombocytopenia, and other hematologic abnormalities. Children with a history of NLE appear to be at increased risk of developing other autoimmune diseases later in life.[30] Mothers of babies with NLE are often asymptomatic and discover their Ro/SSA positivity only after the diagnosis of NLE in their children has been made. Over time, however, many of these women develop signs and symptoms of autoimmune disease, especially Sjögren syndrome, SLE, and undifferentiated connective tissue disease.[25]

Management

Treatment of the rash with topical corticosteroids is unnecessary because it remits spontaneously, and treatment does not impact the likelihood of residual telangiectasia or scarring.[26] Management strategies to prevent or reverse CHB via the administration of systemic steroids to Ro/SSA-positive pregnant women have been evaluated, and at this time, there is no consensus regarding such therapy. A third-degree heart block is irreversible; however, a first- and second-degree block may be reversible with systemic steroid administration.[27] When utilized, betamethasone or dexamethasone should be chosen because these corticosteroids are not inactivated by placental enzymes; however, systemic steroids are associated with fetal risks (see Ch. 22).[25] Retrospective data on SSA/Ro-positive women with SLE suggest that the use of HCQ during pregnancy may reduce the risk of cardiac NLE.[28] All pregnancies with an anti-Ro/SSA-positive mother should be screened regularly for fetal cardiac abnormalities via fetal echocardiography (weekly from weeks 16 to 26, then biweekly until week 34) and an electrocardiogram at birth. Newborns with a normal electrocardiogram at birth are unlikely to develop cardiac NLE. Any newborn with a CHB without structural cardiac abnormalities should be screened for the presence of circulating maternal SSA/Ro antibody, as should the mother. See Table 11.1.

RHEUMATOID ARTHRITIS

Rheumatoid arthritis (RA) is characterized by symmetric, destructive joint inflammation, principally of the hands and feet. In more aggressive disease, the inflammation may manifest extra-articular symptoms, especially in the skin. The disease presents most commonly between the ages of 20 and 40 years, but can occur at any age, and has a female to male incidence ratio of 3:1.

Clinical Features

RA typically begins with nonspecific symptoms such as low-grade fever, fatigue, malaise, and loss of appetite weeks to months before arthritis presents. The arthritis typically begins in the hands or feet. Any other joint may become inflamed, but involvement of the spine is rare. Patients with extra-articular findings tend to have more severe disease. Specific cutaneous pathology includes rheumatoid nodules and Bywater lesions. Rheumatoid nodules (Fig. 11.5A) may form in the lower dermis and subcutis. These are most common in periarticular locations over extensor surfaces such as the olecranon process, the extensor surfaces of the forearms, the dorsal metacarpophalangeal joints, and the Achilles tendon but may develop in viscera as well. Bywater lesions (Fig. 11.5B), small purpuric papules found at the nail fold or on the digital pulp, are found in mild RA without other systemic sequelae and show histopathologic features of leukocytoclastic vasculitis. Rheumatoid neutrophilic dermatitis—a rare, variably symptomatic eruption—can occur in RA and presents with symmetric erythematous papules, plaques, nodules, and urticarial lesions on the extensor surfaces of the extremities or trunk (Fig. 11.5C). It may resemble Sweet syndrome or urticaria. Rheumatoid vasculitis (Fig. 11.5D), a small- to medium-vessel vasculitis, may cause ulcers and livedoid vasculopathy/*atrophie blanche*, especially on the lower legs. Raynaud phenomenon, sicca syndrome, pyoderma gangrenosum, *livedo reticularis*, and keratoconjunctivitis may occur as well.

The effect of pregnancy on skin disease in RA has been poorly studied.[31] Approximately 75% of women with RA, regardless of disease severity at conception, experience improvement of their symptoms during pregnancy, typically by the second trimester.[11,24,32] A reduction in disease activity is believed to be due to an increase in the activity of regulatory T cells subsequent to changes in the hormonal milieu of pregnancy that results in a downregulation of the inflammatory pathways of RA.[32]

Maternal and Fetal Risks

Pregnancy-induced remissions are often short-lived, and the disease often flares following delivery, usually within 6 months. It is not uncommon for patients to present initially with RA during the postpartum period.[11,24,32] Maternal and fetal risks are summarized in the box.[24,32]

Management

Modifications in RA therapy may be necessary for pregnancy. Disease-modifying antirheumatic drugs and immunosuppressants such as methotrexate, leflunomide,

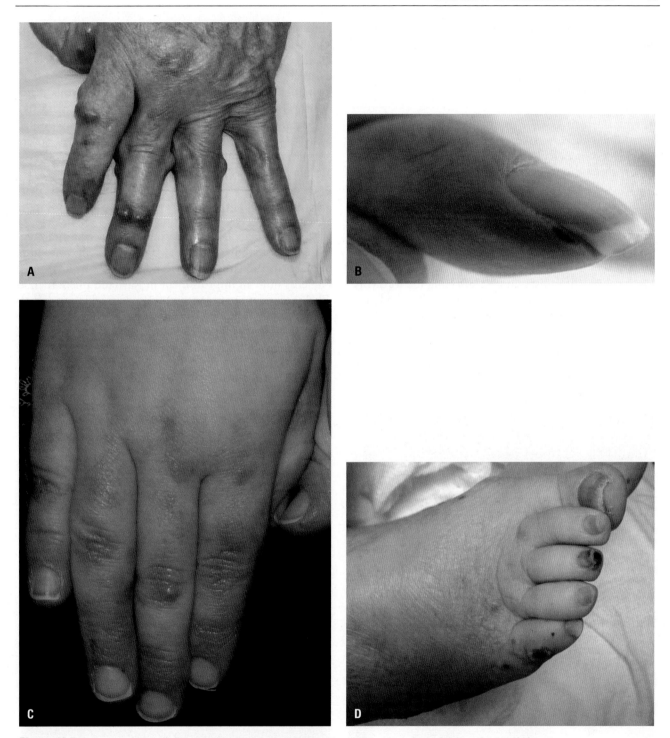

Figure 11.5. Rheumatoid arthritis. **(A)** Rheumatoid nodules. Firm subcutaneous nodules and joint deformity on the hand of a patient with severe long-standing rheumatoid arthritis. **(B)** A Bywater lesion. A small purpuric macule on the nail fold in a patient with rheumatoid arthritis. Bywater lesions are a form of rheumatoid vasculitis. **(C)** Rheumatoid neutrophilic dermatitis presenting with pink papules and patches on the extensor surface of the hand. **(D)** Rheumatoid vasculitis. Dusky red plaque on the lateral foot and necrotic ulcers on the toes and lateral foot.

gold, mycophenolate, and cyclophosphamide could cause fetal harm in pregnancy and should be discontinued prior to conception. Leflunomide undergoes extensive entero-hepatic recirculation and ideally should be discontinued 2 years prior to conception. HCQ can be continued during pregnancy. Flares of disease can be treated with oral corticosteroids, HCQ, and sulfasalazine, but treatment of the cutaneous manifestations during pregnancy is an area requiring further study. Following delivery, a woman may restart her disease-modifying antirheumatic drugs with careful consideration given to the impact on nursing. It is important to closely follow the patient for signs and symptoms of a disease flare following parturition. See Table 11.1.

SYSTEMIC SCLEROSIS

Systemic sclerosis (SSc) (scleroderma) is a fibrosing disorder in which microvascular compromise and fibrosis lead to organ dysfunction in multiple systems. The onset of SSc is most common in the early fifth decade, and so many patients are beyond their childbearing years. The majority of patients with SSc are categorized as having limited SSc (lSSc).

Clinical Features

Skin involvement is distal in lSSc, affecting the forearms, hands, feet, and face. Patients may also have Raynaud phenomenon, sclerodactyly, periungual erythema with dilated tortuous capillary loops, and telangiectases (Figs. 11.6A to 11.6C). Extensive cutaneous fibrosis progressing to the upper arms, shoulders, chest, or abdomen defines diffuse SSc (dSSc) (Fig. 11.6D). Diffuse SSc is marked by an abrupt onset of often pruritic, nonpitting edema of the hands and feet, with or without arthritis, and associated with Raynaud phenomenon. Skin changes progress to firm, tight fibrosis with adherence to subcutaneous structures. The face may develop an expressionless, mask-like appearance, thin lips, and perioral radiating creases called rhagades. Diffuse SSc has a higher incidence of severe systemic involvement (i.e., pulmonary fibrosis or scleroderma renal crisis), especially early in its course.

Maternal and Fetal Risks

There is a paucity of data regarding scleroderma and pregnancy. Most studies have shown that pregnancy has little impact on the course of scleroderma.[33,34] In fact, most patients note an improvement in Raynaud phenomenon likely secondary to pregnancy-related vasodilation,[33,34] although dyspepsia may worsen during pregnancy due to reduced lower esophageal sphincter tone and increased intra-abdominal pressure. It appears that SSc does have an association with small-for-gestational age infants and

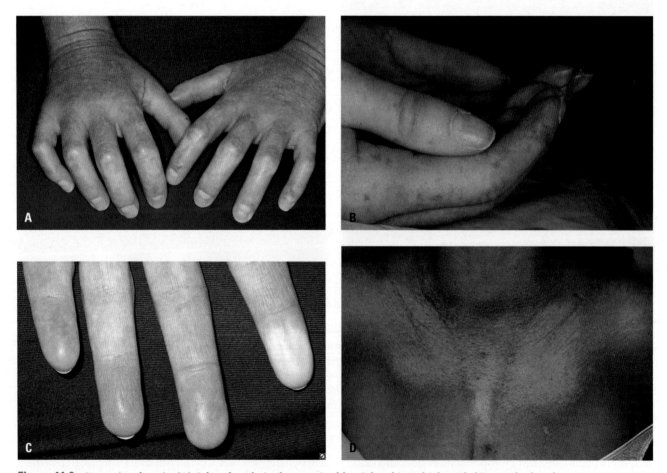

Figure 11.6. Systemic sclerosis. (**A**) Sclerodactyly is characterized by tight, shiny, thickened skin on the hands that results in reduced mobility and tapering of the fingertips. (**B**) Sclerodactyly and numerous telangiectases. (**C**) Raynaud phenomenon. Blue, white, and red fingertips in a patient with systemic sclerosis during an active episode of Raynaud phenomenon. (**D**) Widespread "salt and pepper" hyper- and hypopigmented patches on the chest and shoulders of a patient with diffuse cutaneous systemic sclerosis.

preterm births, and early dSSc (the first 3 to 5 years) is associated with increased rates of miscarriage and fetal demise.[35] Early dSSc is also associated with higher rates of maternal cardiopulmonary and renal complications, including the scleroderma renal crisis.[34] Because mortality rates are significantly elevated in patients with significant pulmonary hypertension, pregnancy should be avoided in these women.[33]

Management

It is important to monitor blood pressure and serum creatinine in pregnancy in order to evaluate for the onset of renal crisis, which has an extremely high mortality rate and can be difficult to distinguish from preeclampsia. The fibrotic plaques can include the perineum and abdomen, particularly in disseminated disease. When the perineum is involved, the skin may lack the necessary elasticity to allow for normal vaginal delivery. If fibrosis is present over the abdomen, it is still considered safe to perform a cesarean delivery, which may require an incision through areas of induration.[33] Therapeutic options for skin thickening are limited. Some improvement in nonpregnant patients has been demonstrated with phototherapy, topical calcineurin inhibitors, and topical calcipotriene; there are no data to support routine use of these agents for scleroderma during pregnancy.[36] Systemic therapies such as methotrexate, mycophenolate mofetil, cyclophosphamide, and D-penicillamine should be avoided in pregnancy. Systemic glucocorticoids should be used with caution because they may precipitate renal crisis. Calcium channel blockers for vasospastic symptoms should be minimized if possible.[33] Angiotensin-converting enzyme (ACE) inhibitors have been associated with fetal/neonatal renal insufficiency in a small number of cases. However, they are efficacious in hypertension and renal crises, and their benefits may outweigh the risks in these cases. H_2-receptor blockers such as ranitidine and cimetidine and proton pump inhibitors such as omeprazole (all are pregnancy category C) appear to be safe in pregnancy for treating gastroesophageal reflux. See Table 11.1.

DERMATOMYOSITIS

Dermatomyositis (DM) primarily affects the skin and/or skeletal muscles. The disease has a bimodal incidence, peaking first in early adolescence, and then again at the beginning of the sixth decade. Only 14% of DM patients are of childbearing age, and, as such, studies of pregnancy in this population are limited.[37]

Clinical Features

Pathognomonic skin findings in DM include Gottron papules and Gottron sign (Fig. 11.7). Gottron papules are shiny, pink, and polygonal and distributed over the

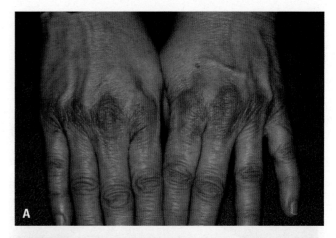

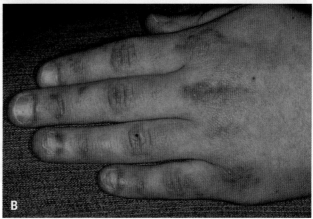

Figure 11.7. Dermatomyositis. **(A)** Erythema of the joints is referred to as a Gottron sign. The skin overlying the metacarpophalangeal joints is involved in this patient. **(B)** Dark pink-purplish papules on the skin over the knuckles are referred to as Gottron papules. This patient also has cuticular hypertrophy, another common finding in patients with dermatomyositis.

dorsum of the knuckles and hands or elbow. A Gottron sign manifests as red to pink macules or patches in a similar distribution. Patients may also develop characteristic but nonspecific pruritic periorbital violet patches and plaques (the "heliotrope rash"), photodistributed red or violet macules with poikiloderma (the "shawl sign"), and periungual erythema with capillary dilation (Fig. 11.8). Less common findings include calcinosis cutis and dystrophic cuticles. The myopathy affects skeletal muscles, and proximal muscle weakness is the most common symptom.

Maternal and Fetal Risks

Case reports and series have detailed DM both flaring and presenting de novo during gestation, including a case with associated respiratory failure.[37–40] For patients experiencing increased disease activity during pregnancy, most cases detail rapid resolution of symptoms following parturition with a slow steroid taper.[39] There are significantly fewer reports detailing flares or new presentations following delivery, and at least one details maternal death.[39]

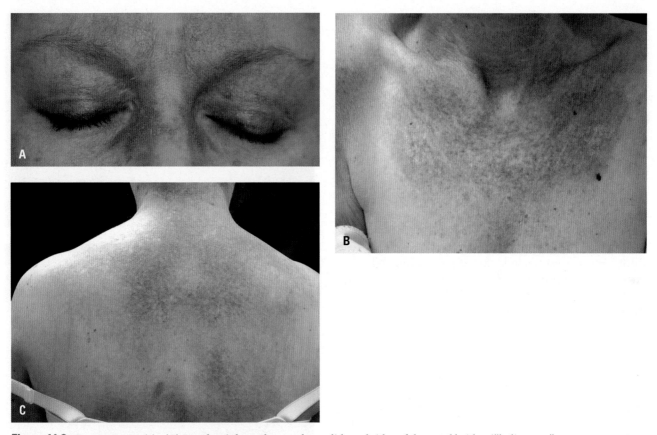

Figure 11.8. Dermatomyositis. (**A**) Purple-pink patches on the eyelids and sides of the nasal bridge ("heliotrope" rash) are classic findings in dermatomyositis. (**B**) Slightly scaly, pink-purple patches and poikiloderma (telangiectases, atrophy, hypo- and hyperpigmentation) on the upper chest. (**C**) Poikiloderma and pink patches on the upper back are referred to as the shawl sign.

A fetal mortality rate as high as 40% in patients with uncontrolled disease has been reported, although data supporting this are weak.[37] The myopathy typically occurs in skeletal muscle and there have been no reports of the uterus being affected.[40] Despite this, there is no consensus yet as to whether DM necessitates cesarean delivery or if vaginal delivery is safe. An assisted vaginal delivery can be required in case of active myositis during labor.

Management

Cutaneous manifestations can be treated with corticosteroids and calcineurin inhibitors. HCQ can be used safely as systemic therapy if topicals fail. Creatine kinase, lactate dehydrogenase, and aldolase, serum markers used to detect myopathy in patients with DM, may be altered by pregnancy. Normal pregnancy may result in slight decreases in creatine kinase during the first trimester and slightly elevated lactate dehydrogenase levels throughout pregnancy. Systemic steroids may be required for myopathy or other systemic manifestations. There are reports of the use of intravenous immunoglobulin (IVIG) as a steroid-sparing agent in pregnancy and for the control of life-threatening respiratory failure.[37–40] More potent immunosuppressants may be necessary under exceptional circumstances but are associated with significant fetal risks. See Table 11.1.

ANTIPHOSPHOLIPID SYNDROME

Antiphospholipid syndrome (APS) is defined by the presence of laboratory abnormalities, including lupus anticoagulant and/or aPL (anticardiolipin and/or anti-β_2-glycoprotein I), plus clinical manifestations, including either pregnancy morbidity or arterial/venous thrombosis (Table 11.2). A diagnosis is often made in women of childbearing age due to pregnancy complications, and careful management of these high-risk pregnancies is critical. Patients with SLE are at increased risk of secondary APS.

Clinical Features

Cutaneous manifestations are nonspecific, but all relate to vaso-occlusive events. Most common among these is *livedo reticularis* (Fig. 11.9A), which occurs in 16% to 25% of patients with APS and is a presenting manifestation in 17% to 40% of cases.[41] Its prevalence is higher in APS associated with SLE than in primary APS (36% versus 16%).[41] It is a mottled, red-blue, retiform, or net-like discoloration

TABLE 11.2	Diagnostic Criteria for Antiphospholipid Antibody Syndrome
Clinical Criteria ■ Must have at least one clinical criterion	■ **Vascular thrombosis** (may be venous, arterial, or small vessel but excludes superficial venous thrombosis) that is confirmed with imaging or histologic evidence ■ **Pregnancy morbidity** (unexplained fetal death at ≥10 weeks' gestation; *or* one or more preterm births before 34 weeks' gestation due to eclampsia, preeclampsia, or placental insufficiency; *or* three or more unexplained pregnancy losses occurring at ≤10 weeks' gestation
Laboratory Criteria ■ Must be within 5 years of clinical event and demonstrated on at least two occasions 12 or more weeks apart	■ **One or more of the following:** ■ IgG &/or IgM anticardiolipin in moderate or high titer ■ IgG of IgM β₂-glycoprotein I antibodies at a titer >99th percentile for the testing laboratory ■ Lupus anticoagulant activity

Ig, immunoglobulin.

resulting from occluded dermal arterioles, which supply a wedge of skin in the shape of an inverted cone. Livedo patterns have been further classified into *reticularis* and *racemosa*. *Livedo reticularis* refers to net-like discoloration with uniform, even, complete rings, or links, whereas *livedo racemosa* refers to a coarse, irregular pattern composed of open rings or links of varying size that may be more generalized (Figs. 11.9B and 11.9C). Some authors have suggested that *livedo racemosa* is more specific for APS than *livedo reticularis* and is associated with the arterial subset of APS.[41,42] *Livedo reticularis* can also be observed as a physiologic response to cold, particularly on the lower legs in children (*cutis marmorata*) and in those with light skin. Its appearance is most suggestive of APS when the discoloration occurs over the trunk or buttocks or in those patients with known LE.[41]

Other cutaneous findings in APS include acute cutaneous necrosis, ulcerations, gangrene, splinter hemorrhages, superficial thrombophlebitis, petechiae, purpura, pseudovasculitis, Degos-like lesions, primary anetoderma, and *atrophie blanche*/livedoid vasculopathy (Fig. 11.10).[41,42] Catastrophic APS is a potentially lethal, quickly progressing multiorgan system coagulopathy, which may result in extensive skin necrosis that resembles purpura fulminans, HELLP (hemolysis, elevated liver enzymes and low platelet) syndrome, or disseminated intravascular coagulation.[41,42] There are no studies specifically addressing the impact of pregnancy on cutaneous manifestations of APS.

Maternal and Fetal Risks

Pregnancy complications include pregnancy-related maternal thromboses (5%), early and severe preeclampsia/eclampsia, placental insufficiency, intrauterine growth restriction (30%), and recurrent pregnancy loss.[8,10,11] The presence of aPL does not always compromise pregnancies, and over 50% of women with known persistent aPL have successful pregnancies without treatment.[43]

Management

There is a lack of large, well-controlled, and prospective trials. Screening for aPL is recommended in women with a history of unexplained arterial/venous thromboembolism, a new embolic event during pregnancy, a history of one or more fetal losses (>10 weeks' gestation), or three or more embryonic losses.[44] Current recommendations support at least low-dose aspirin administration for any patient with APS attempting conception. Heparin or low–molecular-weight heparin (started once intrauterine pregnancy has been confirmed and continued throughout pregnancy) combined with low-dose aspirin should be considered for those patients with aPL who have history of at least one miscarriage or fetal death and may reduce pregnancy loss by 50% (see Table 11.1).[44] The previous intervention is strongly recommended if there is a history of a thrombotic event[45]; however, optimal management is an area of ongoing study. Most authors recommend holding heparin at the onset of labor or 12 hours before a planned induction, but recommendations vary based on the dose of anticoagulation and the patient's risk of thromboembolism. Due to the increased risk of venous thromboembolism in the postpartum period, anticoagulation is generally continued postpartum for a minimum of 6 weeks.

Many authors recommend the following monitoring during pregnancy: baseline serum creatinine, urine protein-to-creatinine ratio, hepatic transaminases, early sonography to establish estimated date of delivery, serial ultrasounds every 3 to 4 weeks during the late second and third trimesters to assess fetal growth and amniotic fluid volume, and umbilical artery Doppler flow analysis in cases of fetal growth restriction.[44] There are no established treatments specifically tailored for cutaneous disease. *Livedo reticularis* tends to not respond to therapy.[41] Ulcerations and livedoid vasculopathy may improve with anticoagulation.

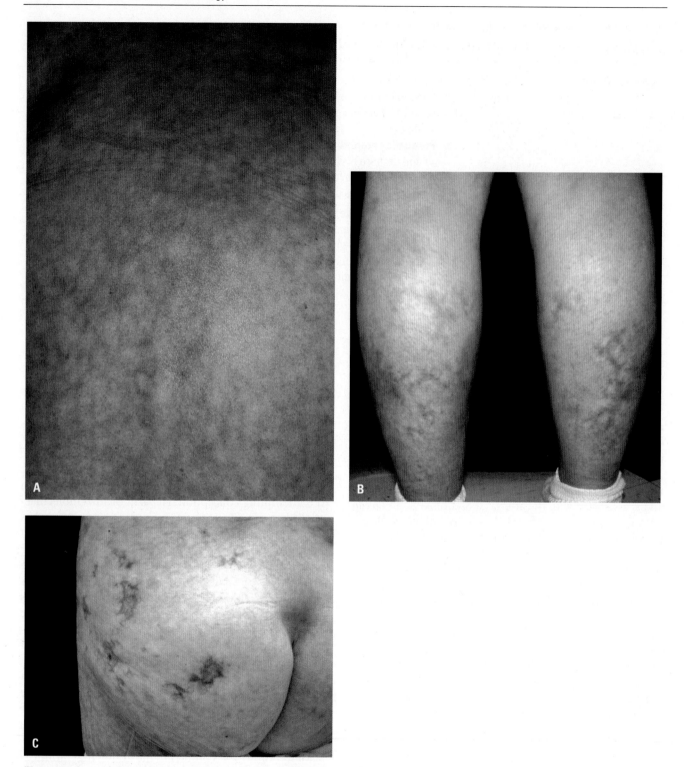

Figure 11.9. Antiphospholipid antibody syndrome. (**A**) *Livedo reticularis*. Red, dusky, even, net/mesh-like macules on the back. (**B**) *Livedo racemosa*. Red, dusky, irregular, unevenly reticulated macules on the lower legs. (**C**) Ulcerated *livedo racemosa*.

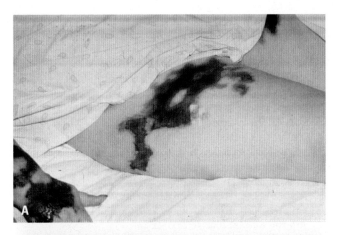

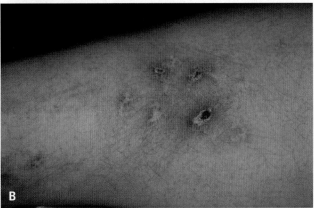

Figure 11.10. Antiphospholipid antibody syndrome. (**A**) Acute cutaneous necrosis. (**B**) Livedoid vasculopathy. Small, painful, crusted ulcers and atrophic white stellate scars with punctuate telangiectases on the lower leg.

MATERNAL RISKS

Systemic lupus: Two- to three-fold ↑ lupus activity (worsening of arthralgias, skin disease, and constitutional symptoms), gestational hypertension, preeclampsia, risks from pharmacologic Rx

Neonatal lupus: ↑ risk of autoimmune disease later in life, ↑ risk of NLE in subsequent pregnancies, risks from pharmacologic Rx

Rheumatoid arthritis: Postpartum flare, ↑ cesarean section, risks from pharmacologic Rx

Systemic sclerosis: ↑ morbidity/mortality from renal crisis, worsened gastroesophageal reflux, risks from pharmacologic Rx

Dermatomyositis: Disease flare, assisted vaginal delivery if active myositis during labor, risks from pharmacologic Rx

Antiphospholipid syndrome: Arterial/venous thrombosis, severe preeclampsia/eclampsia, risks from pharmacologic Rx

FETAL RISKS

Systemic lupus: Preterm delivery, low birth weight, pregnancy loss, stillbirth, premature rupture of membranes; risks from pharmacologic Rx

Neonatal lupus: CHB, cardiomyopathy, hydrops fetalis, subacute cutaneous lupus-like skin rash, thrombocytopenia, hepatobiliary disease, ↑ risk of other autoimmune disease later in life, risks from pharmacologic Rx

Rheumatoid arthritis: Preterm delivery, IUGR, risks from pharmacologic Rx

Systemic sclerosis (limited data): Preterm delivery, IUGR, risks from pharmacologic Rx

Dermatomyositis (limited data): Preterm delivery, IUGR, miscarriage, stillbirth, risks from pharmacologic Rx

Antiphospholipid syndrome: Miscarriage, stillbirth, IUGR, preterm delivery, risks from pharmacologic Rx

CHB, congenital heart block; IUGR, intrauterine growth restriction; NLE, neonatal lupus erythematosus; Rx, treatment.

KEY POINTS

- Approximately 20% of pregnancies with women with SLE result in miscarriage or fetal death, with the highest risk occurring in the second trimester; the risks of preterm delivery, low birth weight, cesarean section, and preeclampsia are also increased; flares of skin disease during pregnancy have been reported in 20% to 90% of patients.

- Neonatal lupus is characterized by any combination of cutaneous, cardiac, hepatobiliary, and/or hematologic manifestations related to transfer of maternal Ro/SSA, La/SSB, or U1RNP autoantibodies.

- Rheumatoid arthritis often improves during pregnancy but frequently flares within the first 6 months' postpartum.

- Data regarding the impact of pregnancy on systemic sclerosis are limited; however, morbidity and mortality from scleroderma renal crisis in pregnancy is very high; Raynaud phenomenon often improves during pregnancy due to vasodilation.

- Dermatomyositis is uncommon in women during childbearing years; it appears that the risk of maternal and fetal complications during pregnancy is correlated with the severity of disease.

- APS may result in pregnancy loss at any point in pregnancy; screening for aPL antibodies is recommended in women with a history of thromboembolism, one or more fetal losses (>10 weeks' gestation), or three or more embryonic losses; anticoagulation improves the likelihood of live births.

REFERENCES

1. Yell JA, Burge SM. The effect of hormonal changes on cutaneous disease in lupus erythematosus. *Br J Dermatol.* 1993;129:18–22.
2. Mintz G, Niz J, Guitierrez G, et al. Prospective study of pregnancy in systemic lupus erythematosus. Results of a multidisciplinary approach. *J Rheumatol.* 1986;13:732–739.

3. Lockshin MD, Reinitz E, Druzin ML, et al. Lupus pregnancy, case-control prospective study demonstrating absence of lupus exacerbation during or after pregnancy. *Am J Med.* 1984;77:893–898.

4. Meehan RT, Dorsey, JK. Pregnancy among patients with systemic lupus erythematosus receiving immunosuppressive therapy. *J Rheumatol.* 1987;14:252–258.

5. Lockshin MD. Pregnancy does not cause systemic lupus erythematosus to worsen. *Arthritis Rheum.* 1989;32:665–670.

6. Tincani A, Faden D, Tarantini M, et al. Systemic lupus erythematosus and pregnancy: a prospective study. *Clin Exp Rheumatol.* 1992;10:439–446.

7. Petri M. Hopkins lupus pregnancy center: 1987 to 1996. *Rheum Dis Clin North Am.* 1997;23:1–13.

8. Clowse, MEB. Lupus activity in pregnancy. *Rheum Dis Clin North Am.* 2007;33:237–252.

9. Doria A, Tincani A, Lockshin M. Challenges of lupus pregnancies. *Rheumatology (Oxford).* 2008;47:iii9–iii12.

10. Boumpas DT, Fessler BJ, Austin HA, et al. Systemic lupus erythematosus: emerging concepts part 2: dermatologic and joint disease, the antiphospholipid antibody syndrome, pregnancy and hormonal therapy, morbidity and mortality and pathogenesis. *Ann Intern Med.* 1995;123:42–53.

11. Keeling S, Oswald A. Pregnancy and rheumatic disease: "by the book" or "by the doc." *Clin Rheumatol.* 2009;28:1–9.

12. Clark CA, Spitzer KA, Nadler JN, et al. Preterm deliveries in women with systemic lupus erythematosus. *J Rheumatol.* 2003;30:2127–2132.

13. Lee HJ, Sinha AA. Cutaneous lupus erythematosus: understanding of clinical features, genetic basis, and pathobiology of disease guides therapeutic strategies. *Autoimmunity.* 2006;39:433–444.

14. Werth V. Clinical manifestations of cutaneous lupus erythematosus. *Autoimmun Rev.* 2005;4:296–302.

15. Gilliam JN, Sontheimer RD. Distinctive cutaneous subsets in the spectrum of lupus erythematosus. *J Am Acad Dermatol.* 1981;4:471–475.

16. Clarke JT, Werth VP. Rheumatic manifestations of skin disease. *Curr Opin Rheumatol.* 2010;22:78–84.

17. Chang AY, Werth VP. Treatment of cutaneous lupus. *Curr Rheumatol Rep.* 2011;13:300–307.

18. Bano S, Bombardieri S, Doria A, et al. Lupus erythematosus and the skin. *Clin Exp Rheumatol.* 2006;24:s26–s35.

19. Parke AL. Antimalarial drugs, systemic lupus erythematosus and pregnancy. *J Rheumatol.* 1998;15:607–610.

20. Wallace DJ. Antimalarial agents and lupus. *Rheum Dis Clin North Am.* 1994;20:243–263.

21. Costedoat-Chalumeau N, Amoura Z, Duhaut P, et al. Safety of hydroxychloroquine in pregnant patients with connective tissue diseases: a study of one hundred thirty-three cases compared with a control group. *Arthritis Rheum.* 2003;48:3207–3211.

22. Christopher V, Al-Chalabi T, Richardson PD, et al. Pregnancy outcome after liver transplantation: a single-center experience of 71 pregnancies in 45 recipients. *Liver Transp.* 2006;12:1138–1143.

23. Tauscher AE, Fleischer AB, Phelps KC, et al. Psoriasis and pregnancy. *J Cutan Med Surg.* 2002;6:561–570.

24. Märker-Hermann E, Fischer-Betz R. Rheumatic diseases and pregnancy. *Curr Opin Obstet Gynecol.* 2010;22:458–465.

25. Lee LA. The clinical spectrum of neonatal lupus. *Arch Dermatol Res.* 2009;301:107–110.

26. Buyon JP, Clancy RM. Neonatal lupus: basic research and clinical perspectives. *Rheum Dis Clin N Am.* 2005;31:299–313.

27. Friedman DM, Kim MY, Copel JA, et al. Prospective evaluation of fetuses with autoimmune-associated congenital heart block followed in the PR interval and dexamethasone evaluation (PRIDE) study. *Am J Cardiol.* 2009;103:1102–1106.

28. Izmirly PM, Kim MY, Llanos C, et al. Evaluation of the risk of anti-SSA/Ro-SSB/La antibody-associated cardiac manifestations of neonatal lupus in fetuses of mothers with systemic lupus erythematosus exposed to hydroxychloroquine. *Ann Rheum Dis.* 2010;69:1827–1830.

29. Lee LA, Sokol RJ, Buyon JP. Hepatobiliary disease in neonatal lupus: prevalence, and clinical characteristics in cases enrolled in a national registry. *Pediatrics.* 2002;109:E11

30. Martin V, Lee LA, Askanase AD, et al. Long-term followup of children with neonatal lupus and their unaffected siblings. *Arthritis Rheum.* 2002;46:2377–2383.

31. Nelson JL, Ostensen M. Pregnancy and rheumatoid arthritis. *Rheum Dis Clin North Am.* 1997;23:195–212.

32. Sayah A, English JC III. Rheumatoid arthritis: a review of the cutaneous manifestations. *J Am Acad Dermatol.* 2005;53:191–209.

33. Steen V. Pregnancy in scleroderma. *Rheum Dis Clin North Am.* 2007;33:345–358.

34. Chakravarty E. Vascular complications of systemic sclerosis during pregnancy. *Int J Rheumatol.* 2010;2010:287248.

35. Steen V. Pregnancy in women with systemic sclerosis. *Obstet Gynecol.* 1999;94:15–20.

36. Zwischenberger BA, Jacobe HT. A systematic review of morphea treatments and therapeutic algorithm. *J Am Acad Dermatol.* 2011;65:925–941.

37. Nozaki Y, Ikoma S, Funauchi M, et al. Respiratory muscle weakness with dermatomyositis during pregnancy: successful treatment with intravenous immunoglobulin therapy. *J Rheumatol.* 2008;35:2289.

38. Yassaee BA, Kovarik C, Werth V. Pregnancy-associated dermatomyositis. *Arch Dermatol.* 2009;145:952–953.

39. Kanoh H, Izumi T, Seishima M, et al. A case of dermatomyositis that developed after delivery: the involvement of pregnancy in the induction of dermatomyositis. *Br J Dermatol.* 1999;141:897–900.

40. Williams L, Chang P, Park E, et al. Successful treatment of dermatomyositis during pregnancy with intravenous immunoglobulin monotherapy. *Obstet Gynecol.* 2007;109:561–563.

41. Frances C. Dermatological manifestations of Hughes' antiphospholipid antibody syndrome. *Lupus.* 2010;19:1071–1077.

42. Weinstein S, Piette W. Cutaneous manifestations of antiphospholipid antibody syndrome. *Hematol Oncol Clin N Am.* 2008;22:67–77.

43. Lockwood CJ, Romero R, Feinberg RF, et al. The prevalence and biologic significance of lupus anticoagulant and anticardiolipin antibodies in a general obstetric population. *Am J Obstet Gynecol.* 1989;161:369–373.

44. American College of Obstetrics and Gynecologists Committee on Practice Bulletins—Obstetrics. ACOG Practice Bulletin No 118: Antiphospholipid syndrome. *Obstet Gynecol.* 2011;117:192–199.

45. Bates SM, Greer IA, Pabinger I, et al. American College of Chest Physicians. Venous thromboembolism, thrombophilia, antithrombotic therapy, and pregnancy: American College of Chest Physicians Evidence-Based Clinical Practice Guidelines, 8th ed. *Chest.* 2008;133:844S–886S.

CHAPTER 12

Metabolic and Bullous Disease

Nicole Fett ■ Victoria P. Werth

INTRODUCTION

Metabolic and bullous diseases rarely occur in pregnancy; however, they have significant effects on maternal and fetal outcomes when they do occur. This chapter will discuss porphyria cutanea tarda, acrodermatitis enteropathica, erythema multiforme, pemphigus vulgaris, pemphigus foliaceus, epidermolysis bullosa acquisita, and linear immunoglobulin (Ig)A dermatosis in the setting of pregnancy, with an emphasis on maternal and fetal risks and management options.

METABOLIC DISEASE

Porphyria Cutanea Tarda

Epidemiology

Porphyria cutanea tarda (PCT), the most common subtype of porphyria, is estimated to occur in 1 out of every 10,000 people.[1]

Etiology

PCT is caused by a decrease in uroporphyrinogen decarboxylase (UROD) activity, either through a genetic mutation (referred to as hereditary or type II PCT) or an acquired deficiency of the enzyme (referred to as sporadic or type I PCT).[2] Hereditary PCT is inherited as an autosomal dominant trait with low penetrance; therefore, a family history may not be elicited.[2] Sporadic PCT makes up over 75% of PCT cases and is associated with alcohol abuse, hepatitis B and C, HIV, iron overload (via transfusions, hemochromatosis, and supplementation), and oral estrogens.[2] Decreased UROD activity results in hepatic accumulation of uroporphyrin, which circulates in plasma and is excreted in the urine.[1]

Clinical Features

Patients present with tense bullae and vesicles on sun-exposed surfaces. Lesions heal with scarring, milia, hyperpigmentation, and hypertrichosis (Fig. 12.1). Less frequently, patients will present with sclerodermoid changes and skin fragility.

Diagnosis

PCT is diagnosed based on abnormal 24-hour urine porphyrin testing. Patients with PCT have elevated urine levels of uroporphyrin and coproporphyrin. Histopathology reveals a noninflammatory subepidermal blister with festooning of the dermal papilla and thickening of the dermal vessel walls (Fig. 12.2).

Maternal and Fetal Risks

Several case reports have detailed the course of PCT in pregnancy.[3-7] Approximately half of these women experienced flares of their PCT during their pregnancies. Anecdotally, PCT is thought to worsen during the first and second trimesters, when estrogen levels are at their highest, and then improve in the last trimester when iron stores are at their lowest and patients are experiencing hemodilution. Two cases were treated with phlebotomy during pregnancy[4,6] and another with low-dose chloroquine (125 mg by mouth twice a week) with good results.[5] A population-based cohort study revealed that mothers with sporadic PCT had two times the odds of having small-for-gestational age infants and those with familial PCT had three times the odds of having a child who experienced perinatal death.[8] However, the study did not control for alcohol use, tobacco use, hepatitis B and C, or HIV status, all of which may be confounders or effect modifiers.[8]

Management

PCT management focuses on avoidance of sun and triggers, such as alcohol consumption and iron supplementation. Patients should be counseled to wear a sunscreen containing zinc oxide or titanium dioxide (which absorbs in the 410-nm wavelengths that induce porphyria) daily. Patients who continue to be symptomatic despite these preventive interventions may undergo two to three phlebotomy sessions or need antimalarial therapy (chloroquine or hydroxychloroquine). Chloroquine (pregnancy category C) dosed at 125 mg by mouth twice a week is the only antimalarial reported as a treatment for PCT during pregnancy. Worldwide, chloroquine is most commonly used as malarial prophylaxis and treatment and is reportedly safe in pregnant women when utilized in this manner (see Ch. 22).[9] Retrospective studies assessing chloroquine safety in pregnant women with autoimmune disease have not found adverse maternal or fetal outcomes.[9] Although hydroxychloroquine has not been reported as a therapy for PCT in pregnancy, the experience from the treatment of autoimmune diseases with hydroxychloroquine indicates that it is safe in pregnancy.[9] Expectant mothers with PCT should also be evaluated for HIV and hepatitis B and C infections, all of which are associated with the disease.

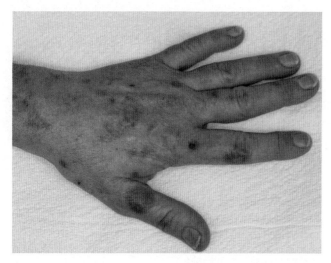

Figure 12.1. Flaccid blisters on the dorsal hands with scarring, milia, and hypertrichosis in porphyria cutanea tarda. (Courtesy of Dr. William Aughenbaugh, University of Wisconsin Hospital and Clinics.)

Acrodermatitis Enteropathica

Epidemiology

Acrodermatitis enteropathica (AE) is very rare, and its incidence in the United States is unknown. AE in the context of pregnancy has been reported very infrequently.

Etiology

AE, a hereditary zinc deficiency, is a rare autosomal recessive disorder caused by a mutation in the *SLC39A4* gene, which encodes a zinc transporter, zip4.[2,10] Zip4 is normally expressed in enterocytes in the duodenum and jejunum and functions to absorb dietary zinc.[2,10] The causative mutation of AE results in impaired dietary zinc absorption. Acquired zinc deficiency secondary to malnutrition is rare. Zinc is required at the catalytic sites of metalloenzymes and, through "zinc fingers," plays an important role in

protein folding, and therefore enzymatic activity.[10] Dietary zinc-depletion animal studies illustrate the importance of zinc in normal mammalian fetal development.[11] Despite these findings, dietary zinc deficiency in humans has not been routinely associated with adverse fetal and neonatal outcomes.[11] Two case-control studies reveal significantly lower zinc levels in mothers and children with neural tube defects and cleft palate compared with controls.[12,13] However, prenatal zinc supplementation trials in zinc-deficient populations have failed to improve outcomes[11]; patients with AE caused by a mutation, and not by severe malnutrition, have severe enough zinc deficiency to result in skin, gastrointestinal, and central nervous system disruptions.

Clinical Features

The cutaneous features of AE and acquired zinc deficiency are identical. Patients present with eczematous pink plaques on acral, anogenital, and periorificial sites (Figs. 12.3 and 12.4). These plaques form vesicles and then desquamate. Untreated AE may also result in alopecia, diarrhea, emotional lability, growth delay, mental slowing, photophobia, hypogonadism, infections, and death.[10]

Diagnosis

The diagnosis requires a high index of suspicion. A measurement of serum zinc should be performed first thing in the morning while fasting.[10] The blood should be drawn in a trace-element free tube (royal blue).[10] Zinc levels should be >70 mg/dL.[10] Unfortunately, cutoffs for a deficiency are not well-defined, and, therefore, zinc levels need to be interpreted within the clinical context. Low levels of serum alkaline phosphate are also supportive of zinc

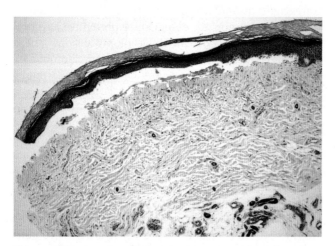

Figure 12.2. A subepidermal blister without inflammatory infiltrate, which is consistent with porphyria cutanea tarda (hematoxylin-eosin, ×10).

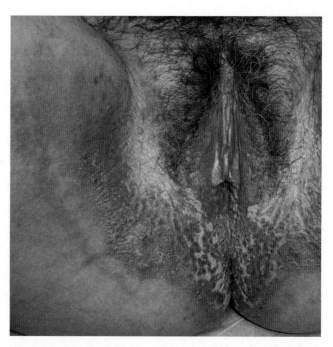

Figure 12.3. Erythematous plaque with superficial desquamation in the anogenital region in a patient with acrodermatitis enteropathica.

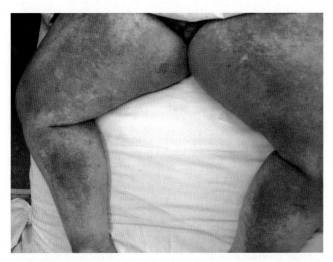

Figure 12.4. Erythema with erosion of the inner thighs in a pregnant patient with acquired (dietary) zinc deficiency. (Courtesy of Dr. Jennifer Jenkins.)

deficiency.[10] Histopathologic features include confluent parakeratosis, a decreased granular layer, epidermal pallor with focal dyskeratosis, vacuolization, balloon degeneration, and psoriasiform hyperplasia (Fig. 12.5). These histopathologic findings are nonspecific, in that they are present in several nutritional deficiencies.

Maternal and Fetal Risks

A case series of seven pregnant women with AE was published in 1981. Three of the patients did not receive treatment for AE. These three cases resulted in one spontaneous abortion, a child with anencephaly, and a child with achondroplastic dwarfism.[14] An additional article reported two pregnancies in a patient with AE.[15] Oral zinc supplementation was provided throughout both pregnancies, and serum zinc levels were monitored very closely during pregnancy. Both pregnancies were uneventful and resulted in healthy offspring.

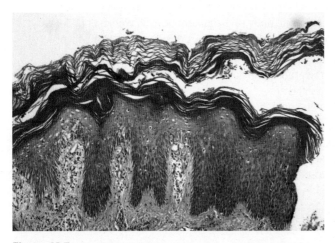

Figure 12.5. Confluent parakeratosis, decreased granular layer, epidermal pallor with focal dyskeratosis, and psoriasiform hyperplasia, which is consistent with acrodermatitis enteropathica (hematoxylin-eosin, ×20).

Management

Patients with characteristic skin findings, low serum zinc levels, and histopathologic findings consistent with a nutritional deficiency should be treated with 3 mg/kg per day of elemental zinc.[2,10] Patients will experience dramatic improvement within 2 to 3 days.

Erythema Multiforme

Epidemiology

The annual incidence of erythema multiforme (EM) is estimated at approximately 1%, with adults aged 20 to 40 years most commonly affected.[16] EM rarely occurs during pregnancy.[17–19]

Etiology

The vast majority of EM occurs in the setting of a herpes simplex virus type 1 (HSV-1) or 2 (HSV-2) infection, with EM lesions appearing 7 to 8 days after an HSV flare and resolving within 2 weeks.[16] EM is most likely caused by a cell-mediated immune process directed against viral antigens deposited in lesional skin.[20] Rarely, medications have been associated with EM, the most common being antibiotics, nonsteroidal anti-inflammatory drugs (NSAIDs), and antiepileptic agents.[16]

Clinical Features

EM presents with symmetric targetoid lesions on the distal extremities, usually with involvement of one mucosal surface (Figs. 12.6 and 12.7). A prodrome of headache, malaise, and myalgia is not uncommon.

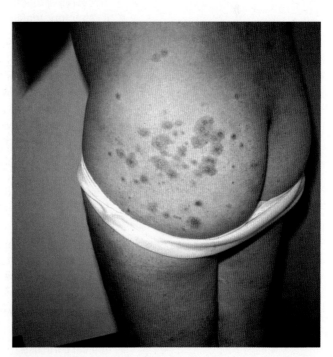

Figure 12.6. Erythema multiforme in a pregnant woman. Note the typical targetoid lesions on the trunk. (Courtesy of Dr. Iris Aronson.)

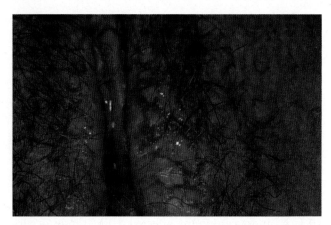

Figure 12.7. Erythema and superficial ulceration on the labia majora in erythema multiforme. (Courtesy of Dr. Joe Brooks.)

Diagnosis

A diagnosis is based on a clinical examination. When the examination is inconclusive, a biopsy should be performed. Histopathologic features include basal cell vacuolar degeneration, necrotic keratinocytes, and an inflammatory infiltrate around blood vessels and the dermal–epidermal junction.

Maternal and Fetal Risks

Patients should be evaluated for HSV infection, given the high morbidity and mortality associated with vertical HSV transmission to the fetus.[21] Pregnant women with EM should undergo serologic testing for HSV and viral identification (Table 12.1).[21] Cross-sectional studies reveal that approximately 48% of pregnant women will have antibodies against HSV-1, and 11% will have antibodies against HSV-2.[21] Because rates of vertical transmission are substantially different in mothers with primary versus recurrent HSV, serologic testing for IgG and IgM is appropriate. Primary HSV infection at the time of delivery carries a rate of vertical transmission between 20% and 50%.[21] For patients with a known HSV infection, acyclovir prophylaxis is recommended from 36 weeks to the time of delivery[21] and has been shown to reduce HSV recurrence at term and to reduce cesarean deliveries. Of note, cesarean delivery is recommended by the American College of Obstetrics and Gynecology in women with active genital

TABLE 12.1	Summary of Management Options
Condition	**Comments**
Porphyria cutanea tarda	■ UV avoidance, protective clothing, daily sunscreen with zinc oxide or titanium dioxide ■ Alcohol avoidance; no iron supplementation ■ Screen for hepatitis B, C, and HIV ■ 2–3 phlebotomy sessions or chloroquine 125 mg twice per week[9] if preventive measures are ineffective ■ If refractory, trial of hydroxychloroquine
Acrodermatitis enteropathica	■ Zinc supplementation (3 mg/kg/d of elemental zinc)[2,10] ■ Eliminate causes of dietary zinc deficiency
Erythema multiforme	■ Serologic testing for HSV antibodies (IgG and IgM) and viral identification (culture, PCR, or DFA) ■ Search for other infectious etiologies; review possible causative medications ■ If HSV positive, provide systemic antiviral treatment from 36 weeks until delivery; if HSV prodrome or HSV signs at time of delivery, consider cesarean delivery
Pemphigus vulgaris	■ Systemic corticosteroids ■ Add azathioprine if required prednisone dose >0.5 mg/kg/d[28,29] ■ Intravenous immunoglobulin G[22] ■ Supportive care for neonatal pemphigus vulgaris
Pemphigus foliaceus	■ Topical corticosteroids ■ Systemic corticosteroids if refractory to topical steroids ■ Add azathioprine if required systemic steroid dose >0.5 mg/kg/d[28,29] ■ Dapsone for disease refractory to steroids[41]
Epidermolysis bullosa acquisita	■ Wound care ■ Dapsone trial if neutrophils predominate in biopsy[45]
Linear IgA dermatosis	■ Wound care ■ Topical corticosteroids ■ Dapsone 50–200 mg/d[46]

DFA, direct fluorescent antibody assay; HIV, human immunodeficiency virus; HSV, herpes simplex virus; Ig, immunoglobulin; PCR, polymerase chain reaction; UV, ultraviolet light.

involvement or HSV prodromal symptoms at the time of delivery (see Ch. 14).[21]

Management

Once an HSV infection is confirmed, treatment with acyclovir is warranted. Possible causative medications should be withdrawn. Local wound care with mouthwashes (either oral rinsing with warm saline or a solution composed of diphenhydramine, Xylocaine, and Kaopectate) can provide relief. Topical steroids may be beneficial but should not be applied on large surface areas in order to minimize systemic absorption. Patients with severe, refractory disease who limit their oral intake may need additional immunosuppressive therapy. Dapsone, antimalarials, and azathioprine have shown a benefit in case reports. Given the lack of evidence with these therapies, they should be used with caution in pregnant patients.

AUTOIMMUNE BULLOUS DISEASE

Pemphigus Vulgaris

Epidemiology

Pemphigus vulgaris (PV) is a very rare disease with an estimated incidence of approximately 1 out of 240,000 people.[22] The average age of disease presentation is in the 40s and 50s, after normal childbearing years, and thus PV in pregnancy is exceedingly rare.[22]

Etiology

PV is caused by autoantibodies against desmoglein 1 and 3. Desmoglein 1 and 3 are desmosomes (bridges that hold cells together) found between keratinocytes in the epidermis. Desmoglein 3 is more closely related to mucous membrane disease. Patients with only anti-desmoglein 1 autoantibodies and no mucosal disease have a different variant of pemphigus, pemphigus foliaceus (PF).

Clinical Features

PV presents with superficial erosions and flaccid blisters of the mucocutaneous surfaces, with a predilection for seborrheic skin areas, such as the face, midchest, and upper back (Figs. 12.8 and 12.9).

Diagnosis

A biopsy of the edge of a new erosion or blister for histopathologic examination and a biopsy of uninvolved skin for direct immunofluorescence (DIF) are required. In addition, enzyme-linked immunosorbent assays (ELISAs) that detect autoantibodies to desmogleins 1 and 3 can be very helpful. Histologically, PV presents with acantholysis (i.e., rounding up and pulling apart of keratinocytes as a result of a loss of cell–cell adhesion, which causes intraepidermal blister formation) (Fig. 12.10). Eosinophils are often abundant. On DIF, IgG stains the intercellular spaces, resulting in a "chicken-wire" pattern.

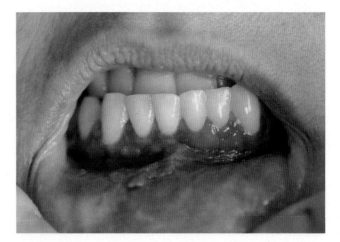

Figure 12.8. Superficial desquamation of the gingivae in pemphigus vulgaris. (Courtesy of Dr. Misha Rosenbach, University of Pennsylvania.)

Maternal and Fetal Risks

A recent literature review of PV occurring prior to or during pregnancy details 49 pregnancies occurring in 38 women.[23] Of the reported cases, 37% of mothers developed PV during their pregnancy and 63% of mothers were diagnosed with PV prior to their pregnancy.[23] Based on reported cases, PV has been associated with an increased risk of stillbirth, infant death, and intrauterine growth restriction (IUGR).[23] All mothers of stillborn infants had severe, refractory PV and were treated with systemic steroids alone or in combination with other immunosuppressive agents during their pregnancies.[23] PV often flares during the first two trimesters (54% of patients), and then again postpartum (44% of patients).[24] Neonatal PV (Fig. 12.11) may result from transplacental transfer of maternal antidesmoglein

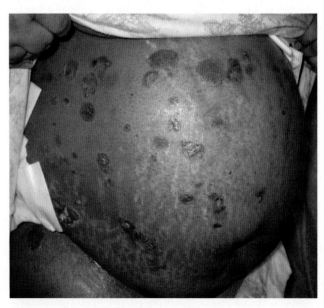

Figure 12.9. Superficial erosions and tense blisters in a pregnant patient with pemphigus vulgaris. (Courtesy of Dr. Aimee Payne, University of Pennsylvania.)

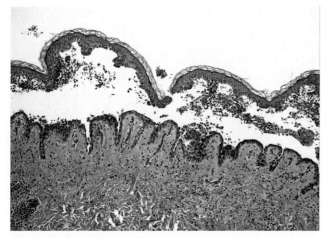

Figure 12.10. An intraepidermal blister with epidermal acantholysis and tomb-stoning of the basal layer (hematoxylin-eosin, ×10). (Courtesy of Dr. Aimee Payne, University of Pennsylvania.)

autoantibodies to the fetus. Neonatal PV is estimated to affect 2% to 45% of infants born to mothers with PV[23,24] and can occur even if the maternal disease is in remission throughout pregnancy and peripartum.[23,25,26] Neonatal PV remits within approximately 2 weeks with supportive care.

Management

Treatment of PV during pregnancy is a challenging balance of risks and benefits. Untreated PV has high morbidity and mortality; however, immunosuppressive agents are not without maternal and fetal risks. Topical steroids can be used for minimal involvement. For more severe disease, the treatment most commonly used during pregnancy is systemic steroids. Systemic steroid use during pregnancy has been associated with an increased risk of oral cleft in the fetus if administered in the first trimester, IUGR, and premature rupture of membranes.[27]

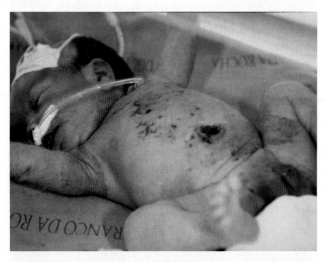

Figure 12.11. Large erosions, denuded areas, and crusts secondary to the healing of bullae on the chest, neck, axillae, thighs, and genital region in neonatal pemphigus. Note the involvement of the oral mucosa. (Courtesy of Dr. Paulo R. Cunha.)

Although no evidence-based studies on the treatment of PV in pregnancy have been published, most authors suggest adding azathioprine as a steroid-sparing agent if a prednisone dose >0.5 mg/kg per day is required for disease control.[23,24] Azathioprine has been used throughout pregnancy without a statistically significant increase in adverse outcomes.[28,29]

A successful outcome with plasmapheresis has also been published,[24,30,31] although plasmapheresis has a higher risk of treatment morbidity and mortality than other PV therapies.[32,33] Approximately 40% of plasmapheresis treatments have an associated complication.[32] In a randomized controlled trial, over 20% of pemphigus patients treated with plasmapheresis died compared to no deaths in the control group.[33] Recently, a case series of eight women with PV successfully treated with intravenous immunoglobulin G (IVIG) throughout 12 pregnancies has been published.[22] One patient was unable to tolerate IVIG secondary to severe, intractable headaches. The remaining seven patients were treated at 1 month intervals throughout pregnancy and for 2 months postpartum without any adverse effects or poor maternal or fetal outcomes.[22] Their children were followed for several years and showed no adverse effects of being exposed to IVIG in utero. The majority of these women used IVIG as monotherapy.[22] This suggests that IVIG may be a safe and effective alternative to systemic steroids and azathioprine.

Pemphigus Foliaceus

Epidemiology

Pemphigus foliaceus (PF) has an estimated incidence of 1 out of 1 million people.[34] Endemic PF (*fogo selvagem*) has an estimated incidence of 50 in 1 million people in endemic areas.[35]

Etiology

PF is caused by autoantibodies against desmoglein 1. There are two forms of PF: endemic PF, also referred to as *fogo selvagem*, and PF. *Fogo selvagem* occurs predominantly in Brazil and Colombia and is thought to be associated with molecular mimicry to an environmental factor, possibly the black fly.

Clinical Features

Superficial erosions (Fig. 12.12) are typically noted in a seborrheic distribution (i.e., on the face, scalp, central chest and upper back), and with an absence of mucosal involvement.

Diagnosis

The evaluation for PF requires a biopsy of the edge of the new erosion or blister for histopathologic examination and a biopsy of uninvolved skin for DIF. Histopathologic features include acantholysis (rounding up and pulling apart of cells in the epidermis) within the granular zone, which causes sloughing of the superficial epidermis (Fig. 12.13) and often conspicuous eosinophils. On DIF, IgG stains the intercellular spaces, resulting in a "chicken-wire" pattern. ELISA can be very helpful in detecting antibodies to desmoglein 1.

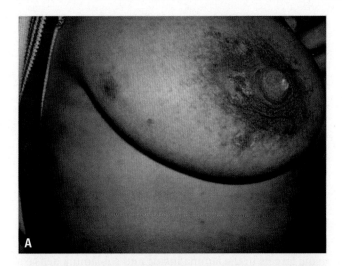

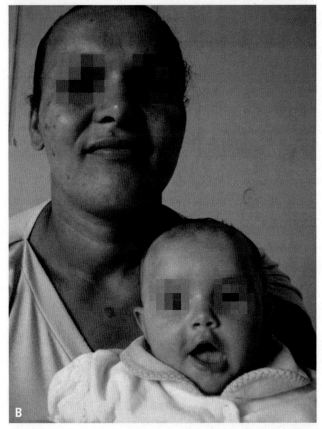

Figure 12.12. (**A**) Superficial flaccid blisters on the breast in a pregnant patient with pemphigus foliaceus. (**B**) The mother (shown in **A**) with active pemphigus foliaceus (healing bullous lesion on the chest) postpartum and the uninvolved infant. (Courtesy of Dr. Paulo R. Cunha.)

Maternal and Fetal Risks

Mothers with endemic PF do well during their pregnancies, and no infants born to mothers with *fogo selvagem* have ever developed clinical features of *fogo selvagem* (see Fig. 12.12B) despite having weakly positive DIFs and anti-desmoglein 1 autoantibodies in their sera.[36] Two infants born to mothers with PF have developed lesions of PF that resolved within 2 weeks.[37,38] Unaffected infants born to mothers with PF have

been found to have positive DIF.[39] In vitro studies have revealed that in adults, desmoglein 1 is present throughout the epidermis and desmoglein 3 is only present at the basal and intermediate basal levels, but in neonates, desmoglein 3 is expressed throughout the epidermis.[40] It is thought that desmoglein 3 expression throughout the epidermis in neonates protects them against neonatal PF.[40]

Management

Treatment is similar to that of PV, although PF is generally more responsive to topical steroids than PV. Therefore, topical steroids should be used as first-line therapy. Systemic steroids are necessary for recalcitrant disease. Azathioprine may be used as a steroid-sparing agent if a prednisone dose >0.5 mg/kg per day is required.[23,24,29,30] Dapsone is an effective systemic steroid-sparing agent and can be used in patients who fail steroids as monotherapy or in combination with systemic steroids.[41] It is considered relatively safe in pregnancy (see Ch. 22).[9]

Epidermolysis Bullosa Acquisita

Epidemiology

Epidermolysis bullosa acquisita (EBA) has an incidence of 1 in 4 million people.[42] There are only three reported cases of EBA occurring during pregnancy.[42–44]

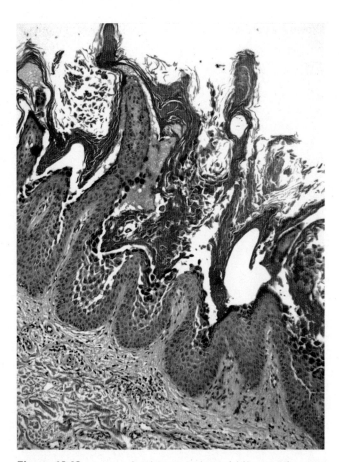

Figure 12.13. A superficial intraepidermal blister with acantholysis consistent with pemphigus foliaceus (hematoxylin-eosin, ×20).

Etiology

EBA is caused by autoantibodies against the noncollagenous N-terminal domain (NC1) of the alpha chain of type VII collagen. These autoantibodies decrease the anchoring fibrils in the lamina densa and cause skin fragility at the dermal–epidermal junction.[42]

Clinical Features

Patients present with blisters and erosions over areas of trauma (dorsal hands, elbows, knees, and feet) that heal with scarring, milia, and dyspigmentation (Fig. 12.14).

Diagnosis

A skin biopsy of a new blister for histopathologic examination and a biopsy of perilesional skin for DIF on salt-split skin are required. In salt-split skin preparations, the immune deposits are typically located on the dermal side of the cleavage, which helps distinguish EBA from bullous pemphigoid (BP). Immunoblotting can detect autoantibodies to the alpha chain of type VII collagen.

Maternal and Fetal Risks

In one of the three reported cases, neonatal EBA occurred shortly after birth and spontaneously remitted after 10 days.[42]

Management

EBA tends to be refractory to steroids and immunosuppressants. Dapsone treatment may be helpful in cases showing a predominance of neutrophils on a skin biopsy.[45]

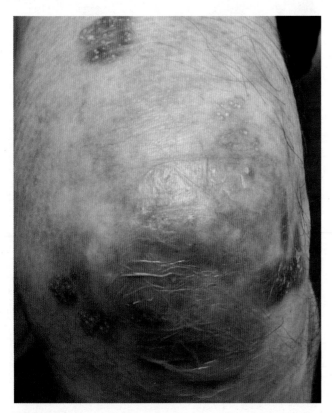

Figure 12.14. Erythematous shiny plaques with milia over extensor surfaces, which are consistent with epidermolysis bullosa acquisita.

Linear IgA Dermatosis

Epidemiology

Linear IgA dermatosis (LAD) is a rare autoimmune disease with a bimodal presentation. LAD is the most common autoimmune blistering disease in childhood, although the exact prevalence is unknown. In adults, the prevalence is estimated to be less than 1 case per 100,000 people. There are few reports of LAD during pregnancy. The largest case series to date collected 12 patients with LAD who experienced a total of 19 pregnancies among them over a 40-year time span.[46]

Etiology

LAD is caused by IgA autoantibodies against several antigenic targets in the lamina lucida and sublamina densa: a 97-kd protein that is a portion of the extracellular domain of the 180-kd BP antigen 2 (BPAg2); a 120-kd antigen portion of BPAg2, BPAg1, and BPA2, a 285-kd target antigen that has not been further characterized; and a 250-kd antigen corresponding to collagen VII. These autoantibodies recruit inflammatory cells, predominantly neutrophils, to the dermal–epidermal junction.

Clinical Features

Patients present with tense blisters, most commonly on the trunk and extremities. Approximately 50% of patients have mucosal involvement as well. The bullae are characteristically grouped in a herpetiform pattern referred to as a "cluster of jewels" (Fig. 12.15). Approximately 50% of children and adults will go into spontaneous remission. Remission rates are close to 100% in drug-induced LAD upon withdrawal of the inciting medication.

Diagnosis

A skin biopsy of a new blister for histopathologic examination and a biopsy of perilesional skin for DIF are required. On DIF, linear IgA staining (90%) along the basement

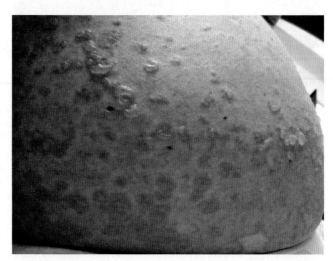

Figure 12.15. Linear IgA dermatosis in pregnancy, presenting with typical tense bullae in annular configurations. (Courtesy of Dr. Karolyn Wanat, University of Pennsylvania.)

membrane zone is noted, which helps differentiate LAD from BP and EBA.

Maternal and Fetal Risks

In the largest series, most patients experienced improvement of LAD throughout their pregnancies and flare in the peripartum period.[46] One of 19 children was born with one blister that quickly remitted spontaneously. One patient delivered early at 38 weeks. One mother had nine children, three of whom were born after the diagnosis of LAD. Her seventh child was born with *patent ductus arteriosus*, and her ninth child was born with a *patent foramen ovale*.[46]

Management

Patients may not require treatment during pregnancy. If treatment is required, topical steroids are the first-line therapy. Dapsone is the best option for disease that is unresponsive to topical steroids or that involves the mucous membranes, but physicians should be vigilant about the medication's possible maternal and neonatal adverse effects. LAD typically responds to dapsone doses ranging from 50 to 200 mg per day.[46]

MATERNAL RISKS

Porphyria cutanea tarda: Disease exacerbation

Acrodermatitis enteropathica: Rash, infections, death (untreated disease)

Erythema multiforme: HSV-related complications, bacterial superinfection of bullous lesions and erosions, vaginal stenosis secondary to bullous vaginal lesions (one case)

Pemphigus vulgaris: Disease exacerbation, maternal death, adverse effects from immunosuppressive medications, vaginal delivery can exacerbate vulvar erosions, cesarean section may heal poorly secondary to erosions and/or systemic steroids

Pemphigus foliaceus: None

Epidermolysis bullosa acquisita: Unknown

Linear IgA dermatosis: Mucosal scarring

FETAL RISKS

Porphyria cutanea tarda: *Sporadic*: Twofold increase in IUGR; *Hereditary*: Threefold increase in perinatal death

Acrodermatitis enteropathica: Spontaneous abortion, congenital defects (anencephaly and achondroplastic dwarfism)

Erythema multiforme: If related to HSV, vertical HSV transmission to infant

Pemphigus vulgaris: Stillbirth, infant death, IUGR, neonatal pemphigus vulgaris

Pemphigus foliaceus: Minimal risk for neonatal PF

Epidermolysis bullosa acquisita: Neonatal disease spontaneously remitted (one report)

Linear IgA dermatosis: Infantile disease (one case); two infants born to same mother with congenital anomalies (one report)

HSV, herpes simplex virus; IUGR, intrauterine growth restriction.

KEY POINTS

- **Porphyria cutanea tarda:** During pregnancy, approximately half of patients will experience exacerbation; treatment during pregnancy centers on sun protection, use of physical-block sunscreens (such as zinc oxide or titanium dioxide), and avoiding triggers

- **Acrodermatitis enteropathica:** Lesions on acral and periorificial sites in mothers and affected infants; can be fatal if untreated; treatment is elemental zinc supplementation

- **Erythema multiforme:** Association with HSV; the pregnant patient should be evaluated for HSV infection, and antiviral treatment should be administered to prevent vertical HSV transmission to fetus

- **Pemphigus vulgaris:** Untreated disease can be fatal; disease increases fetal risks, including stillbirth, perinatal death, IUGR, and neonatal pemphigus; systemic steroids is first-line treatment, azathioprine should be added if required systemic steroid dose >0.5 mg/kg per day; IVIG monotherapy has shown promise

- **Pemphigus foliaceus:** Does not confer a risk to the fetus or infant and can be usually controlled with topical steroids

- **Epidermolysis bullosa acquisita:** Presents with tense blisters and is generally refractory to treatment

- **Linear IgA disease:** May improve in pregnancy, and approximately half of the patients will not require systemic treatment during gestation; dapsone 50 to 200 mg per day is the systemic treatment of choice

REFERENCES

1. Frank J, Poblete-Gutierrez P. Porphyria cutanea tarda—when skin meets liver. *Best Pract Res Clin Gastroenterol.* 2010;24:735–745.
2. Perez-Maldonado A, Kurban AK. Metabolic diseases and pregnancy. *Clin Dermatol.* 2006;24:88–90.
3. Loret de Mola JR, Muise KL, Duchon MA. Porphyria cutanea tarda and pregnancy. *Obstet Gynecol Surv.* 1996;51:493–497.
4. Rajka G. Pregnancy and porphyria cutanea tarda. *Acta Derm Venereol.* 1984;64:444–445.
5. Goerz G, Hammer G. Porphyria cutanea tarda and pregnancy. *Dermatologica.* 1983;166:316–318.
6. Baxi LV, Rubeo TJ Jr, Katz B, et al. Porphyria cutanea tarda and pregnancy. *Am J Obstet Gynecol.* 1983;146:333–334.

7. Urbanek RW, Cohen DJ. Porphyria cutanea tarda: pregnancy versus estrogen effect. *J Am Acad Dermatol.* 1994;31:390–392.

8. Tollanes MC, Aarsand AK, Sandberg S. Excess risk of adverse pregnancy outcomes in women with porphyria: a population-based cohort study. *J Inherit Metab Dis.* 2011;34:217–223.

9. Nosten F, McGready R, d'Alessandro U, et al. Antimalarial drugs in pregnancy: a review. *Curr Drug Saf.* 2006;1:1–15.

10. Maverakis E, Fung MA, Lynch PJ, et al. Acrodermatitis entero-pathica and an overview of zinc metabolism. *J Am Acad Dermatol.* 2007;56:116–124.

11. Gebreselassie SG, Gashe FE. A systematic review of effect of prenatal zinc supplementation on birthweight: meta-analysis of 17 randomized controlled trials. *J Health Popul Nutr.* 2011;29:134–140.

12. Krapels IP, Rooij IA, Wevers RA, et al. Myo-inositol, glucose and zinc status as risk factors for non-syndromic cleft lip with or without cleft palate in offspring: a case-control study. *BJOG.* 2004;111:661–668.

13. Srinivas M, Gupta DK, Rathi SS, et al. Association between lower hair zinc levels and neural tube defects. *Indian J Pediatr.* 2001;68:519–522.

14. Neldner KH, Hambidge KM. Zinc therapy of acrodermatitis enteropathica. *N Engl J Med.* 1975;292:879–882.

15. Brenton DP, Jackson MJ, Young A. Two pregnancies in a patient with acrodermatitis enteropathica treated with zinc sulphate. *Lancet.* 1981;2:500–502.

16. Huff JC, Weston WL, Tonnesen MG. Erythema multiforme: a critical review of characteristics, diagnostic criteria, and causes. *J Am Acad Dermatol.* 1983;8:763–775.

17. Amichai B, Meltzer S. Herpes simplex virus associated erythema multiforme in a prepartum woman without involvement of the newborn. *J Eur Acad Dermatol Venereol.* 2002;16:546.

18. Brown ZA, Ashley R, Douglas J, et al. Neonatal herpes simplex virus infection: relapse after initial therapy and transmission from a mother with an asymptomatic genital herpes infection and erythema multiforme. *Pediatr Infect Dis J.* 1987;6:1057–1061.

19. Nelson M, Confino E, Friberg J, et al. Erythema multiforme in a pregnancy resulting from in vitro fertilization: a case report. *J Reprod Med.* 1988;33:230–231.

20. Brice SL, Krzemien D, Weston WL, et al. Detection of herpes simplex virus DNA in cutaneous lesions of erythema multi-forme. *J Invest Dermatol.* 1989;93:183–187.

21. Westhoff GL, Little SE, Caughey AB. Herpes simplex virus and pregnancy: a review of the management of antenatal and peri-partum herpes infections. *Obstet Gynecol Surv.* 2011;66:629–638.

22. Ahmed AR, Gurcan HM. Use of intravenous immunoglobulin therapy during pregnancy in patients with pemphigus vulgaris. *J Eur Acad Dermatol Venereol.* 2011;25:1073–1079.

23. Kardos M, Levine D, Gurcan HM, et al. Pemphigus vulgaris in pregnancy: analysis of current data on the management and outcomes. *Obstet Gynecol Surv.* 2009;64:739–749.

24. Daneshpazhooh M, Chams-Davatchi C, Valikhani M, et al. Pem-phigus and pregnancy: a 23-year experience. *Indian J Dermatol Venereol Leprol.* 2011;77:534.

25. Tope WD, Kamino H, Briggaman RA, et al. Neonatal pemphigus vulgaris in a child born to a woman in remission. *J Am Acad Dermatol.* 1993;29:480–485.

26. Bonifazi E, Milioto M, Trashlieva V, et al. Neonatal pemphigus vulgaris passively transmitted from a clinically asymptomatic mother. *J Am Acad Dermatol.* 2006;55:S113–S114.

27. Park-Wyllie L, Mazzotta P, Pastuszak A, et al. Birth defects after maternal exposure to corticosteroids: prospective cohort study and meta-analysis of epidemiological studies. *Teratology.* 2000;62:385–392.

28. Ostensen M, Khamashta M, Lockshin M, et al. Anti-inflammatory and immunosuppressive drugs and reproduction. *Arthritis Res Ther.* 2006;8:209.

29. Viktil K, Engeland A, Furu K. Outcomes after anti-rheumatic drug use before and during pregnancy: a cohort study among 150,000 pregnant women and expectant fathers. *Scand J Rheu-matol.* 2012;41:196–201.

30. Goldberg NS, DeFeo C, Kirshenbaum N. Pemphigus vulgaris and pregnancy: risk factors and recommendations. *J Am Acad Dermatol.* 1993;28:877–879.

31. Shieh S, Fang YV, Becker JL, et al. Pemphigus, pregnancy, and plasmapheresis. *Cutis.* 2004;73:327–329.

32. Shemin D, Briggs D, Greenan M. Complications of therapeutic plasma exchange: a prospective study of 1,727 procedures. *J Clin Apher.* 2007;22:270–276.

33. Guillaume JC, Roujeau JC, Morel P, et al. Controlled study of plasma exchange in pemphigus. *Arch Dermatol.* 1988;124:1659–1663.

34. Bastuji-Garin S, Souissi R, Blum L, et al. Comparative epidemi-ology of pemphigus in Tunisia and France: unusual incidence of pemphigus foliaceus in young Tunisian women. *J Invest Derma-tol.* 1995;104:302–305.

35. Warren SJ, Lin MS, Giudice GJ, et al. The prevalence of anti-bodies against desmoglein 1 in endemic pemphigus foliaceus in Brazil. Cooperative Group on Fogo Selvagem Research. *N Engl J Med.* 2000;343:23–30.

36. Rocha-Alvarez R, Friedman H, Campbell IT, et al. Pregnant women with endemic pemphigus foliaceus (Fogo Selvagem) give birth to disease-free babies. *J Invest Dermatol.* 1992;99:78–82.

37. Walker DC, Kolar KA, Hebert AA, et al. Neonatal pemphigus foliaceus. *Arch Dermatol.* 1995;131:1308–1311.

38. Hirsch R, Anderson J, Weinberg JM, et al. Neonatal pemphigus foliaceus. *J Am Acad Dermatol.* 2003;49:S187–S189.

39. Eyre RW, Stanley JR. Maternal pemphigus foliaceus with cell surface antibody bound in neonatal epidermis. *Arch Dermatol.* 1988;124:25–27.

40. Wu H, Wang ZH, Yan A, et al. Protection against pemphigus foliaceus by desmoglein 3 in neonates. *N Engl J Med.* 2000;343:31–35.

41. Gurcan HM, Ahmed AR. Efficacy of dapsone in the treatment of pemphigus and pemphigoid: analysis of current data. *Am J Clin Dermatol.* 2009;10:383–396.

42. Abrams ML, Smidt A, Benjamin L, et al. Congenital epidermoly-sis bullosa acquisita: vertical transfer of maternal autoantibody from mother to infant. *Arch Dermatol.* 2011;147:337–341.

43. Kero M, Niemi KM, Kanerva L. Pregnancy as a trigger of epi-dermolysis bullosa acquisita. *Acta Derm Venereol.* 1983;63:353–356.

44. Kubo A, Hashimoto K, Inoue C, et al. Epidermolysis bullosa ac-quisita exacerbated by systemic estrogen and progesterone treat-ment and pregnancy. *J Am Acad Dermatol.* 1997;36:792–794.

45. Gurcan HM, Ahmed AR. Current concepts in the treatment of epidermolysis bullosa acquisita. *Expert Opin Pharmacother.* 2011;12:1259–1268.

46. Collier PM, Kelly SE, Wojnarowska F. Linear IgA disease and pregnancy. *J Am Acad Dermatol.* 1994;30:407–411.

CHAPTER 13

Bacterial, Fungal, and Parasitic Skin Disease

George Kroumpouzos ■ Noah Craft ■ Dirk Elston

INTRODUCTION

Pregnancy can affect the acquisition and severity of certain bacterial, mycobacterial, fungal, and parasitic infections. Although infectious vaginitis is the most common infection in pregnancy,[1,2] emerging infections, such as those caused by methicillin-resistant *Staphylococcus aureus* (MRSA), are becoming clinically relevant. The effects of pregnancy on infectious processes are related to those of high estrogen levels on the maternal immune system, including a decrease of cellular-mediated immunity, impairment of the activity of natural killer cells, suppression of neutrophil function, and possibly impairment of local antibody responses.[3] Still, the interaction between high estrogen levels and the maternal immune system depends on several attributes of the infectious agent and host, which may lead to disparate outcomes.[3] This chapter focuses on infections with skin manifestations that can be affected by pregnancy and/or have been associated with maternal and/or fetal risks. Management is outlined in Table 13.1.

BACTERIAL INFECTIONS

Skin and Soft Tissue Infections

Skin and soft tissue infections (SSTIs) can be caused by Group A *Streptococcus*, *Staphylococcus aureus*, *Bacteroides* spp., *Clostridium* spp., and *Enterobacteriaceae*. Superficial SSTIs, such as folliculitis, abscesses, mastitis, and cellulitis, are associated with a low risk of complications if treated promptly.[4] Bacterial folliculitis seems to be relatively common in pregnancy (Fig. 13.1). SSTIs often start at superinfected wound sites following procedures, or postpartum secondary to traumatic vaginal birth. Complicated SSTIs associated with an involvement of deep soft tissue are uncommon in pregnancy. These include streptococcal cellulitis, clostridial myonecrosis, and necrotizing fasciitis; can be associated with a high risk of life- and limb-threatening complications; and typically require surgical intervention.[4] Disseminated infection by *Neisseria gonorrhoeae* can be promoted by pregnancy and manifests as an acute arthritis-dermatosis syndrome. Skin lesions are scattered necrotic vesiculopustules (Fig. 13.2); they are due to embolic septic vasculitis and contain gonococci. Asymmetric arthralgia, tenosynovitis, or septic arthritis can be observed; perihepatitis may occasionally develop, whereas endocarditis and meningitis are rare complications.

Infections from *S. aureus* occur with increasing frequency, especially in patients with a coexisting skin disease, such as atopic dermatitis (see Ch. 9, Fig. 9.8). Strains of MRSA, initially reported in the hospital setting, have been increasingly isolated from patients in the community setting. Rectovaginal MRSA colonization rates of 0.5% to 3.5% have been reported in pregnancy.[5] Community-acquired MRSA (CA-MRSA) is becoming increasingly relevant in pregnancy and puerperium, with infections of the breast, buttocks, vulvovaginal area (Fig. 13.3), and groin; MRSA is commonly isolated from vulvar abscesses and is increasing in frequency in breast infections, such as mastitis and abscesses.[6] Only a small percentage of colonized pregnant patients develop clinical manifestations. The risk of vertical transmission to the fetus/neonate is very low, and an increase in early-onset neonatal MRSA infection has not been shown.[6] Antibiotics that have activity against most CA-MRSA strains and that can be considered safe in pregnancy include rifampin, clindamycin (risk of inducible resistance), ciprofloxacin, trimethoprim-sulfamethoxazole (but avoid in the first trimester), and gentamicin; intravenous vancomycin should be reserved for severe soft tissue MRSA infections (safety of antibiotics discussed in Ch. 23).[5] Current data do not support the implementation of large scale screening and decolonization regimens in the obstetric population.[5] MRSA carriage or infection is not a contraindication to breastfeeding; however, a breast abscess may require a temporary cessation of breastfeeding. Draining lesions should be covered to limit infant exposure.

Lyme Disease

Lyme disease is caused in the United States by the spirochete *Borrelia burgdorferi* with ticks of the Ixodidae family (*Ixodes scapularis* and *Ixodes pacific*) serving as vectors of the disease. Early localized disease is characterized by the *erythema chronicum migrans*, a rash that occurs within 1 week of infection but that can develop as late as 16 weeks after the tick bite. The rash expands centrifugally as an erythematous, annular, round to oval, well-demarcated plaque and can reach a diameter of more

TABLE 13.1	**Summary of Management Options**
Type of Infection	**Management Options**
Bacterial	■ SSTIs: Oral or IV antibiotics such as cephalosporins, penicillins, and clindamycin[4]; incision and drainage of abscess; surgical intervention for necrotizing infections ■ Impetigo: Topical mupirocin, oral first-generation cephalosporins, or dicloxacillin ■ Bacterial folliculitis: Topical clindamycin, oral cephalexin, or dicloxacillin[4] ■ Disseminated gonococcal infection: Hospitalization; IV or IM ceftriaxone[43] ■ MRSA: Incision and drainage of abscess; oral antibiotics such as clindamycin or rifampin for mild disease; IV vancomycin for severe invasive disease[5] ■ Lyme disease: Oral amoxicillin or cefuroxime[8]
Mycobacterial	■ Leprosy: Regimen of rifampin, dapsone, and clofazimine[12]; systemic corticosteroids for leprosy reactions and "silent neuritis"[17] ■ Tuberculosis: Regimen of isoniazid, rifampin, ethambutol[19] ■ Atypical mycobacteria: Oral clarithromycin ± other agents (rifampin, ciprofloxacin)[21–24]; rifabutin and ethambutol for *M. marinum*[25]
Fungal	■ Candida: Topical clotrimazole, miconazole, or nystatin[26]; nystatin or amphotericin oral suspension for thrush[27]; amphotericin B for disseminated/systemic infection[26] ■ Dermatophytes: Topical clotrimazole,[26] miconazole, ketoconazole ■ Pityrosporum folliculitis: Topical ketoconazole,[29] ciclopirox[a] ■ Tinea versicolor: Topical ciclopirox,[30] clotrimazole,[a] terbinafine[a] ■ Sporotrichosis: Thermotherapy (localized lesions), amphotericin B[31] ■ Coccidioidomycosis: Amphotericin B[33] ■ Blastomycosis: Amphotericin B[37] ■ Cryptococcosis: Amphotericin B (pulmonary or disseminated disease)[38]
Parasitic	■ Scabies: Permethrin,[39] precipitated sulfur,[b] benzyl benzoate 25%[c] ■ Pediculosis: Permethrin,[42] pyrethrin with piperonyl butoxide,[43] malathion, benzyl alcohol, spinosad ■ Leishmaniasis: Physical modalities such as heat or cryotherapy[44]; amphotericin B for visceral leishmaniasis[46]

[a] Reported as safe in pregnancy (see Ch. 22) and effective in the nonpregnant patient.

[b] Reported as possibly safe in pregnancy (see Ch. 22) but less effective than permethrin.

[c] Approved in Europe but not in the United States (risk of neonatal "gasping syndrome"); the European Guideline for treatment of scabies states that permethrin, benzyl benzoate (applied twice), and sulfur (applied three times) appear to be safe in pregnancy based on limited evidence (level of evidence III; grade B recommendation).

IM, intramuscular; IV, intravenous; MRSA, methicillin-resistant *Staphylococcus aureus*; Rx, therapy; SSTIs, skin and soft tissue infections.

than 30 cm (Fig. 13.4). It may also be accompanied by constitutional symptoms and regional lymphadenopathy. Untreated lesions usually resolve within 3 to 4 weeks. The hematogenous and lymphatic spread of *B. burgdorferi* to distant sites occurs within days to a few weeks after the infection, leading to the early-disseminated stage, which shows skin manifestations, involvement of musculoskeletal and neurologic systems, and cardiac involvement in a small fraction (≤8%) of patients. Manifestations of the late-stage disease can occur months to years after the initial infection.

Transplacental transmission of *B. burgdorferi* is rare[7,8]; however, the existence of congenital borreliosis syndrome remains unproven. Markowitz et al. studied 19 cases of Lyme disease,[9] and reported adverse fetal outcome in five patients, including syndactyly, cortical blindness,

intrauterine fetal death, prematurity, and rash. The trimester of acquisition and the therapy administered were not related to the outcome. Other studies, however, did not confirm fetal risks.[10,11] Pregnant patients should avoid tick-infested areas and remove any ticks as soon as recognized. After a tick bite, the skin should be observed up to 30 days for signs of an infection. Recommendations for therapy during pregnancy are similar to those for nonpregnant patients, with the exception of avoiding tetracyclines. There is no evidence for treating asymptomatic women who are found to be seropositive for Lyme antibodies in gestation. Prophylactic antibiotics are not required for tick bites when there are no signs of infection, although some practitioners prescribe amoxicillin in cases with prolonged (>48 hours) tick attachment in endemic regions.[8] Early-stage disease can be treated

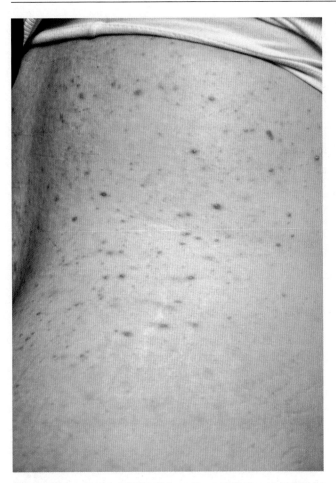

Figure 13.1. Bacterial folliculitis at 29 weeks' gestation: Florid presentation with extensive papulopustules on the trunk. Lesions had persisted for 10 weeks and responded to treatment with clindamycin 1% gel.

in pregnancy with a 3-week course of oral amoxicillin 500 mg three times daily[8]; cefuroxime axetil is an alternative for amoxicillin-allergic patients. Intravenous therapy should be considered for a late-stage disease. There is no evidence that Lyme disease can be transmitted through breastfeeding.

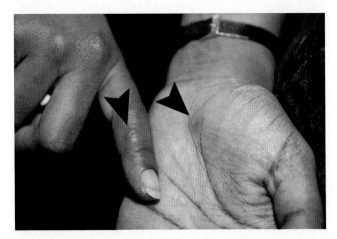

Figure 13.2. Gonococcemia is characterized by scattered necrotic or hemorrhagic vesiculopustules on the distal extremities; here, pustules are shown on the palm and index finger *(arrows)*.

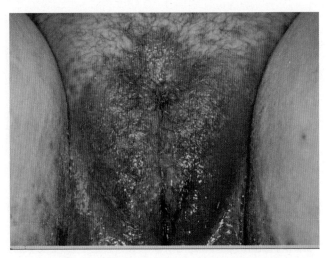

Figure 13.3. An infection of the vulvovaginal area and groin with methicillin-resistant *Staphylococcus aureus*, with intense erythema and pustules, associated with oozing and tenderness. (Courtesy of Dr. Joe Brooks.)

MYCOBACTERIAL INFECTIONS

Leprosy

The pregnancy status is associated with a relative decrease in cellular immunity, which allows *Mycobacterium leprae* to proliferate.[12] The decrease in protective cell-mediated immunity may account for a high rate of relapse of the disease and reactional states during pregnancy.[13] Early studies showed an exacerbation of leprosy during pregnancy or within the first 6 months of lactation (Fig. 13.5)[14]; however, ethnic differences may exist because leprosy exacerbation was not confirmed in a Latin American population.[15] Leprosy reactions may be triggered by pregnancy: type 1

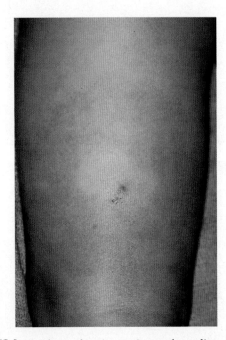

Figure 13.4. *Erythema chronicum migrans*, the earliest skin manifestation of Lyme disease, is an erythematous, annular, round to oval, well-demarcated plaque that shows centrifugal expansion.

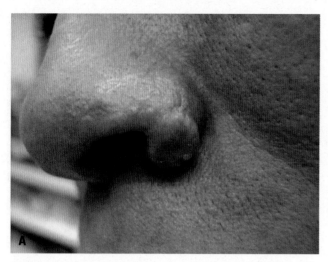
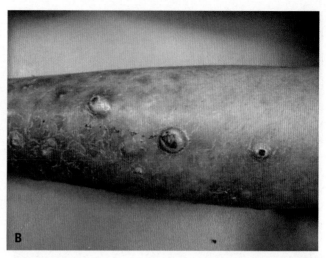

Figure 13.5. Lepromatous leprosy in pregnancy: Exophytic nodules are shown (**A**) on the nose and (**B**) the leg. (Courtesy of Dr. Jennifer Jenkins.)

(reversal) reactions maximally occur postpartum,[13] when the cell-mediated immunity returns to prepregnancy levels, and type 2 reactions (*erythema nodosum leprosum*) may occur throughout pregnancy (Fig. 13.6) and lactation.[16] The increased incidence of disease exacerbation and leprosy reactions has been associated with early loss of motor and/or sensory nerve function secondary to overt, and also "silent" neuritis.[17] Cases of "silent neuritis" predominantly occurred 6 to 9 months after delivery, especially in patients with borderline leprosy.[17] Careful sensory hand screens at 1- to 3-month intervals after delivery have been recommended.[12]

Multidrug therapy of rifampin, dapsone, and clofazimine, similar to that administered in the nonpregnant patient, is the treatment of choice during pregnancy[12]; the safety of these medications is summarized in Chapter 22, Table 22.6. Leprosy reactions should be treated with oral corticosteroids[17] but not thalidomide, which is contraindicated in pregnancy. Vigilance for "silent neuritis" in the postpartum period must be maintained, and treatment with systemic steroids should be instituted promptly.[12] Patients with leprosy should be counseled about the effects of pregnancy on the disease before they become pregnant, and pregnancies should be planned

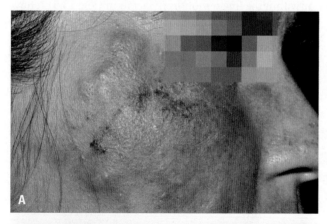
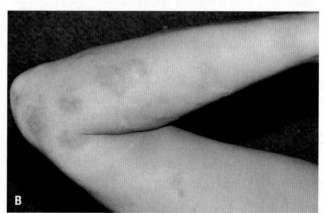
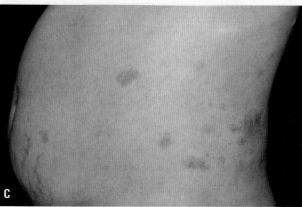

Figure 13.6. A leprosy type 2 reaction (*erythema nodosum leprosum*) in a patient with lepromatous leprosy in the third trimester. Inflammatory plaques and nodules are shown (**A**) on the face, (**B**) the upper extremity, and (**C**) the trunk. (Courtesy of Dr. Joel Lastoria.)

when the disease is well controlled. Leprosy has been associated with increased fetal mortality, prematurity, and low birth weight,[14] risks proportionate to the bacterial load (higher in lepromatous type). Approximately 20% of children born to mothers with leprosy will develop the disease by puberty. Transplacental transmission is rare, and the risk is higher with untreated, multibacillary (lepromatous) disease.[18]

Tuberculosis

Tuberculosis (TB) is caused by *Mycobacterium tuberculosis* and, less often, *Mycobacterium bovis* and *Mycobacterium africanum*. Extrapulmonary involvement is seen mainly in advanced HIV infection (>60% of the cases). The presentation of TB in pregnant women is similar to that in nonpregnant women.[19] Cutaneous TB is rare and has been only exceptionally reported in pregnancy.[20] Pregnancy does not affect the course of TB, and congenital TB has been uncommon. The disease is unlikely to have fetal effects if the mother has been on effective treatment in pregnancy. However, there has been an increase in obstetric morbidity and fetal risks in cases with late diagnosis, incomplete treatment, and in those with advanced pulmonary lesions.[19] Mild fetal risks have been reported in extrapulmonary TB that was not confined to the lymph nodes.[19] The active disease should be treated aggressively in pregnancy with a regimen of isoniazid, rifampin, pyrazinamide, and ethambutol[19]; streptomycin should be avoided. Most antituberculous drugs are compatible with breastfeeding.

Atypical Mycobacterial Infections

There have been only sparse reports of atypical mycobacterial infections in pregnancy that were not associated with adverse fetal effects. The physiologic suppression of cellular immune response in pregnancy may predispose pregnant patients to an infection with rapidly growing mycobacteria, such as *Mycobacterium chelonae* and *Mycobacterium fortuitum*.[21] *M. chelonae* sepsis from long-term use of an intravenous catheter,[22] and two cases of infection with *M. fortuitum*[23] have been reported in pregnancy (Fig. 13.7). Oral clarithromycin was effective in the case of *M. chelonae* and a combination with ciprofloxacin in a case of *M. fortuitum*.[21] A Buruli ulcer secondary to an infection by *Mycobacterium ulcerans* was treated in pregnancy with oral clarithromycin and rifampin.[24] A case of fish tank granuloma from *Mycobacterium marinum*[25] did not respond to clarithromycin. The patient was then successfully treated with rifabutin and ethambutol; however, these antibiotics have been associated with significant maternal and fetal risks.

FUNGAL INFECTIONS

Candidiasis

Vulvovaginal candidiasis is discussed in Chapter 14 (see Fig. 14.18). Nonvaginal localized candidiasis, such as that affecting intertriginous areas (candida intertrigo), can be

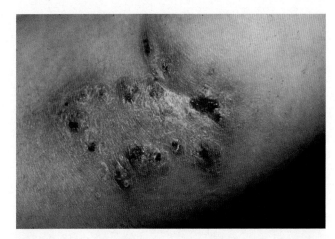

Figure 13.7. An infection from *Mycobacterium fortuitum*: Tender erythematous nodules at the site of inoculation; crusted draining sinuses and abscesses are also shown.

treated in pregnancy with topical antifungal agents such as clotrimazole, miconazole, and nystatin.[26] Disseminated or systemic candidiasis is uncommon in the immunocompetent pregnant patient and can be safely treated with intravenous amphotericin B.[26] Oral candidiasis (thrush) in the immunocompetent patient can be treated with nystatin or amphotericin oral suspension.[27] In the immunocompromised patient, oral suspension of nystatin for 7 to 14 days can be tried first; nevertheless, systemic antifungal treatment with intravenous amphotericin B may be required because of the high relapse rate observed with topical treatment.

Dermatophytoses

The onset of dermatophytic infections such as tinea corporis and tinea pedis (Fig. 13.8) in pregnancy has been reported, but these infections were not as prevalent as candida vaginitis and tinea versicolor in a recent study.[1] Majocchi granuloma can develop in women who shave their legs and who have tinea pedis or onychomycosis (Fig. 13.9). Topical azoles such as clotrimazole and miconazole can be safely used for dermatophytoses in pregnancy.[26] Treatment of onychomycosis during pregnancy is not recommended. Majocchi granuloma, tinea capitis, and bullous tinea often fail to respond to topical treatment. However, treatment with oral antifungals (most are pregnancy category C; see Ch. 22, Table 22.7) is associated with risks, and when oral antifungals are required, one should make an effort to administer them as late in pregnancy as possible.

When critical for the health of the mother, the choice of drugs should be discussed with the obstetrician.

Tinea Versicolor and *Pityrosporum* Folliculitis

Pityrosporum folliculitis and pityriasis (tinea) versicolor, both caused by yeasts of the genus *Malassezia*, can develop in pregnancy.[1] There have been sparse reports of *Pityrosporum* folliculitis in pregnancy[1,28,29]; however, the condition may

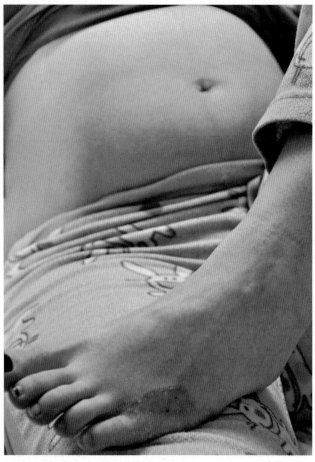

Figure 13.8. Tinea pedis at 32 weeks' gestation: Pruritic erythematous plaque with a scaly, expanding rim and central clearing on the dorsolateral aspect of the foot. The infection had persisted for 2 months and was treated satisfactorily with clotrimazole cream.

be underdiagnosed because of similarities with bacterial folliculitis, pruritic folliculitis of pregnancy, and acne. The infection typically presents with monomorphous follicular papulopustules on the upper trunk (see Ch. 21, Fig. 21.10). Tinea versicolor is relatively common in pregnancy[1]; in a

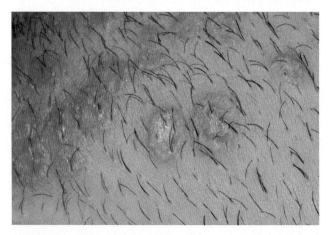

Figure 13.9. Majocchi granuloma, usually due to *Trichophyton rubrum*, represents an infection of the hair follicle with seconday rupture and is characterized by perifollicular pustules and granulomas. Here, shown in the suprapubic area.

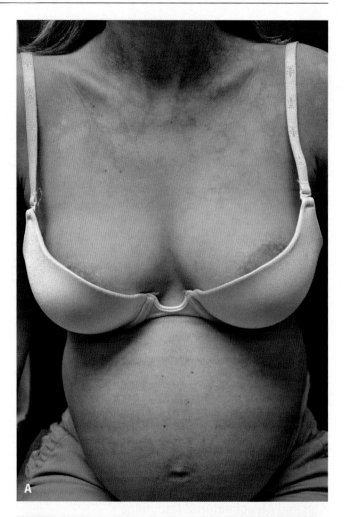

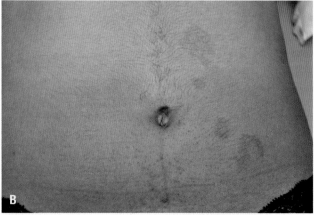

Figure 13.10. Tinea versicolor. **(A)** Hypopigmented patches with annular borders forming geographic configurations on the upper chest, shoulders, and neck. **(B)** Lesions can be hyperpigmented in patients of color; here, shown at 6 weeks' gestation.

recent study, the frequency of tinea versicolor in pregnancy (Fig. 13.10) was not different from that reported in a general population living in temperate climates, but a higher degree of colonization by *Malassezia* was noted at the end of pregnancy and postpartum.[30] The effect of warm temperature on increased colonization was noted only in the first trimester. In the same study, affected pregnant patients required a long topical treatment to achieve mycologic and clinical cure, but they were disease free 6 months after delivery. Treatment of tinea versicolor in pregnancy is not required, but if lesions are symptomatic, topical ciclopirox is a safe option[30]; topical clotrimazole and terbinafine are alternative options (both are pregnancy category B).

Subcutaneous Mycoses

Sporotrichosis is a subcutaneous mycosis caused by *Sporothrix schenckii* (Fig. 13.11). The course of sporotrichosis in pregnancy was reported in two studies relevant to zoonotic epidemics in Brazil.[31,32] Cats were the main link in the epidemiologic chain. There was a predominance of the lymphocutaneous form (>80%), with fixed sporotrichosis being less common. No fetal risks were reported. Of 17 patients, 10 were treated effectively with local heat (thermotherapy), 2 patients received amphotericin B, 1 received terbinafine, and 2 received itraconazole after delivery. If the lesions are small and localized, conservative treatment with thermotherapy is appropriate until the time of delivery, when the clinical course and serology can be reevaluated.[31] For more extensive lesions, amphotericin B seems to be the safest option.

Systemic Mycoses

Downregulation of the T-cell responses in pregnancy facilitates the development of dimorphic mycoses, such as coccidioidomycosis and blastomycosis. **Coccidioidomycosis** is caused by the mold *Coccidioides immitis* (Fig. 13.12). Primary infection of the respiratory tract secondary to inhalation occurs in the vast majority of the cases. Dissemination to skin and other organs depends on several host factors, including immunosuppression and pregnancy. Although coccidioidomycosis is a rare occurrence in pregnancy, it is often disseminated and severe[33]; pregnancy is a risk factor for disseminated coccidioidomycosis.[34,35] Disseminated disease (meninges > skin > bone) is associated with the trimester of pregnancy, with the highest risk seen in the third

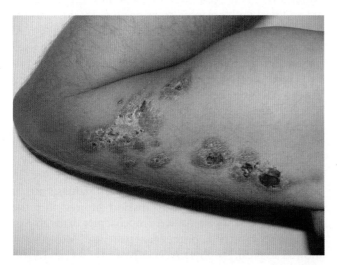

Figure 13.11. Sporotrichosis: A typical presentation of crusted, ulcerated plaques and nodules along the path of lymphatic drainage ("sporotrichoid" pattern). (Courtesy of Dr. Mayra Ianhez.)

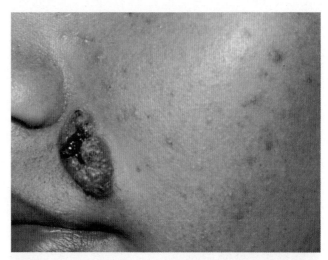

Figure 13.12. Coccidioidomycosis: An inflamed, verrucous, partially ulcerated plaque. The face is the most common site of involvement. The disseminated infection shows solitary or multiple papules, nodules, verrucous plaques, abscesses, and sinus tracts. Primary cutaneous disease is rare and develops from direct inoculation into the skin through trauma. (Appears with permission of VisualDx. © Logical Images, Inc, www.visualdx.com.)

trimester and postpartum, and in those of African American descent.[33] Presence of erythema nodosum, one of the cutaneous manifestations of the disease, has been associated with a positive outcome.[36] Vertical transmission to the fetus has been disputed despite some evidence of intrauterine acquisition. Transmission to the neonate is thought to be secondary to aspiration of vaginal secretions. Untreated disseminated disease during pregnancy has been almost invariably fatal. Overall, 64% of mothers and 69% of infants survived,[33] but most of the deaths occurred in the era before the availability of antifungal drugs. Improved maternal and fetal outcomes have been associated with early disease recognition and prompt treatment with amphotericin B.

Blastomycosis is caused by the mold *Blastomyces dermatitidis*. Primary infection initially involves the lungs, and secondary cutaneous dissemination is common (Fig. 13.13). Blastomycosis can cause severe systemic illness in pregnancy, including, in most cases, involvement of the lungs as well as the skin (25%), bone, and the genitourinary and central nervous systems.[37] Amphotericin B is the drug of choice. In a retrospective analysis of 19 cases, there were no maternal deaths and amphotericin B was successfully administered in 13 patients (11 prepartum and 2 postpartum). Some cases showed spontaneous resolution postpartum without treatment. Two newborns, born to mothers who did not receive treatment, died of congenital blastomycosis; however, the placental status was unknown.

Cryptococcosis is caused by *Cryptococcus neoformans* and occurs predominantly in the immunocompromised patient (opportunistic mycosis). Primary cutaneous disease secondary to inoculation of the fungus through trauma is rare. Maternal morbidity includes meningitis and pulmonary involvement. Patients with progressive pulmonary disease or dissemination require systemic antifungal therapy; amphotericin B is the treatment of choice.[38] The fetal outcome

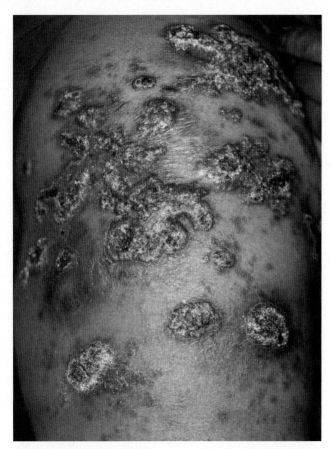

Figure 13.13. Blastomycosis: Well-demarcated, verrucous papules and plaques with scale crust; many lesions show central ulceration. Pustules are common in the borders of the lesions. Lesions tend to occur on exposed skin and heal with cribriform scarring. (Appears with permission of VisualDx. © Logical Images, Inc, www.visualdx.com.)

depends on effective treatment of the maternal infection.[38] Although infection of the placenta has been documented, the risk of congenital cryptococcosis is low. Neonates may acquire an invasive pulmonary infection through aspiration.

PARASITIC INFECTIONS

Scabies is caused by the mite *Sarcoptes scabiei* var. *hominis*, an obligate human parasite (Fig. 13.14). The prevalence of scabies in pregnancy has not been systematically studied.[39] In a study of 505 pregnant patients with pruritic dermatoses, six cases of scabies were identified, which represents approximately 22% of all infections in the study.[40] Permethrin 5% cream (pregnancy category B) can be tried first; alternative treatment options are shown in Table 13.1, and safety of antiparasitic agents is summarized in Chapter 22, Table 22.10. There have been sparse reports of **pediculosis** in pregnancy. An association between pediculosis pubis and pregnancy[41] has not been confirmed. Shaving the hair represents a safe alternative but may not be acceptable to many women. Combing and mineral oil or styling-gel can be tried first for head lice. Permethrin can be the

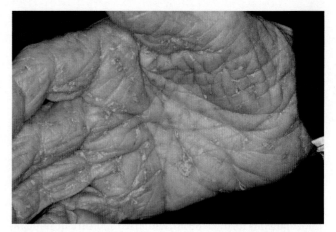

Figure 13.14. Scabies: Intensely pruritic crusted and/or excoriated papules on the palm. Areas that are typically affected and may show pathognomonic scabietic burrows include the interdigital webs of the hands, flexural aspect of the wrists, axillae, postauricular areas, the waist/belt area, the umbilicus, the genitalia, the nipples/areolae, ankles, and the feet.

initial pharmacologic treatment[42]; however, topical pyrethrin with piperonyl butoxide (pregnancy category C),[43] and malathion (pregnancy category B) can also be used. Malathion should not be used during lactation because of the potential for neonatal respiratory depression. Newer agents, including benzyl alcohol and spinosad (both are pregnancy category B), have less accumulated data.

Leishmaniasis

Leishmaniasis is caused by intracellular protozoan parasites of the genus *Leishmania*, which are transmitted by the bite of the sand fly, with canines and rodents serving as reservoirs. Old World cutaneous leishmaniasis is caused by *Leishmania tropica complex*, whereas New World leishmaniasis is caused by *Leishmania mexicana complex* or the *Leishmania Viannia* subgenus. Lesions at bite sites start as papules that can become nodular and eventually ulcerate and heal with atrophic scarring (Fig. 13.15). Chronic lesions occur in a small fraction of patients. Widespread lesions can occur, especially in the immunocompromised patient. Mucocutaneous leishmaniasis is caused by *Leishmania braziliensis* complex and, in addition to skin lesions, mucosal lesions can develop, especially in the naso-oropharyngeal area. Visceral leishmaniasis (kala azar) is caused by *Leishmania donovani*, *Leishmania infantum*, or *Leishmania chagasi*, and manifests with constitutional symptoms, lymphadenopathy, and hepatosplenomegaly.

A retrospective, case-control study that involved 26 pregnant patients with cutaneous leishmaniasis in an area with *L. braziliensis* transmission showed that the lesions in pregnant patients were much larger than those in age- and sex-matched nonpregnant patients.[44] Most lesions showed atypical, exophytic/vegetative features (Fig. 13.16), which contrasts with the typical presentation of a well-demarcated ulcer with raised borders. This presentation is

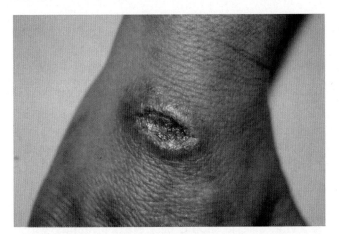

Figure 13.15. Cutaneous leishmaniasis: Lesions at bite sites become ulcerated and show raised borders with a crusted center. Here, shown on the hand of a pregnant Brazilian patient that became infected during an outbreak of American (New World) leishmaniasis in a rural area of the State of Sao Paulo, Brazil. (Courtesy of Dr. Paulo R. Cunha.)

also supported by larger skin lesions during pregnancy in a C57BL/6 mouse,[45] which was attributed to downregulation of Th1 cytokines in pregnancy. There was a high rate of preterm births and stillbirths in untreated patients in the study,[44] which needs to be confirmed. Because spontaneous postpartum resolution of skin lesions has been reported, the value of several treatments for *L. braziliensis* in pregnancy cannot be assessed, especially because standard treatments (pentavalent antimonials) are potentially abortogenic. Physical modalities, such as local hyperthermia and cryotherapy, are safe in gestation; successful treatment with cryotherapy in pregnancy is shown in Figure 13.17. Visceral leishmaniasis has been associated with a risk of vertical transmission to the fetus, especially with treatment failure. Amphotericin B is the safest treatment for visceral

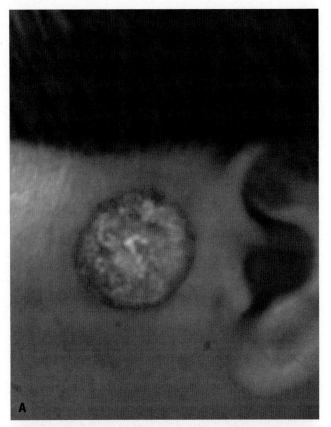

A

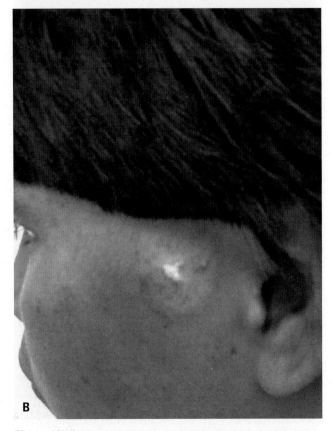

B

Figure 13.17. Cutaneous leishmaniasis. **(A)** The lesion shown in the third trimester, prior to cryotherapy. **(B)** The lesion shown after cryotherapy that was performed in pregnancy. Excellent response with mild postinflammatory hypopigmentation. (Courtesy of Dr. Raimunda Sampaio.)

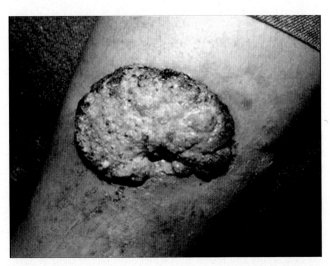

Figure 13.16. Lesions of leishmaniasis in pregnancy can be larger than those seen in the nonpregnant patient and show exophytic/vegetative features. (Courtesy of Dr. Raimunda Sampaio.)

leishmaniasis in pregnancy[46] and may be also useful in an extensive mucocutaneous disease.

Skin manifestations of **toxoplasmosis** are not affected by pregnancy, but this infection has been associated with serious fetal risks. Congenital toxoplasmosis has been associated with chorioretinitis, hearing loss, developmental delays, and other fetal malformations. Guidelines on the prevention and treatment of toxoplasmosis in pregnancy have been published.[47]

MATERNAL RISKS

Bacterial infections: Sepsis; life- and limb-threatening complications with complicated SSTIs (rare); arthritis and other serious risks from disseminated gonococcal infection; risks from Lyme disease similar to nonpregnant patients

Mycobacterial infections: Exacerbation of leprosy and leprosy reactions, "silent neuritis"; risks from tuberculosis and atypical mycobacteria similar to nonpregnant patients; risks from pharmacologic Rx

Fungal infections: ↑ mortality with disseminated coccidioidomycosis; risks from blastomycosis and cryptococcosis similar to nonpregnant patients

Parasitic infections: Leishmaniasis associated with more exophytic/vegetative, larger lesions; risks from pharmacologic Rx

FETAL RISKS

Bacterial infections: Vertical transmission of MRSA to fetus (rare); transplacental transmission of Lyme disease (rare); fetal adverse effects in Lyme disease debated

Mycobacterial infections: Leprosy associated with ↑ fetal mortality, prematurity, ↓ birth weight, development of disease by puberty, transplacental transmission (rare)

Fungal infections: Vertical transmission to fetus with candida vaginitis (rare); transmission to neonate at delivery (coccidioidomycosis, cryptococcosis)

Parasitic infections: Vertical transmission to the fetus in visceral leishmaniasis; ↑ rate of preterm delivery and stillbirths in untreated cutaneous leishmaniasis (one study)

MRSA, methicillin-resistant *Staphylococcus aureus*; Rx, treatment; SSTIs, skin and soft tissue infections; ↑, increased; ↓, decreased.

KEY POINTS

- Bacterial infections, such as folliculitis and infections from methicillin-resistant *Staphylococcus aureus* are relatively common during gestation but are not associated with any substantial maternal or fetal risks if treated promptly.

- Nonvulvovaginal candidiasis, dermatophyte infections, *pityrosporum* folliculitis, and tinea versicolor are encountered less often than candida vaginitis in gestation; they can be safely treated with topical antifungal agents.

- Leprosy can exacerbate during pregnancy or within the first 6 months of lactation, and leprosy reactions are triggered by pregnancy, with a type 2 reaction being associated with an increased maternal risk of "silent neuritis" postpartum; multidrug regimens are similar to those of nonpregnant patients, and systemic steroids should be used for leprosy reactions.

- Lyme disease should be treated promptly with amoxicillin or cefuroxime; amphotericin B is the safest systemic antifungal agent for systemic mycoses; permethrin is treatment of choice for scabies and pediculosis in pregnancy.

- Lesions of cutaneous leishmaniasis in pregnancy are larger and often exhibit atypical, exophytic/vegetative features; a conservative therapeutic approach is recommended as spontaneous postpartum resolution can occur, and physical modalities such as local hypothermia or cryotherapy can be tried first.

- Fetal risks have been documented mainly in leprosy, untreated visceral leishmaniasis, and toxoplasmosis; a late diagnosis and/or incomplete or irregular treatment increases the fetal risks in tuberculosis; ineffective treatment increases the fetal risks in cryptococcosis.

REFERENCES

1. Kumari R, Jaisankar TJ, Thappa DM. A clinical study of skin changes in pregnancy. *Indian J Dermatol Venereol Leprol.* 2007; 73:141.
2. Sever JL, Ellenberg JH, Ley A, et al. Incidence of clinical infections in a defined population of pregnant women. *Prog Clin Biol Res.* 1985;163B:317–326.
3. Styrt B, Sugarman B. Estrogens and infection. *Rev Infect Dis.* 1991;13:1139–1150.
4. Gravett CA, Gravett MG, Martin ET, et al. Serious and life-threatening pregnancy-related infections: opportunities to reduce the global burden. *PLoS Med.* 2012;9:e1001324. doi:10.1371/journal.pmed.1001324
5. Beigi RH. Clinical implications of methicillin-resistant *Staphylococcus aureus* in pregnancy. *Curr Opin Obstet Gynecol.* 2011;23: 82–86.
6. Torres M, Moayedi S. Gynecologic and other infections in pregnancy. *Emerg Med Clin North Am.* 2012;30:869–884.
7. Weber K, Bratzke HJ, Neubert U, et al. *Borrelia burgdorferi* in a newborn despite oral penicillin for Lyme borreliosis during pregnancy. *Pediatr Infect Dis J.* 1988;7:286–289.
8. Walsh CA, Mayer EW, Baxi LV. Lyme disease in pregnancy: case report and review of the literature. *Obstet Gynecol Surv.* 2007;62:41–50.
9. Markowitz LE, Steere AC, Benach JL, et al. Lyme disease during pregnancy. *JAMA.* 1987;255:3394–3396.

10. Weber K, Pfister HW. Clinical management of Lyme borreliosis. *Lancet.* 1994;343:1017–1020.

11. Williams CL, Strobino BA. Lyme disease transmission during pregnancy. *Contemp Ob/Gyn.* 1990;35:48–64.

12. Lyde CB. Pregnancy in patients with Hansen disease. *Arch Dermatol.* 1997;133:623–627.

13. Duncan ME, Pearson JMH, Ridley DS, et al. Pregnancy and leprosy: the consequences of alterations of cell-mediated and humoral immunity during pregnancy and lactation. *Int J Lepr.* 1982;50:425–435.

14. Duncan ME. An historical and clinical review of the interaction of leprosy and pregnancy: a cycle to be broken. *Soc Sci Med.* 1993;37:457–572.

15. Ulrich M, Zulueta AM, Caceres-Dittmat G, et al. Leprosy in women: characteristics and repercussions. *Soc Sci Med.* 1993;37:445–456.

16. Duncan ME, Pearson JMH. The association of pregnancy and leprosy. III. Erythema nodosum leprosum in pregnancy and lactation. *Lepr Rev.* 1984;55:129–142.

17. Duncan ME, Pearson JMH. Neuritis in pregnancy and lactation. *Int J Lepr Mycobact Dis.* 1982;50:31–38.

18. Duncan ME, Melsom R, Pearson JM, et al. A clinical and immunological study of four babies of mothers with lepromatous leprosy, two of whom developed leprosy in infancy. *Int J Lepr Other Mycobact Dis.* 1983;51:7–17.

19. Ormerod P. Tuberculosis in pregnancy and the puerperium. *Thorax.* 2001;56:494–499.

20. Figueroa Damian R, Arredondo Garcia JL. [Tuberculosis in the pregnant woman]. *Ginecol Obstet Mex.* 1992;60:209–216.

21. Safdar A. Clinical microbiological case: infection imitating lymphocutaneous sporotrichosis during pregnancy in a healthy woman from the South-eastern USA. *Clin Microbiol Infect.* 2003;9:244–246.

22. Katz VL, Farmer R, York J, et al. Mycobacterium chelonae sepsis associated with long-term use of an intravenous catheter for treatment of hyperemesis gravidarum. A case report. *J Reprod Med.* 2000;45:581–584.

23. Katayama I, Nishioka K, Nishiyama S. Mycobacterium fortuitum infection presenting as widespread cutaneous abscess in a pregnant woman. *Int J Dermatol.* 1990;29:383–384.

24. Dossou AD, Sopoh GE, Johnson CR, et al. Management of *Mycobacterium ulcerans* infection in a pregnant woman in Benin using rifampicin and clarithromycin. *Med J Aust.* 2008;189:532–533.

25. Tan EK, Gibson JL, Gallagher AP. A pregnant woman with fish tank granuloma. *J Obstet Gynaecol.* 2008;28:802–803.

26. Sobel JD. Use of antifungal drugs in pregnancy: a focus on safety. *Drug Saf.* 2000;23:77–85.

27. Huang DB, Ostrosky-Zeichner L, Wu JJ, et al. Therapy of common superficial fungal infections. *Dermatol Ther.* 2004;17:517–522.

28. Heymann WR, Wolf DJ. *Malassezia (pityrosporum)* folliculitis occurring during pregnancy. *Int J Dermatol.* 1986;25:49–51.

29. Parlak AH, Boran C, Topçuoglu MA. Pityrosporum folliculitis during pregnancy: a possible cause of pruritic folliculitis of pregnancy. *J Am Acad Dermatol.* 2005;52:528–529.

30. Zampino MR, Osti F, Corazza M, et al. Prevalence of pityriasis versicolor in a group of Italian pregnant women. *J Eur Acad Dermatol Venereol.* 2007;21:1249–1252.

31. Costa RO, Bernardes-Engemann AR, Azulay-Abulafia L, et al. Sporotrichosis in pregnancy: case reports of 5 patients in a zoonotic epidemic in Rio de Janeiro, Brazil. *An Bras Dermatol.* 2011; 86:995–998.

32. Ferreira CP, do Valle AC, Freitas DF, et al. Pregnancy during a sporotrichosis epidemic in Rio de Janeiro, Brazil. *Int J Gynaecol Obstet.* 2012;117:294–295.

33. Crum NF, Ballon-Landa G. Coccidioidomycosis in pregnancy: case report and review of the literature. *Am J Med.* 2006;119:993. e11–e17.

34. Calderón Garcidueñas AL, Piña Osuna K, Cerda Flores RM. [A clinical and pathological study of coccidioidomycosis and pregnancy in four Mexican women]. *Ginecol Obstet Mex.* 2004;72: 450–454.

35. Barbee RA, Hicks MJ, Grosse D, et al. The maternal immune response in coccidioidomycosis. Is pregnancy a risk factor for serious infection? *Chest.* 1991;100:709–715.

36. Arsura EL, Kilgore WB, Ratnayake SN. Erythema nodosum in pregnant patients with coccidioidomycosis. *Clin Infect Dis.* 1998;27:1201–1203.

37. Lemos LB, Soofi M, Amir E. Blastomycosis and pregnancy. *Ann Diagn Pathol.* 2002;6:211–215.

38. Ely EW, Peacock JE Jr, Haponik EF, et al. Cryptococcal pneumonia complicating pregnancy. *Medicine (Baltimore).* 1998;77: 153–167.

39. Judge MR, Kobza-Black A. Crusted scabies in pregnancy. *Br J Dermatol.* 1995;132:116–119.

40. Ambros-Rudolph CM, Müllegger RR, Vaughan-Jones SA, et al. The specific dermatoses of pregnancy revisited and reclassified: results of a retrospective two-center study on 505 pregnant patients. *J Am Acad Dermatol.* 2006;54:395–404.

41. Hart G. Factors associated with pediculosis pubis and scabies. *Genitourin Med.* 1992;68:294–295.

42. Hollier LM, Workowski K. Treatment of sexually transmitted diseases in women. *Obstet Gynecol Clin North Am.* 2003;30: 751–775, vii–viii.

43. Centers for Disease Control and Prevention. Sexually Transmitted Diseases Guidelines. *Morb Mort Wkly Rep.* 2010:59.

44. Morgan DJ, Guimaraes LH, Machado PR, et al. Cutaneous leishmaniasis during pregnancy: exuberant lesions and potential fetal complications. *Clin Infect Dis.* 2007;45:478–482.

45. Krishnan L, Guilbert LJ, Russell AS, et al. Pregnancy impairs resistance of C57BL/6 mice to Leishmania major infection and causes decreased antigen-specific IFN-gamma response and increased production of T helper 2 cytokines. *J Immunol.* 1996; 156:644–652.

46. Kumar A, Mittal M, Prasad S. Treatment of leishmaniasis in pregnancy. *Int J Gynaecol Obstet.* 2001;72:189–190.

47. Franco A, Ernest JM. Parasitic infections. In: James DK, Steer PJ, Weiner CP, et al., eds. *High-Risk Pregnancy: Management Options.* 4th ed. Philadelphia, PA: Elsevier Saunders; 2011:543–562.

Viral and Sexually Transmitted Disease

Farhan Khan ■ Rana M. Mays ■ Joe Brooks ■ Stephen K. Tyring

INTRODUCTION

Viral and sexually transmitted diseases pose significant maternal and fetal risks. Prevention and prompt treatment of such infections are of utmost importance in order to eliminate congenital and neonatal disease and risks, such as spontaneous abortion. Any febrile infectious disease may precipitate uterine activity and lead to premature delivery. This chapter focuses on infections with mucocutaneous manifestations that pose maternal and/or fetal risks and reviews the clinical manifestations, risks, and management during pregnancy. Maternal and fetal risks from viral diseases are listed in the respective box.

VIRAL DISEASES

Herpes Simplex Virus

Herpes simplex virus (HSV) affects 22% of pregnant females in the United States.[1] HSV belongs to the Alphaherpesviriniae subfamily of Herpesviridae, which includes HSV-type 1 (HSV-1), HSV-type 2 (HSV-2), and varicella-zoster virus (VZV). Genital herpes is typically caused by HSV-2, whereas orolabial herpes is most commonly attributed to HSV-1; however, an increasing proportion of genital herpes cases are due to HSV-1 (Fig. 14.1).[2] HSV infections are classified into primary, nonprimary first episode, and recurrent.

Clinical Features

HSV typically presents as painful, grouped vesicles on an erythematous base and, occasionally, lymphadenopathy (see Figs. 14.1 and 14.2A). Vesicles rupture into shallow ulcers. It is difficult to distinguish a primary from a nonprimary or recurrent infection, but lesions occur between 2 to 14 days after exposure and may appear larger and more abundant in a primary infection. Prodromal burning, pain, or paresthesia may be experienced as well as systemic flulike symptoms such as headache, malaise, and myalgia. The clinical diagnosis of genital herpes is challenging because lesions and symptoms may not always be present. Also, lesions may appear at different stages (vesicles, pustules, ulcers) and in various locations including the vulva, perineum, buttocks, vagina, or cervix (Fig. 14.2).

Diagnosis

Virus or antigen detection is possible in active lesions. Viral cell culture is the gold standard with approximately 100% specificity and a sensitivity of 30% to 95%. HSV can be diagnosed in fresh vesicles by a Tzanck smear or direct fluorescent antibody assays (DFA); however, the sensitivity for these methods has a wide range (i.e., 73% to 100% and 41% to 70%, respectively). DFA is often the initial diagnostic test because it has a rapid turnaround time and can differentiate between HSV and VZV. Polymerase chain reaction (PCR) is the most sensitive method for HSV detection in cerebrospinal fluid.[3] Because HSV can present atypically and 70% of infected pregnant women are asymptomatic, identifying serum antibodies against type-specific glycoproteins (gG1 from HSV-1 and gG2 from HSV-2) helps to identify seropositive women and/or partners. The sensitivity of these tests for HSV-2 ranges between 80% and 98% with a specificity ≥96%.[4] Confirmatory testing by Western blot may be indicated as a first-line diagnostic test, if a recent HSV infection is suspected.

Maternal and Fetal Risks

See Maternal and Fetal Risks in the *Viral Diseases* box. HSV may be acquired in utero (5%), peripartum (85%), or postpartum (10%). HSV acquired in utero may result in vesicular skin lesions, microcephaly, hydrocephalus, and chorioretinitis. Peripartum and postpartum disease is classified as localized, central nervous system (CNS), or disseminated disease (Fig. 14.3) Nearly one-third of neonates with HSV will have CNS disease and one-fourth will have disseminated disease with a combined mortality rate of 68%.[5] Primary HSV during pregnancy may result in more severe maternal disease such as disseminated HSV, which may result in the death of the mother and fetus.

Management

Pharmacologic treatment is shown in Table 14.1. It is unknown whether antiviral therapy of the pregnant patient's contacts, suppressive or episodic, decreases HSV transmission to pregnant patients. The current recommendations aim to avoid all forms of sexual contact with partners known to have herpes. Additionally, neither the routine screening of pregnant women nor the routine antepartum HSV cultures for active recurrent disease are recommended.[2] When administered at or after 36 weeks'

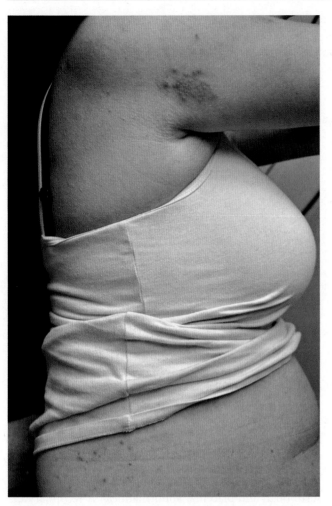

Figure 14.1. Herpes simplex virus 1 infection on the arm, which developed at 27 weeks' gestation. (Courtesy of Dr. George Kroumpouzos.)

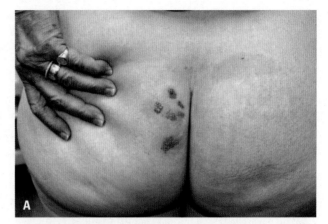

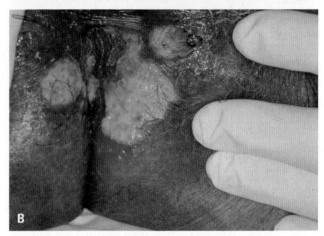

Figure 14.2. **(A)** A herpes simplex virus (HSV) infection: Discrete grouped vesicles on an erythematous base. Recurrent disease occurs on the labia minora/majora and buttocks. **(B)** A chronic HSV-2 infection associated with ovarian carcinoma: Well-demarcated superficial erosions involving the vulva and perineum. (Courtesy of Dr. Dirk Elston.)

gestation, both valacyclovir and acyclovir were shown to reduce HSV recurrence at term and to reduce the frequency of cesarean deliveries.[2] The incidence of neonatal herpes after starting antiviral therapy remains unknown. Currently, antiviral therapy in HSV-seropositive women without a history of genital herpes is not recommended.[4]

According to the American College of Obstetrics and Gynecology (ACOG), a cesarean delivery is indicated in women with active genital lesions or prodromal symptoms, including vulvar pain and burning during delivery. A cesarean delivery is not recommended for women with a history of herpes but no active genital lesions at delivery as well as women with active nongenital lesions.[4] No studies have evaluated whether antiviral treatment is superior to cesarean delivery in reducing the incidence of neonatal HSV infection.

Human Papillomavirus

Human papillomavirus (HPV) causes several types of warts, including common (Fig. 14.4) and genital warts (*condylomata acuminata*) (Fig. 14.5). Over 40 serotypes of HPV may affect the genital area, but the two most relevant

categories are those that cause cervical cancer (i.e., serotypes 16, 18, 31, and 33) and those that cause genital warts (serotypes 6 and 11). It is estimated that more than half of sexually active individuals become infected with HPV in their lifetime; however, most may be asymptomatic and

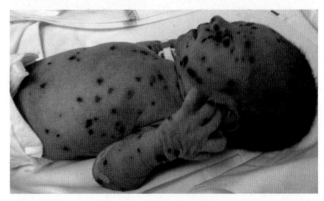

Figure 14.3. Disseminated neonatal herpes secondary to herpes simplex virus 2: Erosions and ulcerations are noted. (Courtesy of Dr. Iria Neri.)

TABLE 14.1	Treatments for Herpes Simplex[2] and Varicella[12] Infections	
Indication	**Acyclovir**	**Valacyclovir**
Primary disease	400 mg PO tid × 7–10 d	1 g PO bid × 7–10 d
Recurrent disease	400 mg PO tid × 5 d *or* 800 mg PO bid × 5 d	500 mg PO bid × 3 d *or* 1 g PO daily × 5 d
Suppressive therapy	400 mg PO tid from 36 wks' gestation until delivery	500 mg PO bid from 36 wks' gestation until delivery
Severe or disseminated disease	5–10 mg/kg IV q8h × 2–7 d, then oral Rx as in primary disease to complete 10 d	
Active varicella	800 mg PO 5 ×/d × 7 d	1 g PO tid × 7 d
Severe varicella (i.e., varicella pneumonia)	10–15 mg/kg IV q8h × 7–10 d	

bid, twice daily; d, day; IV, intravenous; PO, by mouth; q8h, every 8 hours; Rx, treatment; tid, three times daily; wks, weeks.

self-limited.[4] The prevalence of HPV during pregnancy varies between 5.4% and 68%.[6]

Clinical Features

Most HPV infections are asymptomatic, unrecognized, or subclinical in patients. The typical papules can appear flesh-colored, pink, or hyperpigmented with rough surfaces and may appear flat, papular, or pedunculated. They occur more commonly around the introitus but can occur at multiple sites within and around the anogenital tract such as the cervix, urethra, perineum, or intrarectal (see Fig. 14.5). Genital warts may proliferate and become more friable during pregnancy.[4] Condylomata acuminata can rarely develop on extragenital regions (Fig. 14.6).

Diagnosis

A diagnosis is usually made by visual inspection and can be confirmed by biopsy for atypical lesions. Acetic acid staining (3% to 5%) allows for the detection of HPV

changes by turning infected epithelial lining white upon application; however, this is not specific for HPV infection. Although HPV DNA testing is available, the Centers for Disease Control and Prevention (CDC) do not recommend routine DNA testing.[4]

Maternal and Fetal Risks

Women with condylomata acuminata, particularly those with extensive disease, are at increased risk for a cesarean delivery. Oncogenic HPV strains are associated with preterm birth and placental abnormalities.[7] A secondary infection from bacterial trapping in larger masses may lead to fetal infection in utero, a premature rupture of membranes, and chorioamnionitis. Also, cases of congenital anogenital and conjunctival warts have been reported.[8] The HPV types 6 and 11 that are associated with genital warts also cause recurrent respiratory papillomatosis in the neonate, a chronic disease characterized by proliferation of squamous papillomas in the respiratory tract.[9] In children, 50% of

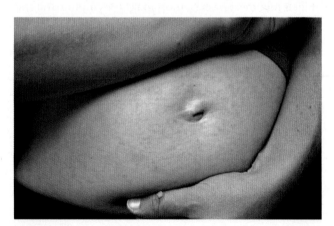

Figure 14.4. Common warts on the right forearm and left thumb that developed in the second trimester; there was no history of warts prior to gestation. (Courtesy of Dr. George Kroumpouzos.)

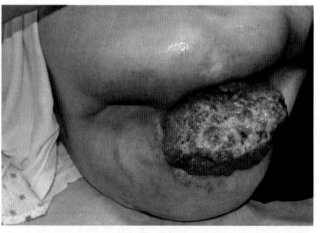

Figure 14.5. Condylomata acuminata of the vulva: A tumorous, verrucous mass protruding from the vulva and extending onto the perineum.

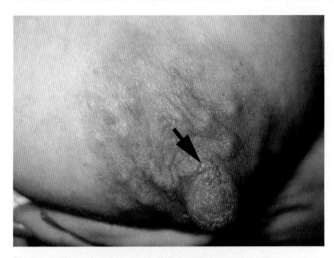

Figure 14.6. Condyloma acuminatum *(arrow)* on the nipple in a pregnant patient. (Courtesy of Dr. Patricia Cristodor.)

respiratory papillomatosis cases have a maternal history of genital warts with possible vertical transmission.[9]

Management

Cryotherapy is the first-line treatment for common warts in pregnancy; a limited application of squaric or salicylic acid is likely safe. An abnormal Pap smear during pregnancy warrants colposcopic evaluation, but urgent treatment depends on the extent of the disease. If no lesions are present or cervical intraepithelial neoplasia 1 is found, treatment is not recommended.[4] Topical imiquimod, sinecatechins, podophyllin, podofilox, and cantharidin should not be used in pregnancy. Cryotherapy is the first-line therapeutic option for genital warts during pregnancy; trichloroacetic acid has an acceptable safety profile but is less effective. The judicious use of laser modalities has been successful. HPV vaccines are not recommended during pregnancy and should be put on hold if a woman becomes pregnant during a series.[10] A cesarean delivery is indicated only when pelvic outlet obstruction results from genital warts or if vaginal delivery would cause extreme bleeding.[4] To date, there is no evidence that a cesarean delivery can prevent respiratory papillomatosis in offspring.[11]

Varicella-Zoster Virus

VZV causes varicella (chickenpox) and herpes zoster (shingles). Because of widespread vaccination, chickenpox occurs in approximately 5% of women of childbearing age, and the incidence of primary VZV during pregnancy is even lower. Unlike varicella, herpes zoster is not thought to cause severe adverse effects during pregnancy.

Clinical Features

A prodrome of constitutional symptoms including fever, malaise, and chills precedes the exanthem. The exanthem is characterized by pruritic lesions appearing at different stages of evolution, including erythematous papules, vesicles, pustules, and crusts. The exanthem classically starts on the head

and descends to the trunk; lesions may rapidly transform from one stage to the next. Herpes zoster (reactivation of latent VZV) starts with a prodrome of localized burning and pain in a unilateral and dermatomal distribution (Fig. 14.7). During the active phase, erythematous papules appear, which progress to vesicles and bullae, subsequently developing crust. New papulovesicles may appear as other lesions resolve. Postherpetic neuralgia may develop and lasts weeks to years after cutaneous involvement has resolved.

Diagnosis

This is based on history and clinical presentation; however, immunofluorescence may be used to detect the VZV antigen or enzyme-linked immunosorbent assay (ELISA) can be used to detect the VZV antibody. Serologic testing can be performed in pregnant women with no history of chickenpox who have been exposed; however, the sensitivity of such tests is low. Viral PCR of cord blood or fetal serologies, immunoglobulin (Ig)M within the first month of life, or IgG persisting beyond the seventh month of life are all suggestive of intrauterine VZV infection. Thus, a high index of suspicion and physical exam findings still remain a key to diagnosis during the prenatal period.

Maternal and Fetal Risks

Current evidence suggests that the infection does not cause first trimester spontaneous abortion; however, intrauterine growth restriction and low birth weight are nearly universal.[12] Other risks are shown under Maternal and Fetal Risks in the *Viral Diseases* box. VZV infection occurring during the first 20 weeks carries a 2% risk of congenital varicella syndrome, whereas neonatal varicella suggests that infection occurred late in pregnancy.[13] **Congenital varicella syndrome** is a rare and devastating complication and is thought to be a result of a combination of disseminated in utero infection and a poor host–virus interaction to establish latency. The neonate can present with skin lesions and limb and muscle hypoplasia. Other severe manifestations include neurologic impairment ranging from seizures to mental retardation, microphthalmia, chorioretinitis, cataracts, and abnormalities of the

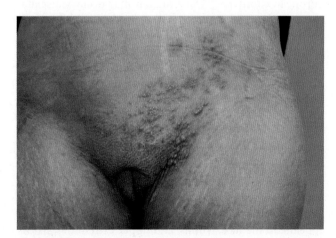

Figure 14.7. Herpes zoster: Grouped vesicles on an erythematous base in a dermatomal (L1) distribution.

gastrointestinal and genitourinary systems.[13] **Neonatal varicella** can develop secondary to transplacental transmission through an ascending infection or through the neonatal respiratory tract. A neonatal infection within the first 10 to 12 days of life suggests an intrauterine infection, whereas infection after this time indicates a neonatal infection. Neonatal mortality is low unless the neonate is born <28 weeks' gestation or weighs <1,000 g and is thought to result from inadequate passive immunity against VZV.[12] Case series of maternal varicella during pregnancy show a risk of **infant zoster** in the first or second year of life.[13]

Maternal pneumonia occurs in up to 20% of VZV-infected pregnant patients. It has a higher mortality in pregnant women than in the general population and constitutes the majority of morbidity associated with adult varicella. The risk to the mother increases with increasing gestational age. Symptoms typically begin 3 to 5 days after the appearance of the rash and may progress, with the most severe cases requiring mechanical ventilation.[12]

Management

See Table 14.1.[12] If a pregnant woman is exposed to varicella, varicella-zoster immunoglobulin (VZIG) administered at time of exposure or up to 96 hours later may prevent or lessen the severity of the illness.[12] There is evidence to support concomitant VZIG and oral antivirals to treat VZV in pregnancy. The dose of VZIG typically given is 125 mg per 10 kg to a maximum of 625 mg, and the duration of action is unknown.[12] Intravenous acyclovir should be administered to infants who develop VZV within the first 2 weeks of life. VZIG should be given to infants born to mothers who develop varicella 5 days before to 2 days after delivery. If VZV symptoms persist despite VZIG administration, the neonate should be started on a course of acyclovir.[12]

HIV

HIV-1 and -2 subtypes cause AIDS. The majority of HIV infections in the United States are caused by HIV-1, whereas HIV-2 is common in West Africa and some European countries.[4] Transmission may occur via sexual contact, blood products, or from mother to child. Each year, more than 2 million HIV-positive women become pregnant worldwide, and approximately 600,000 babies are infected with HIV.[14] Per CDC guidelines, all pregnant women should be tested for HIV at the first prenatal visit and again during the third trimester.[4]

Clinical Features

Although symptoms can be nonspecific, acute retroviral syndrome develops in 50% to 80% of patients acutely infected with HIV.[4] The syndrome is characterized by fever, malaise, lymphadenopathy, pharyngitis, headache, and rash in 30% to 50% of patients. The rash is maculopapular and appears on the face, trunks, and upper extremities; palms and soles can also be affected.[15] Associated skin disorders include eosinophilic folliculitis, molluscum contagiosum

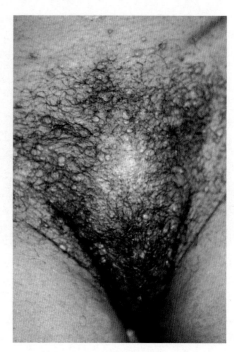

Figure 14.8. Molluscum contagiosum in an HIV-positive female: Typical umbilicated papules are shown.

(Fig. 14.8), Kaposi sarcoma (see Ch. 15, Fig. 15.11), VZV infections, and genital warts; these have been less common since the introduction of antiretroviral therapy (ART).

Diagnosis

HIV is diagnosed by serologic tests that detect antibodies to HIV-1 and HIV-2 and by virologic tests that detect HIV antigens or RNA. Rapid enzyme immunoassay screening enables a presumptive diagnosis, which must be confirmed by antibody testing with Western blot or indirect immunofluorescence assay, or HIV-1 RNA assay virologic testing. Virologic testing can also be used to identify acute infection in persons negative for HIV antibody.[4]

Maternal and Fetal Risks

Perinatal transmission is the primary fetal risk. Without intervention and antiretroviral drugs, 15% to 20% of infants born to HIV-infected mothers will become infected with HIV, and 12% to 14% of infants who breastfeed into their second year of life will become infected.[4] Risk factors for perinatal transmission include increased viral load, duration of ruptured membranes, mode of delivery (cesarean section or vaginal), low birth weight, and smoking. Current observations do not support an adverse effect of pregnancy on the natural course of HIV. However, opportunistic infections acquired during pregnancy can run a more aggressive course when compared with the course in nonpregnant HIV-infected women.[16,17]

Management

Management includes counseling, ART, cesarean delivery, and avoidance of breastfeeding. With intervention and ART, the risk of HIV transmission to infants can be

TABLE 14.2	**Management Options for Other Viral Diseases**[a]
Disease	**Management**
Rubella[19]	■ Screen for rubella immunity during first antenatal visit; MMR vaccine should not be given during pregnancy; however, inadvertent vaccination is not an indication for termination of pregnancy. ■ Discuss termination with serologic confirmation of disease in first trimester. ■ Evaluation for fetal infection by invasive procedure; if confirmed or suspected, fetal monitoring is recommended.
Measles[19]	■ MMR vaccine should be avoided in pregnancy. ■ Consider immunoglobulin administration within 6 days of suspected infection.
Parvovirus B19 (erythema infectiosum)[20]	■ After 20 weeks' gestation, monitor fetus for hydrops via ultrasound; if hydrops develops, periumbilical blood sampling to diagnose extent of fetal anemia; consider intrauterine transfusion if anemia.
Enterovirus infection[22]	■ Monitor neonatal for peripartum transmission of echovirus infection.

[a] Treatment of acute maternal infection is generally symptomatic.

MMR, measles, mumps, and rubella.

reduced to <2%. If ART is required, it should be initiated or continued regardless of gestational age. The benefits, risks, and goals of therapy should be discussed with the mother if ART is initiated during the first trimester. Nucleoside/nucleotide reverse transcriptase inhibitors (NRTI/NtRTI) are the backbone therapy for ART. For treatment-naïve patients, recommended combinations include the baseline NRTI zidovudine-lamivudine and an add-on protease inhibitor such as lopinavir/ritonavir. Additionally, zidovudine is a recommended add-on regardless of previous regimen because studies have shown high placental drug levels with a concomitant decreased viral transmission.[17,18] A scheduled cesarean delivery is recommended for women not receiving ART or zidovudine prophylaxis and those with levels >1,000 copies per milliliter to reduce the risk of vertical transmission. Women who present in labor with no prior therapy should receive intravenous zidovudine. The standard of care, regardless of maternal ART, is to provide infant prophylaxis with 6 weeks of intravenous zidovudine. In order to avoid neonatal HIV-1 transmission postpartum, the CDC recommends against breastfeeding.[18]

OTHER VIRAL DISEASES

Rubella, measles, parvovirus B19 (fifth disease), and enteroviruses pose a significant threat to the fetus and mother, although the routine measles, mumps, and rubella (MMR) vaccination has virtually eradicated the risk of rubella and measles in the United States, with only occasional endemic outbreaks. Other viral infections that are associated with maternal and fetal risks but that do not present with an exanthem include hepatitis and cytomegalovirus infections. Management options are summarized in Table 14.2.

Rubella

Rubella is a relatively uncommon viral infection caused by an RNA virus (*Rubivirus* of the Togaviridae family) and manifests with an exanthem.

Clinical Features

Symptoms occur about 14 days after exposure before the onset of the exanthem. The exanthem, a diffuse reticulated maculopapular eruption, starts on the face and spreads onto the trunk and arms (Fig. 14.9). It may be preceded

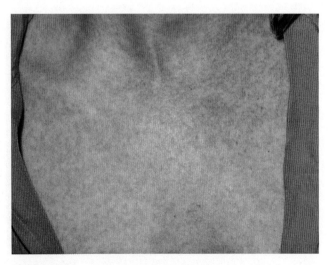

Figure 14.9. A reticulated maculopapular eruption of rubella. (Appears with permission of VisualDx. © Logical Images, Inc.)

by constitutional symptoms, malaise, or low-grade fever associated with lymphadenopathy. Other symptoms include headache, sore throat, cough, and conjunctivitis; however, subclinical illness has been reported in up to 50% in some series.[19] The most severe manifestation in older children and adults is arthritis, which can persist for up to 1 month postinfection.

Diagnosis

The virus can be detected within 3 days of suspected exposure and up to 1 week after resolution of the exanthem; thus, patients can be infectious for up to 14 days. Nucleic acid tests and viral cultures are also available. A fourfold increase in viral antibody titers between the initial infection and the resolution of symptoms is also diagnostic. The virus can be isolated from the blood, urine, nasal secretions, or cerebrospinal fluid.

Maternal and Fetal Risks

Congenital rubella syndrome is the most severe. The risk for transmission is highest at 11 weeks of gestation and decreases during the remainder of pregnancy; congenital rubella infection is rare during the second or third trimester. The syndrome is associated with low birth weight, meningoencephalitis, thrombocytopenia, purpura, and bony radiolucencies. These complications tend to resolve with minimal sequelae; however, the more severe permanent anomalies of congenital rubella syndrome include cardiac defects such as patent ductus arteriosus, cataracts, iris hypoplasia, microphthalmos, retinopathy, mental retardation, developmental delay, microcephaly, and sensorineural hearing loss.

Management

A routine antenatal MMR vaccination is the most appropriate means to prevent transmission. Women of childbearing age should not become pregnant within 28 days of vaccination; however, a pregnancy should not be terminated if it occurs within that time. Currently, there are no approved therapies for the treatment of suspected or confirmed rubella infection during pregnancy, and immunoglobulin administration in acute infection is controversial.[19]

Measles

Measles is caused by an RNA virus of the Paramyxoviridae family. The virus is transmitted via droplet inhalation with a peak incidence in late winter to early spring.

Clinical Features

Symptoms begin 10 to 12 days after exposure and consist of a prodrome of fever, malaise, cough, conjunctivitis, and coryza, which last 2 days. The pathognomonic Koplik spots (gray-white ulcerations on the buccal mucosa) appear toward the end of the prodrome and last for approximately 24 hours. As the Koplik spots resolve, a morbilliform eruption appears, starting on the face (Fig. 14.10A) and progressing onto the trunk and extremities (Fig. 14.10B).[19]

Diagnosis

If an infection is suspected, antibody titers should be measured via ELISA or a hemagglutination inhibition test. The detection of the virus or viral cultures from nasopharyngeal secretions, saliva, urine, or blood can be performed as well. Samples should be obtained within 7 to 10 days. An IgM assay is also available and requires a collection of clinical samples within 72 hours of the onset of the morbilliform eruption.[19]

Maternal and Fetal Risks

See Maternal and Fetal Risks in the *Viral Diseases* box. The disease is not associated with birth defects.

Management

The routine MMR vaccination remains the most effective preventative strategy. Intramuscular measles immunoglobulin may be injected within 6 days of suspected infection at a dose of 0.25 ml/kg with a maximum dose of 15 ml. This intervention will not prevent infection but can

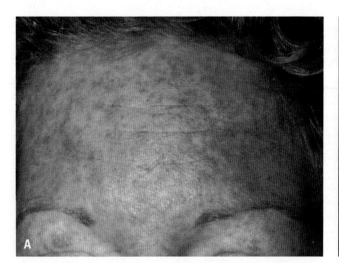 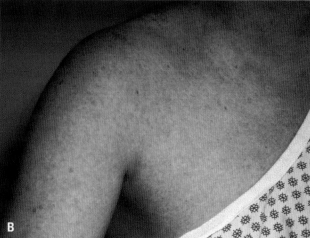

Figure 14.10. A morbilliform eruption of measles. (**A**) Onset on the face. (**B**) Extension onto the chest and arm. (Appears with permission of VisualDx. © Logical Images, Inc.)

reduce the severity and onset of symptoms so that MMR can be administered after pregnancy or the termination of pregnancy.[19] It may also decrease the risk of neonatal measles if maternal infection is close to parturition.

Parvovirus B19

Parvovirus B19 causes fifth disease (erythema infectiosum). Infection often occurs from droplet inhalation from an infected individual.

Clinical Features

The characteristic "slapped cheek" exanthem, consisting of bright red erythema of the cheeks that is noted in children, is subtle or absent in adults. The presentation is subtle in adults with constitutional symptoms and acute symmetric arthropathy (30% to 60%), which is the primary manifestation; however, the disease can be asymptomatic. Up to 50% of infected pregnant patients are asymptomatic. A morbilliform eruption involving the trunk and extremities (Fig. 14.11) may develop in both pediatric and adult patients; it often shows central clearing, thus taking on a "lacy"/reticulated appearance.

Diagnosis

It is established through blood titers of anti-B19 IgG and IgM antibodies that can be detected with radioimmunoassay or ELISA. A fourfold rise in IgG antibody titers measured 4 weeks apart establishes the diagnosis. Anti-B19 IgM alone is suggestive of infection within the previous 2 to 4 months, but a false negative can occur in the window when IgM levels fall and IgG production starts. PCR can be used to diagnose an in utero infection from amniotic fluid.

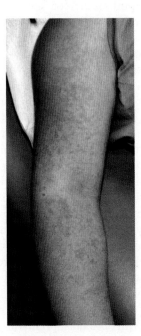

Figure 14.11. A parvovirus B19 infection: Morbilliform eruption of the upper extremities.

Maternal and Fetal Risks

Vertical transmission to the fetus ranges from 30% to 50%, and spontaneous abortion occurs in 5% to 10% of cases infected prior to 20 weeks' gestation. Infection at ≥20 weeks is associated with a negligible risk of spontaneous abortion.[20] Most miscarriages occur between 20 and 28 weeks' gestation. Other risks include low birth weight and fetal hydrops, which can lead to fetal death.

Management

Patient counseling about the risk of fetal loss is warranted prior to 20 weeks' gestation. After 20 weeks' gestation, if infection is suspected or confirmed, periodic ultrasound examinations to monitor the development of fetal hydrops are recommended. If hydrops develops and is accompanied by fetal anemia, intrauterine transfusion can be considered because it has been associated with better outcomes.[20]

Enteroviruses

Herpangina and hand, foot, and mouth disease (HFMD) are common diseases caused by coxsackievirus; the former can be caused also by echovirus. Transmission occurs via fecal–oral or respiratory route in case of herpangina and direct contact for HFMD.

Clinical Features

Herpangina presents with small tender vesicles and erosions in the posterior pharynx, uvula, tonsils, and soft palate accompanied by a fever, sore throat, and enlarged cervical lymph nodes; an exanthem is typically absent. HFMD presents with fever, malaise, and painful erosive stomatitis that affects the tongue, buccal mucosa, palate, uvula, and anterior tonsillar pillars. A maculopapular or vesicular exanthem ensues over 1 to 2 days and primarily affects the palms and soles.

Diagnosis

Both herpangina and HFMD are diagnosed clinically. If desired, throat swabs and blood can be tested for the presence of the virus.

Maternal and Fetal Risks

See Maternal and Fetal Risks in the *Viral Diseases* box.[21] Newborns who acquire coxsackievirus infection in the perinatal period can develop at 3 to 7 days of age severe fulminant multisystem disease, including meningoencephalitis and the failure of several systems secondary to the absence of the protecting maternal antibody. The severity of neonatal infection ranges from asymptomatic viral shedding to rapidly fatal disease.[22]

Management

Herpangina and HFMD are self-limited and managed symptomatically.

NONVIRAL SEXUALLY TRANSMITTED DISEASES

The CDC and ACOG recommend universal screening at the first prenatal visit for syphilis and chlamydia; screening high-risk women for gonorrhea is also recommended.[23] ACOG recommends screening for syphilis at 32–26 weeks, and CDC, during the third trimester and at delivery, for patients at high risk for syphilis.[4] Risk factors of contracting syphilis, chlamydia, and gonorrhea in women include older age and African American race for syphilis, and younger age (<25 years) and African American race for chlamydia and gonorrhea.[23] As per CDC guidelines, patients at increased risk for chlamydia (see above; also, having a new or multiple sexual partners) should be retested in the third trimester to prevent maternal postnatal and neonatal complications.[4]

Syphilis

Syphilis is caused by the spirochete *Treponema pallidum*.

Clinical Features

The primary lesion develops at the site of inoculation as a firm, painless ulcer with indurated borders (chancre) (Fig. 14.12A), typically 3 to 4 weeks after exposure. The

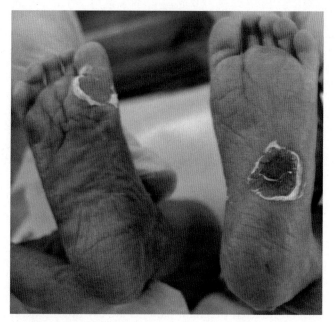

Figure 14.13. Congenital syphilis: Bullous lesions on the soles. (Courtesy of Dr. Iria Neri.)

chancre is rarely detected in women because it commonly occurs in the internal genital tract. Secondary syphilis develops anytime after the primary chancre resolves, and presents as a generalized maculopapular or papulosquamous exanthem that typically involves the palms and soles (Fig. 14.12B); mucosal ulcers and aphthae are also noted.[24] Secondary syphilis shows a wide spectrum of mucocutaneous manifestations, including condylomata lata in the anogenital area, patchy alopecia, and hypopigmented macules.[25] Tertiary (late) syphilis, a consequence of untreated syphilis, is rare.

Congenital syphilis is divided into early (within the first 2 years of life) and late (presenting in the child or adolescent).[24] The most common manifestations of early congenital syphilis are prematurity and low birth weight (10% to 40% of infants), hepatomegaly with or without splenomegaly (33% to 100%), a rash (40%), and bone changes (75% to 100%)[26]; intense crying and thrombocytopenia may also occur. As in secondary syphilis, lesions involve palms and soles, but lesions in congenital syphilis tend to be more erosive and often bullous (pemphigus syphiliticus) (Fig. 14.13). Other skin findings include mucosal plaques, hemorrhagic rhinitis ("snuffles"), condylomata lata, and radial periorificial fissures. Late congenital syphilis may manifest as interstitial keratitis, sabre tibia (Saber shins), gummas (locally destructive lesions in skin and other organs), Clutton joints (painless synovitis and effusions of the knees or elbows), Hutchinson teeth, Parrot nodes, saddle nose, frontal bossing, and changes in the eye examination.[24]

Depending on the stage of syphilis, anywhere from 40% to virtually 100% of infants born to untreated mothers are affected, with 50% born prematurely or stillborn.[23] Because the transplacental transmission of *T. pallidum* is high, the severity is greater if infection is acute and presents earlier in the pregnancy; mother-to-child transmission

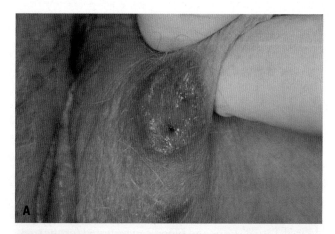

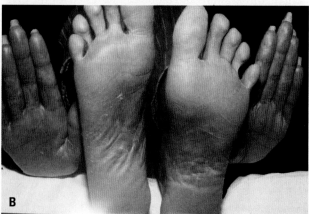

Figure 14.12. (**A**) Primary syphilis: A firm, painless ulcer (chancre) with indurated borders. (**B**) Secondary syphilis showing macular and papulosquamous lesions on the palms and soles.

approaches 100% if infection occurs prior to the seventh month of gestation. Third trimester disease has a lower incidence of transmission, whereas infection 3 to 6 weeks prior to labor is associated with a risk of perinatal but not placental transmission. Additionally, older maternal age is associated with less risk of fetal transmission.[24] Primary (chancre) and secondary syphilis have high rates of vertical transmission because the lesions contain numerous spirochetes; the risk is highest with primary exposure (70% to 100%) but only about 10% from early latent syphilis.[25]

Diagnosis

Diagnosis in the primary stage requires a direct examination of the chancre laboratory confirmation, which may include direct immunofluorescence (sensitivity >90%), dark-field microscopy, and various staining methods. Secondary syphilis presents with more extensive mucocutaneous involvement. Diagnosis is confirmed with serologic tests including Venereal Disease Research Laboratory (VDRL) and rapid plasma reagin (RPR), which are used to screen for the diagnosis and follow-up after treatment. Treponemal-specific tests include the fluorescent treponemal antibody absorption (FTA-ABS) and the *T. pallidum* hemagglutination assay (TPHA), which are used to specifically confirm infection with *T. pallidum*. Neonatal IgM indicates an active infection because maternal IgM does not cross the placenta.[24,26]

Maternal and Fetal Risks

Infection of the fetus can occur as early as 9 to 10 weeks' gestation during primary or secondary syphilis. Fetal risks include spontaneous abortion, prematurity, infant death, and congenital syphilis (see previous).

Management

See Table 14.3. As per CDC, a course of penicillin administered 4 weeks or more before delivery is considered adequate for the prevention of congenital syphilis.[4] If VDRL is positive, a course equivalent to tertiary syphilis protocol should be initiated.

TABLE 14.3 Treatments for Nonviral Sexually Transmitted Diseases[8]	
Infection	**Treatment**
Syphilis	Dose of penicillin[a]
Primary, secondary, early latent (acquired <1 year previously)	BP 2.4 million units IM[b] *or* PP 1.2 million units IM daily × 10 days
Late latent, tertiary	BP 3 doses of 2.4 million units IM at 1-wk intervals *or* PP 1.2 million units IM daily × 20 days
Neonate with no signs of disease born to mother with treated syphilis[c]	BP 50,000 units/kg IM
Neonate with proven or highly probable disease, or born to mother with untreated early syphilis	Aqueous crystalline penicillin G 50,000 units/kg IV q12h × 7 d then q8h × 3 d (100,000–1,500,000 units/kg/d for a total of 10 d) *or* PP 50,000 units/kg IM daily × 10 d
Chlamydia	Azithromycin 1 g PO *or* amoxicillin 500 mg PO tid × 7 d *or* erythromycin base 500 mg PO daily × 7 d *or* 250 mg PO daily × 14 d *or* erythromycin ethylsuccinate 800 mg PO daily × 7 d *or* 400 mg PO daily × 14 d
Gonorrhea	Ceftriaxone 250 mg IM or other third-generation cephalosporin[d]
Trichomoniasis	Metronidazole 2 g PO
Bacterial vaginosis	Metronidazole 250 mg PO tid *or* 500 mg PO bid × 7 d *or* clindamycin 300 mg PO bid × 7d
Candidiasis	Miconazole 2% *or* clotrimazole 1% *or* terconazole 0.4% cream daily for 7 d

[a] The Centers for Disease Control and Prevention (CDC) recommends penicillin desensitization in the case of a penicillin allergy.[4] Alternative regimens in penicillin-allergic patients include azithromycin 500 mg PO daily × 10 d *or* ceftriaxone 1 g IM or IV daily × 10 to 14 days. These are included in World Health Organization guidelines but are not recommended by the CDC (limited data).

[b] Based on clinical experience, some authors recommend a second 2.4 million unit intramuscular dose administered 1 week after the initial dose.

[c] Treatment is optional if the neonate's serum nontreponemal antibody titer < fourfold the maternal titer, and if the mother was fully treated before the pregnancy and if nontreponemal titers remained low and stable before and throughout the pregnancy.[4]

[d] Alternative regimens for patients who cannot tolerate cephalosporins include azithromycin 2 g PO and spectinomycin 2 g IM (not available in the United States). Current guidelines suggest judicious use of azithromycin because of a risk of *N. gonorrhoeae* resistance.

bid, twice daily; BP, benzathine penicillin; d, day; IM, intramuscular; IV, intravenous; PO, by mouth; PP, procaine penicillin; q8h, every 8 hours; tid, three times daily; wk, week.

Chlamydia trachomatis

The obligate intracellular organism *Chlamydia trachomatis* serotypes D through K is the cause of the most common sexually transmitted bacterial infection worldwide.

Clinical Features

Infection is asymptomatic in 50% to 88% of patients. When symptomatic, the most common features are dysuria, dyspareunia, urinary urgency, vaginal discharge, and bleeding. In women, an untreated infection may lead to pelvic inflammatory disease (PID), ectopic pregnancy, and tubal infertility.

Diagnosis

The gold standard for diagnosis is a cell culture, although this test is not universally available and is time-consuming. A nucleic acid amplification test (NAAT) of a vaginal swab or a urine sample (ideally 15 to 50 ml of first void) is preferred over other tests, such as enzyme immunoassays, direct immunofluorescence, or nucleic acid hybridization tests, because of its high sensitivity (90% to 97%) and specificity (99%).[27]

Maternal and Fetal Risks

See Maternal and Fetal Risks in the *Nonviral Sexually Transmitted Diseases* box.[27] A recent acquisition of the infection has been associated with increased fetal risks. Treatment reduces the risks of premature rupture of membranes and preterm labor. Acute PID during the second and/or third gestational months has been associated with congenital heart defects.[28] It is estimated that 20% to 60% of infants born to women with untreated infections develop conjunctivitis or pneumonia.[29]

Management

See Table 14.3. Repeat testing to document chlamydial eradication 3 weeks after completion of therapy is recommended; additionally, infected pregnant women that receive therapy in the first trimester should be retested 3 months after treatment.[4] Neonatal conjunctivitis is treated with erythromycin base or ethylsuccinate 50 mg/kg per day, orally divided into four doses for 14 days; it is not effectively treated/prevented with topical antibiotic therapy, such as erythromycin ointment.[4]

Gonorrhea

Gonorrhea is caused by the gram-negative diplococcus *Neisseria gonorrhoeae*.

Clinical Features

Gonorrhea presents as an asymptomatic vulvovaginitis and cervicitis in 80% of infected women. Like chlamydia, a prolonged and untreated infection predisposes a patient to PID, infertility, or tubal ectopic pregnancy.

Diagnosis

Vaginal swabs show gram-negative diplococci within polymorphonuclear leukocytes (Fig. 14.14); the finding provides an immediate preliminary diagnosis, especially in

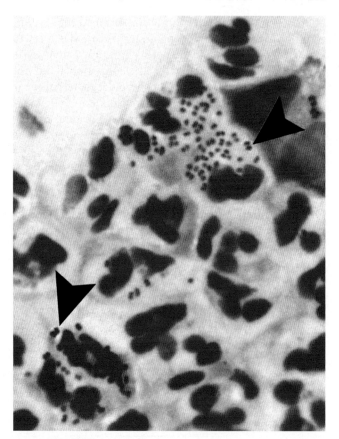

Figure 14.14. Gonorrhea: Gram-negative diplococci *(arrows)* in polymorphonuclear leukocytes. (Courtesy of Dr. Stephen Lyle.)

symptomatic patients. The gold standard for diagnosing gonorrhea is a culture on a selective media (Thayer-Martin) or PCR. The most common diagnostic method in the United States is the NAAT, which uses less invasive collection methods without sacrificing sensitivity.[30,31]

Maternal and Fetal Risks

Gonorrhea is associated with a wide spectrum of maternal and fetal[24] and neonatal risks (see box *Maternal and Fetal Risks of Nonviral Sexually Transmitted Diseases*).[4,32]

Management

Ceftriaxone is the most effective treatment, but cefixime may also be used (see Table 14.3).[23] Gonococcal conjunctivitis (ophthalmia neonatorum) is effectively prevented with a single application of erythromycin 0.5% ophthalmic ointment. For infants with ophthalmia neonatorum or for those at increased risk, a single dose of ceftriaxone 25 to 50 mg/kg intravenously or intramuscularly (dose not to exceed 125 mg) is recommended.[30]

Vaginitis

Infectious vaginitis is the most common infection in pregnancy. The most common causes of vaginal discharge, trichomoniasis, bacterial vaginosis (BV), and candida vulvovaginitis are discussed in the following.

Trichomoniasis

Trichomoniasis is a vaginal infection due to a sexually transmitted, flagellated anaerobic protozoan, *Trichomonas vaginalis*.

Clinical Features

Up to 30% of infected women may be asymptomatic; however, up to 50% exhibit an abundant discharge characterized by purulence, foamy consistency, and foul-smelling odor. Other symptoms include pruritus, vulvar irritation, and hyperemic mucosa with reddish plaques, giving rise to a "strawberry cervix." Dysuria and polyuria may also be present.

Diagnosis

Identifying mobile, flagellated protozoa (trichomonads) on a wet-mount preparation (sensitivity 58% to 82%) establishes the diagnosis (Fig. 14.15). The protozoan exhibits a stereotypical continuous movement. A culture is appropriate with repeatedly negative smears.[24] Commercially available rapid tests on vaginal secretions have shown sensitivity >83% and specificity >97%.[4] Alternatively, recent nucleic-acid based amplification diagnostic tests utilizing vaginal or endocervical swabs or urine have shown excellent efficacy.[33,34] Other features suggestive of trichomoniasis are leukocyte counts greater than the epithelial cell number, a positive whiff test, and vaginal pH >5.4. Pap smears that are positive for *Trichomonas* should be treated but should not be relied upon for diagnosis.[24]

Maternal and Fetal Risks

See Maternal and Fetal Risks in the *Nonviral Sexually Transmitted Diseases* box.[24] Metronidazole treatment has not been shown to reduce risks.[4]

Management

Metronidazole therapy (see Table 14.3).[4]

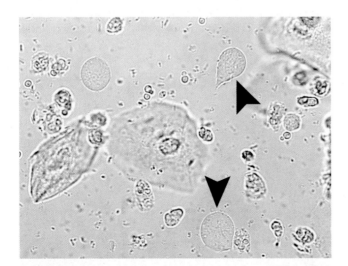

Figure 14.15. A wet-mount preparation of trichomoniasis shows trichomonads *(arrows)* that are characteristically lemon shaped; jerky motility is required for identification. (Courtesy of Seattle STD/HIV Prevention Training Center.)

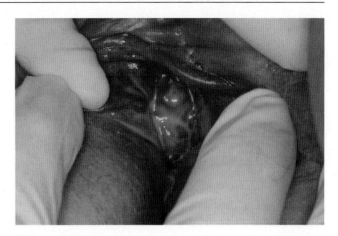

Figure 14.16. Bacterial vaginosis: The typical discharge of white-gray color with creamy consistency.

Bacterial Vaginosis

Bacterial vaginosis (BV) is caused by an overgrowth of anaerobic bacteria, including *Gardnerella vaginalis*, *Bacteroides sp.*, *Mobiluncus sp.*, *Mycoplasmas*, and *Peptostreptococcus*. The infection is generally a result of vaginal flora alterations, including a decrease in acidophilus *Lactobacillus*. This enables an overgrowth of these bacterial species. In some studies, BV is the most common cause of vaginal discharge in women of reproductive age with a prevalence of 10% to 15% and is associated with African American race, smoking, sexual activity, and vaginal douching.[35] BV during pregnancy has a higher incidence (20%) than asymptomatic bacteriuria and infections from *Neisseria gonorrhoeae*, *Chlamydia trachomatis*, and *Trichomonas vaginalis*.

Clinical Features

BV can be asymptomatic in up to 50% of infected women. Symptomatic women have a typical discharge of white-gray color, creamy consistency (Fig. 14.16), and foul-smelling odor that is particularly worse after sexual intercourse or menstruation. Patients do not generally complain of pruritus or inflammation.[24]

Diagnosis

Any three of the following four Amsel criteria must be fulfilled[36]: (1) thin homogeneous vaginal discharge, usually white-gray in color and adherent to vaginal walls, (2) vaginal pH >4.5, (3) a positive whiff test (the development of a fishy odor with addition of 10% KOH to vaginal discharge), and (4) the presence of clue cells (i.e., vaginal epithelial cells with numerous adherent coccobacilli visualized on a wet-mount preparation) (Fig. 14.17) or Gram stain.

Maternal and Fetal Risks

See Maternal and Fetal Risks in the *Nonviral Sexually Transmitted Diseases* box.[37] Evidence does not suggest any benefit in treating asymptomatic BV to prevent preterm birth.[38] Several studies have evaluated the treatment of BV in asymptomatic pregnant women who are at high or low risk for preterm delivery (i.e., a previous preterm

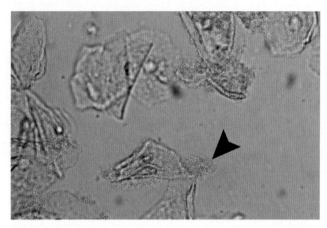

Figure 14.17. A wet-mount preparation of bacterial vaginosis. The *arrow* shows clue cells (i.e., anaerobic bacteria on the periphery of an epithelial cell).

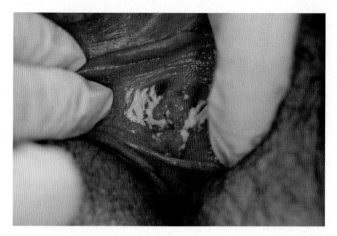

Figure 14.18. Candidiasis: Vulvovaginitis with white-cheesy discharge. Vaginal erythema with white plaques on the mucosa.

delivery, a low prepartum weight) and showed inconsistent results regarding a reduction of adverse outcomes in both groups.[4]

Management

Treatment is recommended for symptomatic disease (see Table 14.3).[24] CDC guidelines do not support routine screening for BV during pregnancy.[4]

Vulvovaginal Candidiasis

Candida vaginitis has been reported in 17% to 50% of pregnant women[39]; of those, 10% to 40% are asymptomatic, and the incidence of symptomatic vaginitis increases with the duration of gestation.[40] *Candida albicans* is the most common of the *Candida* species to cause vulvovaginal candidiasis, being identified in 80% to 90% of cases. Pregnancy results in changes to the vaginal environment that favors the growth of fungi; increased glycogen content in the vaginal epithelium creates an acidic medium and lowers the pH.[24] Factors that also favor the overgrowth of *Candida* include poorly controlled diabetes, obesity, the use of antibiotics, oral contraceptives, corticosteroids and other immunosuppressive medications, synthetic or poorly ventilated clothing that increases humidity, poor hygiene, contact with allergens/irritants, multigravida status, and immunodeficiency states.

Clinical Features

Vulvovaginal pruritus may be associated with a white, thick, and odorless discharge (Fig. 14.18) as well as vulvar hyperemia and edema. The subsequent scratching and itching may result in fissures and maceration of the skin. Other symptoms include dysuria and dyspareunia.

Diagnosis

Direct microscopic visualization of hyphae, pseudohyphae (Fig. 14.19), and although less specific, the detection of birefringent spores in 10% KOH solution or wet-mount preparation confirms a diagnosis (sensitivity 65% to 85%). Unlike BV and trichomoniasis, the vaginal pH in

vulvovaginal candidiasis is normal (4.0 to 4.5). Culture in Sabouraud or Nickerson agar may be utilized when microscopic visualization is difficult or recurrently negative in symptomatic women with a normal vaginal pH.[24]

Maternal and Fetal Risks

See Maternal and Fetal Risks in the *Nonviral Sexually Transmitted Diseases* box. *Candida albicans* can be cultured from up to 50% of neonates born to infected mothers.[41] Neonatal candidiasis can result from passage of the infant through an infected birth canal, and congenital candidiasis can result from an ascending infection in utero. The latter is characterized by generalized skin lesions that appear within 12 hours of delivery.[41]

Management

See Table 14.3.[4] An infection in pregnant patients is regarded as a complication and requires a more extensive treatment course than nonpregnant patients. A 1-week course of a topical azole is effective. There is preliminary evidence that topical antifungal therapy may prevent preterm birth in patients with asymptomatic vaginal candidiasis.[42]

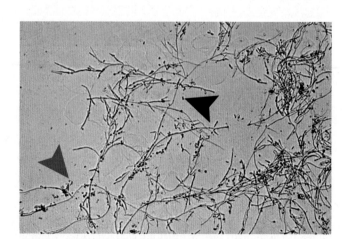

Figure 14.19. A wet-mount preparation of vaginal secretions of candidiasis shows pseudohyphae, yeast cells *(blue arrow)*, and tiny budding yeasts *(black arrow)*.

VIRAL DISEASES

Maternal Risks

HSV: Disseminated disease (encephalitis, hepatitis, coagulopathy, thrombocytopenia, leucopenia, death)

Varicella: Pneumonia

HPV: Cervical cancer

HIV: Opportunistic infection

Rubella: Encephalitis, bleeding, arthritis (rare)

Measles: Pneumonia, encephalitis, death (rare)

Enteroviruses: Upper respiratory aggravation, myocarditis, aseptic meningitis

Parvovirus B19: Aplastic crisis in patients with hemoglobinopathy

Fetal Risks

HSV: Spont abortion, prematurity, congenital/neonatal herpes, neurologic complications, microcephaly, hydrocephalus, chorioretinitis

Varicella: IUGR, LBW, congenital varicella syndrome, fetal death, neonatal varicella, neonatal herpes zoster

HIV: HIV infection

HPV: Genital wart, recurrent respiratory papillomatosis, PROM, chorioamnionitis

Rubella: Congenital rubella syndrome (transient and permanent anomalies), IUGR

Measles: Prematurity, spont abortion (case series), stillbirth, neonatal measles (pneumonia, death)

Enteroviruses: LBW, prematurity, small-for-gestational age infants, spont abortion, neonatal infection (variable severity)

Parvovirus B19: Fetal anemia (self-limited), spont abortion or stillbirth, hydrops fetalis, thrombocytopenia, cardiac failure, LBW

HPV, human papillomavirus; HSV, herpes simplex virus; IUGR, intrauterine growth restriction; LBW, low birth weight; PROM, premature rupture of membranes; spont, spontaneous.

NONVIRAL SEXUALLY TRANSMITTED DISEASES

Maternal Risks

Syphilis: Same as in nonpregnant patient

Chlamydia trachomatis: Pelvic inflammatory disease, ectopic pregnancy, tubal infertility, postpartum endometritis

Gonorrhea: Bartholinitis, perihepatitis, arthritis, endocarditis, endometritis, infertility

Bacterial vaginosis: Postpartum endometritis

Trichomoniasis: Symptomatic aggravation, dysuria, polyuria

Candida vaginitis: Symptomatic aggravation, dysuria, dyspareunia

Fetal/Neonatal Risks

Syphilis: Abortion, prematurity, infant death, early congenital syphilis, late syphilis

Chlamydia trachomatis: Prematurity, PROM, LBW, neonatal conjunctivitis, neonatal pneumonia

Gonorrhea: Prematurity, PROM, fetal death, IUGR, neonatal disease (conjunctivitis, septicemia, arthritis, abscesses in scalp, pneumonia, meningitis, endocarditis, and stomatitis)

Bacterial vaginosis: Preterm labor, PROM, intra-amniotic infection, LBW

Trichomoniasis: PROM, preterm labor, LBW

Candida vaginitis: Preterm birth, chorioamnionitis (rare), congenital candidiasis (rare), neonatal sepsis

IUGR, intrauterine growth restriction, LBW, low birth weight; PROM, premature rupture of membranes.

KEY POINTS

- HSV and VZV infections pose serious maternal and fetal risks, which necessitate prompt acyclovir or valacyclovir therapy; the administration of varicella-zoster immunoglobulin to the seronegative mother within 96 hours postexposure may be beneficial.

- Pregnancy does not alter the course of HIV disease; however, opportunistic infections may run a more aggressive course; zidovudine-lamivudine is a backbone therapy in HIV-positive pregnant patients; zidovudine should be administered to the neonate for up to 6 weeks.

- Routine screening for human papillomavirus during pregnancy is not required; cryotherapy is a safe therapeutic option; surgical removal should be reserved for growing lesions that lead to obstruction of the birth canal; in such cases, cesarean delivery is recommended.

- Viral infections, including measles, mumps, rubella, and enteroviruses have been associated with serious maternal and fetal/neonatal risks.

- The mainstay of therapy for all stages of syphilis during pregnancy is penicillin; fetal risks include spontaneous abortion, prematurity, infant death, and congenital syphilis.

- Gonorrhea is associated with a wide spectrum of maternal and fetal increased risks and is treated with ceftriaxone; chlamydia is the most common sexually transmitted bacterial infection but can be safely treated with macrolides.

- Trichomoniasis and symptomatic bacterial vaginosis can be treated with oral metronidazole, and vulvovaginal candidiasis can be treated with topical azoles.

REFERENCES

1. Baker DA. Consequences of herpes simplex virus in pregnancy and their prevention. *Curr Opin Infect Dis.* 2007;20:73–76.
2. ACOG Practice Bulletin. Clinical management guidelines for obstetrician-gynecologists. No. 82, June 2007. Management of herpes in pregnancy. *Obstet Gynecol.* 2007;109:1489–1498.

3. Anzivino E, Fioriti D, Mischitelli M, et al. Herpes simplex virus infection in pregnancy and in neonate: status of art of epidemiology, diagnosis, therapy and prevention. *Virol J.* 2009;6:40.

4. Centers for Disease Control and Prevention. Sexually Transmitted Diseases Guidelines. *Morb Mort Wkly Rep.* 2010:59.

5. Kimberlin DW. Neonatal herpes simplex infection. *Clin Microbiol Rev.* 2004;17:1–13.

6. Arena S, Marconi M, Ubertosi M, et al. HPV and pregnancy: diagnostic methods, transmission and evolution. *Minerva Ginecol.* 2002;54:225–237.

7. Zuo Z, Goel S, Carter JE. Association of cervical cytology and HPV DNA status during pregnancy with placental abnormalities and preterm birth. *Am J Clin Pathol.* 2011;136:260–265.

8. Ferenczy A. HPV-associated lesions in pregnancy and their clinical implications. *Clin Obstet Gynecol.* 1989;32:191–199.

9. Derkay CS, Wiatrak B. Recurrent respiratory papillomatosis: a review. *Laryngoscope.* 2008;118:1236–1247.

10. Forinash AB, Yancey AM, Pitlick JM, et al. Safety of the HPV bivalent and quadrivalent vaccines during pregnancy. *Ann Pharmacother.* 2011;45:258–262.

11. Silverberg MJ, Thorsen P, Lindeberg H, et al. Condyloma in pregnancy is strongly predictive of juvenile-onset recurrent respiratory papillomatosis. *Obstet Gynecol.* 2003;101:645–652.

12. Lamont RF, Sobel JD, Carrington D, et al. Varicella-zoster virus (chickenpox) infection in pregnancy. *BJOG.* 2012;118:1155–1162.

13. Smith CK, Arvin AM. Varicella in the fetus and newborn. *Semin Fetal Neonatal Med.* 2009;14:209–217.

14. Rigopoulos D, Gregoriou S, Paparizos V, et al. AIDS in pregnancy, part II: treatment in the era of highly active antiretroviral therapy and management of obstetric, anesthetic, and pediatric issues. *Skinmed.* 2007;6:79–84.

15. Khambaty MM, Hsu SS. Dermatology of the patient with HIV. *Emerg Med Clin North Am.* 2010;28:355–368.

16. Ahmad H, Mehta NJ, Manikal VM, et al. Pneumocystis carinii pneumonia in pregnancy. *Chest.* 2001;120:666–671.

17. Rigopoulos D, Gregoriou S, Paparizos V, et al. AIDS in pregnancy, part I: epidemiology, testing, effect on disease progression, opportunistic infections, and risk of vertical transmission. *Skinmed.* 2007;6:18–23.

18. Recommendations for the use of antiretroviral drugs in pregnant HIV-1 infected women for maternal health and intervention to reduce perinatal HIV transmission in the United States. HHS Panel on antiretroviral guidelines for adults and adolescents panel roster. AIDSInfo.nih.gov. http://aidsinfo.nih.gov/guidelines/html/3/perinatal-guidelines. Updated February 12, 2013. Accessed March 2, 2012.

19. White SJ, Boldt KL, Holditch SJ, et al. Measles, mumps, and rubella. *Clin Obstet Gynecol.* 2012;55:550–559.

20. Giorgio E, De Oronzo MA, Iozza I, et al. Parvovirus B19 during pregnancy: a review. *J Prenat Med.* 2010;4:63–66.

21. Chen YH, Lin HC, Lin HC. Increased risk of adverse pregnancy outcomes among women affected by herpangina. *Am J Obstet Gynecol.* 2010;203:49.e1–e7.

22. Modlin JF. Echovirus infections in newborn infants. *Pediatr Infect Dis.* 1988;7:311–312.

23. Koumans EH, Rosen J, van Dyke MK, et al. Prevention of mother-to-child transmission of infections during pregnancy: implementation of recommended interventions, United States, 2003–2004. *Am J Obstet Gynecol.* 2012;206:158.e1–158.e11.

24. Costa MC, Demarch EB, Azulay DR, et al. Sexually transmitted diseases during pregnancy: a synthesis of particularities. *An Bras Dermatol.* 2011;85:767–782.

25. Singh AE, Romanowski B. Syphilis: review with emphasis on clinical, epidemiologic, and some biologic features. *Clin Microbiol Rev.* 1999;12:187–209.

26. Saloojee H, Velaphi S, Goga Y, et al. The prevention and management of congenital syphilis: an overview and recommendations. *Bull World Health Organ.* 2004;82:424–430.

27. Kalwij S, Macintosh M, Baraitser P. Screening and treatment of *Chlamydia trachomatis* infections. *BMJ.* 2010;340:c1915.

28. Acs N, Banhidy F, Puhó EH, et al. Possible association between acute pelvic inflammatory disease in pregnant women and congenital abnormalities in their offspring: a population-based case-control study. *Birth Defects Res A Clin Mol Teratol.* 2008;82:563–570.

29. Hammerschlag MR, Cummings C, Roblin PM, et al. Efficacy of neonatal ocular prophylaxis for the prevention of chlamydial and gonococcal conjunctivitis. *N Engl J Med.* 1989;320:769–772.

30. Woods CR. Gonococcal infections in neonates and young children. *Semin Pediatr Infect Dis.* 2005;16:258–270.

31. Johnson RE, Newhall WJ, Papp JR, et al. Screening tests to detect *Chlamydia trachomatis* and *Neisseria gonorrhoeae* infections—2002. *MMWR Recomm Rep.* 2002;51:1–38.

32. Jones DE, Brame RG, Jones CP. Gonorrhea in obstetric patients. *J Am Vener Dis Assoc.* 1976;2:30–32.

33. Hardick A, Hardick J, Wood BJ, et al. Comparison between the Gen-Probe transcription-mediated amplification *Trichomonas vaginalis* research assay and real-time PCR for Trichomonas vaginalis detection using a Roche LightCycler instrument with female self-obtained vaginal swab samples and male urine samples. *J Clin Microbiol.* 2006;44:4197–4199.

34. Huppert JS, Mortensen JE, Reed JL, et al. Rapid antigen testing compares favorably with transcription-mediated amplification assay for the detection of *Trichomonas vaginalis* in young women. *Clin Infect Dis.* 2007;45:194–198.

35. Goldenberg RL, Klebanoff MA, Nugent R, et al. Bacterial colonization of the vagina during pregnancy in four ethnic groups. Vaginal Infections and Prematurity Study Group. *Am J Obstet Gynecol.* 1996;174:1618–1621.

36. Amsel R, Totten PA, Spiegel CA, et al. Nonspecific vaginitis. Diagnostic criteria and microbial and epidemiologic associations. *Am J Med.* 1983;74:14–22.

37. Guaschino S, De Seta F, Piccoli M, et al. Aetiology of preterm labour: bacterial vaginosis. *BJOG.* 2006;113:S46–S51.

38. McDonald HM, Brocklehurst P, Gordon A. Antibiotics for treating bacterial vaginosis in pregnancy. *Cochrane Database Syst Rev.* 2007:CD000262.

39. Hopsu-Havu VK, Grönroos M, Punnonen R. Vaginal yeasts in parturients and infestation of the newborns. *Acta Obstet Gynecol Scand.* 1980;59:73–77.

40. Sobel JD. Epidemiology and pathogenesis of recurrent vulvovaginal candidiasis. *Am J Obstet Gynecol.* 1985;152:924–935.

41. Winton GB. Skin diseases aggravated by pregnancy. *J Am Acad Dermatol.* 1989;20:1–13.

42. Roberts CL, Rickard K, Kotsiou G, et al. Treatment of asymptomatic vaginal candidiasis in pregnancy to prevent preterm birth: an open-label pilot randomized controlled trial. *BMC Pregnancy Childbirth.* 2011;11:18.

CHAPTER 15

Skin Tumors

Emily Tierney ▪ George Kroumpouzos ▪ Gary Rogers

INTRODUCTION

Pregnancy is associated with changes in benign tumors.[1] Epidermal and vascular tumors and tumors of fibrous or neural tissue can develop or increase in size during gestation. Of women, 10% experience a darkening of melanocytic nevi in the first trimester[2]; however, several studies, including dermoscopy studies, demonstrate only transient mild changes in benign nevi during gestation. More substantial changes have been reported in dysplastic nevi (DN).[3] The prognosis of advanced stage malignant melanoma (MM) arising in pregnancy has not been adequately clarified. This chapter reviews benign and malignant tumors with a focus on nevi and MM. Controversies and the management of these tumors in pregnancy are discussed.

BENIGN TUMORS

A wide spectrum of benign tumors has been reported to change in pregnancy. An increase in the number of epidermal tumors, such as seborrheic keratoses and skin tags, has been documented.[1] **Seborrheic keratoses** may develop in pregnancy or become darker (Fig. 15.1). **Dermatosis papulosa nigra**, a condition characterized by a large number of minute papules with a histopathology of seborrheic keratoses, becomes prominent in pregnancy with the development of new lesions (Fig. 15.2). Skin tags (*molluscum fibrosum gravidarum*) may develop in pregnancy and often regress postpartum (see Ch. 5, Fig. 5.10). Among pregnant women with skin tags and acanthosis nigricans, 40% had gestational diabetes, whereas only 12.3% of pregnant women free of both skin tags and acanthosis nigricans developed gestational diabetes (odds ratio 4.8).[4]

Tumors of fibrous tissue, such as dermatofibromas and collagenomas, can develop in pregnancy. There are several reports of **dermatofibroma** developing during pregnancy. In one report, the development of multiple dermatofibromata was attributed to the altered immunity of pregnancy, which is supported by an association with immunosuppressive therapy.[5] Cases of eruptive **collagenomas** in pregnancy have been reported.[6] Vascular tumors such as hemangioma, pyogenic granuloma (*granuloma gravidarum*) (see Ch. 4, Figs. 4.12 to 4.14), and hemangioendothelioma can increase in size and number in pregnancy; glomus tumors can become tender in gestation.

Neurofibromas can increase in size and number in gestation (see Ch. 16). Plexiform neurofibromas may grow dramatically in pregnancy and occasionally shrink postpartum. A case of bilateral segmental neurofibromatosis, in which the lesions increased in size and darkened during gestation, was reported.[7]

Melanocytic Nevi

Melanocytic nevi may increase in size or erupt during pregnancy[8]; fast growth of nevi has been reported. Clinical evidence has long suggested that melanocytes are estrogen responsive. Estrogen receptor beta (ERβ) is the predominant estrogen receptor in melanocytic cells from all types of nevi.[9] Enhanced positivity for ERβ in normal nevi, with the exception of congenital nevi, during pregnancy was noted as compared with nonpregnant controls; increased ERβ was seen also in DN.[9] The proliferative action of estrogen on the melanocyte cycle was suggested by a study that showed an increased number of mitoses, *superficial micronodules of pregnancy* (clusters of large, HMB45-positive, epithelioid melanocytes with prominent nucleoli abundant pale eosinophilic cytoplasm, and occasional fine melanosomes) and a trend toward increased Ki-67 proliferation index in dermal nevi in pregnancy.[10] The authors indicated that these features are common in pregnancy and stressed the absence of atypical mitotic figures, pleomorphism, an increased nuclear to cytoplasmic ratio, and a lack of maturation.

Clinical and Histopathologic Features

Studies by Foucar et al.[11] and Sanchez, Figueroa, and Rodriguez[2] correlated changes in nevi reported by pregnant women with histologic features. In the former, one-third of patients noted a change in pigmented lesions during pregnancy, but most lesions were not nevi. In the latter, 10% of pregnant patients reported changes in pigmented lesions, such as darkening and an increase in size, especially on the trunk (Fig. 15.3) and mostly in the first trimester. In both studies, histopathologic features of nevi in pregnancy were not significantly different than in the nonpregnant state. A prospective study using photography by Pennoyer et al. showed that only 6.2% of nevi changed in diameter from the first to third trimester, and there was no change in the mean size.[12]

Ellis performed the only study documenting clinical and histologic changes in pregnant women with dysplastic nevus syndrome (DNS); nonpregnant patients

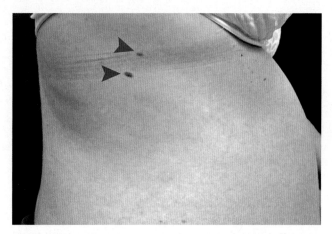

Figure 15.1. Seborrheic keratoses *(arrows)* developed during pregnancy in this patient.

on sex steroid hormones were also included.[3] The rate of clinical change was 3.9-fold higher when patients with DNS were pregnant (Fig. 15.4) than when they were not. No differences were observed regarding oral contraceptives or hormone supplements. Biopsies were performed on one-third of nevi, which were observed to change on examination. The rate of change of histologically dysplastic nevi during pregnancy was twofold higher compared with the interval when these patients with DNS were not pregnant. One MM occurred during pregnancy.

Dermoscopic Features

In a study by Zampino et al.,[13] dermoscopic parameters, total dermoscopic score (TDS) according to the ABCD rule (asymmetry, border irregularity, color, diameter), and size of nevi were evaluated during the first and third trimesters, and at 6 months' postpartum. Dermoscopic changes were mild, and none of the lesions warranted a biopsy. A decrease in global pigmentation and a less prominent pigmented

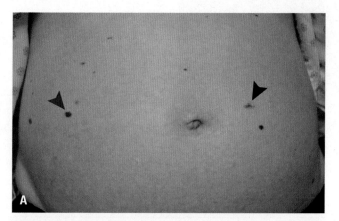

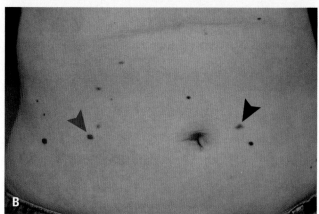

Figure 15.3. Benign nevi on the abdomen. **(A)** Lesions shown with *arrows* became larger during gestation (shown in third trimester) as a result of abdominal expansion; lesion shown with *blue arrow* also became slightly darker in gestation. **(B)** Both nevi returned to their original prepregnancy condition at 5 months' postpartum.

network were observed over the course of pregnancy and postpartum. However, globules increased at the periphery of the lesion (Fig. 15.5) in four nevi throughout pregnancy, in two only in the third trimester, and in two during the first trimester and postpartum. Vascular structures increased

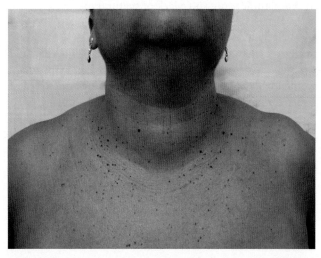

Figure 15.2. Dermatosis papulosa nigra is shown in a pregnant Brazilian patient. Numerous new minute lesions developed in pregnancy. (Courtesy of Dr. Tania Cestari.)

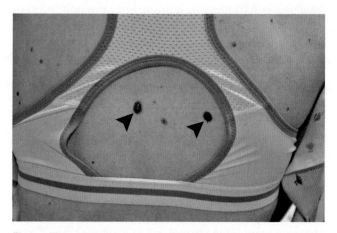

Figure 15.4. A pregnant patient with dysplastic nevus syndrome. The large lesions on the middle of the back *(arrows)* became more exophytic and the rim of pigmentation became darker during gestation.

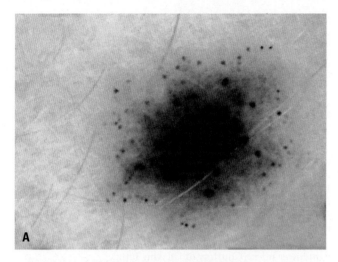

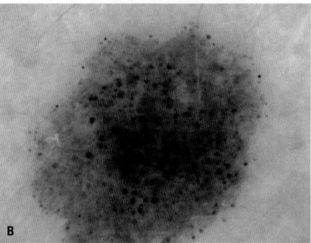

Figure 15.5. Dermoscopy of an abdominal nevus (**A**) at 5 months' gestation and (**B**) at 9 months' postpartum. Growth of the nevus was noted in the third trimester but not postpartum. This nevus shows a globular pattern. Note in image **B** the symmetric enlargement due to previous abdominal distention during gestation. Also, more globules are seen at the periphery, which can be a consequence of the thinning/expansion of the nevus, so that deep nests are pushed against the basal membrane, simulating junctional nests; alternatively, this can reflect recent growth. (Courtesy of Dr. Alin Tatu.)

in number during pregnancy and regressed postpartum. Mean TDS increased during pregnancy and subsequently decreased from the third trimester to postpartum. No significant changes were noted in the size of the nevi. These changes were transient: nevi recovered their prepregnancy appearance after delivery.[13]

Another study included changes from multiple anatomic areas and showed an increase in diameter in 20.6% of nevi during pregnancy; 65% of nevi that increased in size were located in anatomic areas susceptible to expansion (i.e., front of the body, legs) (Fig. 15.6).[14] Mean TDS was significantly greater in the third trimester compared to the first trimester. A study using digital dermoscopy showed that the pigment network becomes more prominent throughout pregnancy, and in lesions with a globular pattern, the

globules become darker; these changes return to their original condition within 1 year after delivery.[15] Finally, a study that used a spectrophotometric cutaneous analysis did not reveal significant changes in the appearance of nevi in pregnancy.[16] While these studies indicate that dermoscopic changes in nonatypical nevi are mild and transient and are noticed primarily in areas of expansion, there is a lack of dermoscopic studies on atypical nevi in pregnancy. Whether dermoscopic changes in DNs, such as those shown in Figure 15.7, have biologic significance remains to be clarified.

Management

Management is summarized in Table 15.1, and in pregnancy, is essentially no different than in the nonpregnant patient. If a single nevus shows significant change and/or the change is out of proportion to changes seen in other nevi, it needs to be biopsied. Some authors recommend

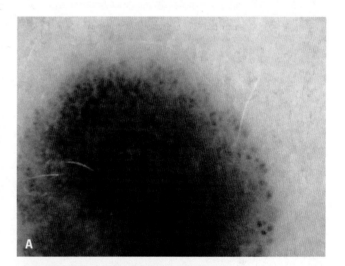

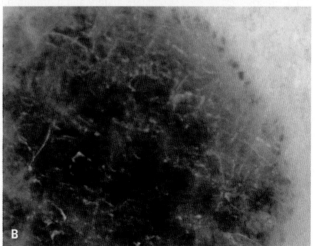

Figure 15.6. Dermoscopy of an abdominal nevus (**A**) at 6 months' gestation and (**B**) at 9 months' postpartum. Note in image **B** the symmetric enlargement, the absence of major architectural changes, and the thicker pigment network on the right lower side. There are a few globules at the right upper side of the periphery. The light color is due to abdominal distention with subsequent thinning of the nevus and pressure of the nevocytic nests down to the basal membrane. (Courtesy of Dr. Alin Tatu.)

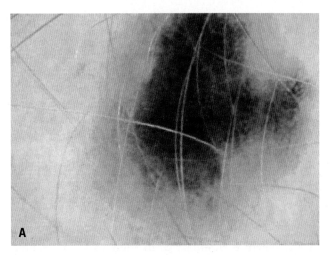
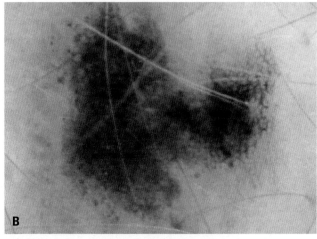

Figure 15.7. Dermoscopy pictures of a dysplastic nevus (**A**) at 4 months' gestation and (**B**) at 9 months' postpartum. Note the asymmetric enlargement; the architectural disorder; the thicker, irregular pigment network; and the presence of peripheral irregular globules on the left upper and right lower sides. (Courtesy of Dr. Alin Tatu.)

TABLE 15.1	Summary of Management Options for Melanocytic Nevi and Malignant Melanoma
Melanocytic Nevi	
Evaluation	■ Thorough personal and family history ■ Complete body skin examination ■ Dermoscopy by experienced physician
Consultation	■ Review changes of benign and atypical nevi in pregnancy ■ Recommend biopsy (if indicated)
Treatment	■ Biopsy of significantly changing nevi or nevi changing out of proportion to others ■ Re-excision of biopsy-proven DN may be postponed to postpartum unless biopsy shows severe atypia ■ Excision of fast-growing nevi ■ Excision if biopsy shows MM (see the following) ■ Clinical follow-up of nevi with minor changes that were not biopsied
Malignant Melanoma	

Evaluation	■ Complete history and thorough examination
	■ Pathology with special attention on Breslow thickness, ulceration, and mitoses
	■ SLNB, preferably without isosulfan blue dye,[36] for tumor stage ≥ T1b if thickness >0.75 mm[33]
	■ Evaluation for distant metastases:
	  ■ Stage < IIB: No scans needed in the absence of clinical suspicion
	  ■ Stage IIB/IIIA: CXR with appropriate shielding and u/s of abdomen/liver
	  ■ Stage > IIIA: Head MRI + PET/CT with an explanation of fetal risks (MRI safer than CT after first trimester)[34]

Consultation	■ Review stage and maternal and fetal prognosis ■ Review risks associated with Rx options
Treatment: Stage I/II	■ WLE with margin determined by Breslow depth under local anesthesia[34] ■ CLND if SLNB is positive[38]
Treatment: Stage III	■ WLE of primary MM (as previous) ■ TLND[38]
Treatment: Stage IV	■ Conservative excision; submit any remaining tissue for *BRAF* mutation analysis ■ Elective termination and tailored Rx (first trimester)[38] ■ Tailored Rx and induction when fetus is viable (second trimester)[38] ■ Induction when fetus is viable and tailored Rx (third trimester)[38] ■ Postpartum examination of placenta[34]

CLND, complete lymph node dissection; CT, computed tomography; CXR, chest X-ray; DN, dysplastic nevus; MM, malignant melanoma; MRI, magnetic resonance imaging; PET, positron emission tomography; Rx, treatment; SLNB, sentinel lymph node biopsy; TLND, therapeutic lymph node dissection; u/s, ultrasound; WLE, wide local excision.

only a clinical follow-up in patients presenting with darkening of multiple nevi because MM is more likely in a single changing lesion than in multiple lesions simultaneously. However, referral to dermatology is advisable and can help reduce patient anxiety. Minor changes in size, especially on areas susceptible to expansion, such as the abdomen, should be recognized, which may help minimize unnecessary biopsies. Excision typically is the recommended treatment for fast-growing nevi.

MALIGNANT MELANOMA

Epidemiology

MM is the most common malignancy in pregnancy and lactation, accounting for 31% and 24% of all malignancies diagnosed, respectively.[17] The incidence of melanoma in pregnancy ranges between 2.8 and 8.5 cases per 100,000 women.[18,19]

Hormonal Influences

Epidemiologic data show a higher survival rate in women compared to men with metastatic disease and in premenopausal compared to postmenopausal women, implicating that endogenous estrogens may play a protective role in MM. Nevertheless, the role of estrogens in MM remains unclear. Expression of ERβ (the predominant ER in the skin that antagonizes the proliferative action of ERα) decreases progressively with increased Breslow thickness and results in more invasive MMs[20]; thus, MMs with an increased level of ERβ expression and conversely decreased ERα expression may be associated with an improved prognosis. These studies implicate ERβ as an important factor in MM progression. In the study by Kvaskoff et al.,[21] which assessed the role of endogenous ovarian produced hormones on MM risk, risk of MM was reduced in women with ≥15 years at menarche, irregular menstrual cycles, <48 years at menopause, and shorter ovulatory life. MM risk increased with parity, the number of pregnancies, and miscarriages. These findings may suggest a reduced MM risk associated with an overall shorter ovulatory life span. However, an effect of parity on MM risk has been less conclusive in other studies.

Clinical Features

Clinical features, including the type and distribution, are not different than those in the nonpregnant patient.[22] Features of nodular and superficial spreading melanoma are shown in Figures 15.8 and 15.9, respectively.

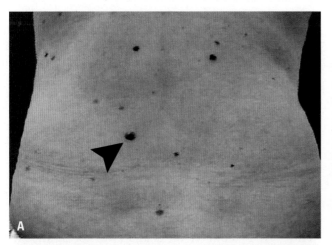

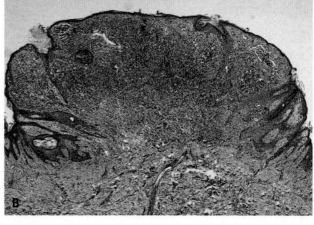

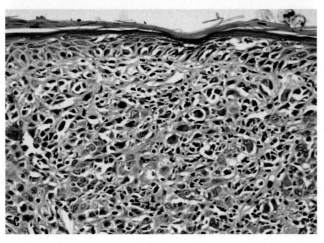

Figure 15.8. (**A**) A nodular melanoma (*arrow*) in a 38-year-old pregnant patient. The tumor developed during gestation in a preexisting nevus. (**B**) Histopathology shows contiguous vertical growth of atypical melanocytes in the dermis. Breslow depth was 2 mm, Clark level III, lymphocytic infiltrate was present in and around the tumor, and mitoses 2/mm² (hematoxylin-eosin, ×10). (**C**) A higher magnification shows atypical melanocytes with predominantly epithelioid morphology, which exhibit a great variation in size and shape. There are uniformly atypical nuclei, mitotic figures, and an absence of maturation (hematoxylin-eosin, ×20).

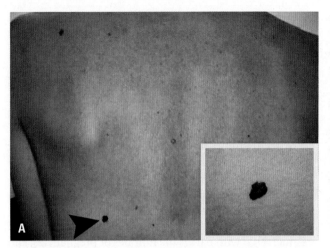 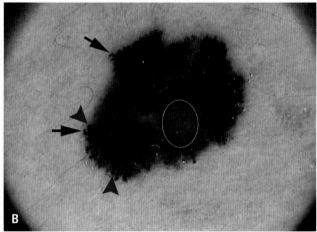

Figure 15.9. (**A**) A superficial spreading melanoma *(arrow)* in a 32-year-old pregnant patient. The inset shows a close view of the tumor. A histopathology showed a Breslow depth of 0.6 mm, and Clark level III. (**B**) Dermoscopy showed an asymmetric pigmented lesion exhibiting irregular streaks *(blue arrows)*, irregular dots/globules *(red arrows)*, and blue-white structures *(white circle)*, a constellation of features that is consistent with melanoma. (Courtesy of Dr. Fernando Augusto de Almeida.)

Histopathologic Features

Three studies have shown thicker MMs in pregnancy[23-25]; however, most studies, including large population studies, did not show an increased tumor thickness for MM in pregnancy.

Maternal Prognosis

Herein, we present groups of studies with three separate conclusions about the impact of pregnancy on the prognosis of MM: (1) pregnant patients develop thicker MMs than nonpregnant controls[23,24]; however, when depth is controlled for, pregnancy has no effect on survival; (2) pregnancy has no effect on prognosis[18,19,22,26-28]; and (3) pregnancy has an adverse effect on MM prognosis (when controlling for tumor depth and other factors).[17,25,28,29] These studies are summarized in Table 15.2.

Thicker melanomas are either not associated with worse overall survival[24] or there is no effect on survival after correcting for tumor thickness.[23] The study by Slingluff et al.[25] showed thicker tumors in pregnancy and shortened disease-free intervals (DFIs), but there was no effect on overall survival. As shown in Table 15.2, most studies on clinically localized MM[22,23,24,26,29] did not show an effect of pregnancy on survival. Therefore, the evidence does not support recommending a delay in childbearing for these patients.

The largest population studies to date[17,18,27] merit a comment. The study by O'Meara et al.,[18] which used data from the California Cancer Registry (1991 to 1999), showed no difference in the pregnancy-associated incidence, distribution of disease stage, or tumor thickness in pregnant versus nonpregnant controls.[18] Pregnancy had no impact on survival, and neonatal outcomes were not affected. Small numbers of women with advanced MM

and the inability to capture MM occurring in pregnancies that were lost or terminated prior to 20 weeks limited the conclusions primarily to women with localized MM.

A retrospective cohort by Lens et al.,[27] which used data from the Swedish National and Regional Registries, showed no statistically significant difference in overall survival between pregnant and nonpregnant groups; the authors' subsequent analysis showed that cause-specific survival is not affected.[30] Pregnancy status after a diagnosis of MM was not a significant predictor of survival. The group also performed a pooled analysis of 10 case-control studies (1966 to 2007) and found a lack of association between MM risk and pregnancy.[19] Interestingly, their data suggest a protective effect of hormones on MM risk where women with higher parity ($\geq$5 live births) had moderately lower MM risk compared with nulliparous women.[19]

Finally, the study by Stensheim et al.,[17] which used data from the Cancer and Medical Birth Registries of Norway, showed a borderline increase in cause-specific survival in patients diagnosed with MM in pregnancy (hazards ratio [HR] = 1.52); however, the analysis was not adjusted for tumor thickness, and after adjusting for body site, there was no increase in cause-specific survival (HR, 1.45, 95% confidence interval [CI], 0.96 to 2.21).[30] The aforementioned large population studies show that survival in MM developing in pregnancy is not affected by gestation. However, because these studies included relatively small numbers of patients with stage III/IV disease, it is premature to conclude about the prognosis of this stage of MM.

Fetal prognosis

Although placental metastasis from maternal cancer is very rare, MM is the most common malignancy to metastasize to the placenta and fetus. The largest review reported 87 cases of placental and/or fetal metastasis, and

TABLE 15.2	Studies on the Prognosis of Melanoma Arising in Pregnancy[a]	
First Author (ref)	**Pregnant Pts (Stage)/Nonpregnant MM Controls**	**Findings**
Thicker Melanomas in Pregnancy; No Effect on Prognosis or No Effect After Correcting for Tumor Thickness[b]		
MacKie et al.[23c]	92 pts with stage I/II MM and 296 controls	No effect on DFI or survival after correcting for tumor thickness
Travers et al.[24]	45 pts (stage stated as "clinically localized") and 420 controls	Trend toward better survival in pregnant MM pts
Pregnancy Has No Effect on Prognosis		
Daryanani et al.[26]	46 pts with stage I/II and 368 controls	No difference in 10-year DFI and 10-year survival between groups
Wong et al.[22]	66 pts with stage I MM and 619 controls	No differences in tumor location, histologic features and 5-year survival between groups
O'Meara et al.[18]	412 pts; MM diagnosed during or within 1 year of pregnancy (all stages) and 2,451 controls	No difference in stage, tumor thickness or prognosis between pt and control groups
Lens et al.[27]	185 pts (stage not stated; 7/65 had Breslow depth >4 mm) and 5,348 nonpregnant controls	No difference in survival between pt and control groups
Lens et al.[19]	Pooled analysis of 10 case-control studies (2,391 pts and 3,199 controls)	Pregnancy does not affect survival
Adverse Effect of Pregnancy on Prognosis		
Slingluff et al.[25]	100 pts (all stages) and 86 controls	Thicker MMs ($P = .05$), ↑ metastatic disease ($P = .008$) but no difference in OS between groups
Trapeznikov et al.[28]	102 pts (all stages) and 599 nonlactating controls	↓ 10-year survival in pts compared to controls ($P < .05$)
Reintgen et al.[29]	58 pts (stage I) and 585 controls (became pregnant within 5 years of MM)	↓ DFI in pts compared to controls ($P = .04$)
Stensheim et al.[17]	160 pts (stage not stated; Breslow depth available for 55% of pts) and 4,460 controls	Slightly ↑ risk of cause-specific death (HR, 1.52) in pts

[a] Table includes only studies of ≥45 patients.

[b] Group also includes study by Slingluff et al. (shown in lower third of the table).

[c] There were 143 who completed their pregnancy before MM; 85 were diagnosed/treated before pregnancy; and 68 were diagnosed between pregnancies.

DFI, disease-free interval; HR, hazard ratio; MM, malignant melanoma; OS, [MM1]; pts, patients; ↑, increased; ↓, decreased.

27 of these cases (31%) were secondary to MM.[31] The fetus was affected in 6 out of 27 cases (22%; or 50% to 60% of tumors with fetal involvement), and 5 out of 6 infants died of the disease. The fetal involvement is always associated with at least a microscopic invasion of the placenta.[32] The increased production of growth factors during pregnancy and vascularity of the placenta may promote metastasis. Maternal outcome is fatal, with most deaths occurring within 7 months of placental and/or fetal metastasis. Placentas of women with known or suspected metastatic MM should be examined grossly and histologically after delivery. Neonates delivered with concomitant placental involvement should be considered a high-risk population.[31] Systemic evaluations and close follow-ups are recommended, and several diagnostic tests have been proposed.[31–32] Infant disease-free survival to 1 year may be associated with an absence of metastatic involvement.[32]

Pregnancy After a Diagnosis of Melanoma

There are no standard recommendations regarding the length of time to wait before becoming pregnant after a diagnosis of MM. If recurrence develops during pregnancy, it may be disastrous both medically and emotionally for the patient and there are potential fetal risks. Tumor thickness is the single most important predictor of recurrence. MacKie et al.[23] showed that the 5-year recurrence rate for tumors <1.5 mm was <10%, but the 5-year mortality rate for tumors 1.5 to 3.5 mm thick was 30%, and >50% for tumors >3.5 mm thick. The authors recommended that the time to wait before becoming pregnant should be based on tumor thickness, evidence of vascular spread, and body site.

MacKie et al.[23] also indicated that 83% of recurrences in stage II occurred within 2 years of initial treatment and recommended that patients with stage I/II disease wait 2 years after surgery before becoming pregnant. Along the same lines, Schwartz, Mozurkewich, and Johnson[33] suggested that patients with thin MMs wait 2 years, whereas patients with thicker lesions wait 3 to 5 years before becoming pregnant. Most authors concur that the recommendation about how long to wait before becoming pregnant after a diagnosis of melanoma should be made on a case-by-case basis, depending primarily on the risk of recurrence (tumor thickness) and the age of the patient, which affects the potential to conceive.

Management

The evaluation of a patient developing MM in pregnancy is shown in Table 15.1. Consultation should include a discussion about the necessary diagnostic workup, the stage and the prognosis, as well as maternal and fetal risks, including those secondary to diagnostic procedures, chemotherapy, and immunotherapy. A recommendation for avoiding oral contraceptives or hormone replacement therapy after the diagnosis of MM[33] is not supported by case-control studies.[34] The consultation for patients with stage IV disease should include the risk of fetal metastasis, which carries a poor prognosis.

The most powerful prognostic factor in clinically localized melanoma is the status of the sentinel lymph node biopsy (SLNB) (recommended for stage ≥T1b if thickness >0.75 mm). SLNB uses a preoperative intradermal injection of technetium-99m (^{99m}Tc)-sulfur colloid and an intraoperative, intradermal injection of blue dye around the tumor.[35] Radiopharmaceuticals used in SLNB deliver doses <5 mGy, which are considered harmless for the fetus (see Ch. 24).[34] However, allergic reactions to isosulfan blue dye have been reported (≤2%), and the incidence of a life-threatening anaphylactic reaction is 0.7% to 1.1%.[36] To prevent these complications, Schwartz et al.[33] proposed the use of radiocolloid alone for SLNB in the first trimester. The authors also suggested that wide local excision and SLNB with blue dye may be delayed until after delivery in women who are in the second half of pregnancy and who have undergone narrow excision of their primary MM with clear histologic margins.[29] Along the same lines, some authors propose postponing SLNB until after delivery for MM at low risk for nodal involvement stages (T1b to T2b).[37] Other staging procedures are shown in Table 15.1. A magnetic resonance imaging (MRI) scan can be used when other nonionizing diagnostic procedures do not suffice, but because it carries a risk of tissue overheating, it should not be used in the first trimester.

Treatment requires a multidisciplinary approach, especially if SLNB is required. For stage I/II disease (no lymph node involvement or distal metastasis), treatment is the same as in a nonpregnant patient. Complete excision under local anesthesia with margins determined by Breslow depth is recommended. The indication for a complete lymph node dissection after SLNB or therapeutic lymph node dissection for regional metastatic MM (stage III disease) does not differ from nonpregnant patients[38]; the former procedure has no proven effect on overall survival. In a disease presenting with distant metastases (stage IV), tailored treatment is recommended, as well as an induction of labor when the fetus is viable (see Table 15.2). Termination of pregnancy can be offered to stage IV patients in the first trimester but is not recommended as it does not, by itself, affect the outcome of MM in the mother[34] and the risk of fetal metastasis is remote.

In stage III/IV disease, less aggressive therapy may be advisable in order to prevent fetal adverse effects with little gain for the mother[34]; survival for pregnant patients treated with chemotherapy (3 to 8 months) did not differ from that of nonpregnant patients who received such therapy. If the patient decides for chemotherapy or radiation, waiting and inducing delivery at 34 weeks prior to the beginning of therapy should be considered,[39] because the perinatal mortality at 34 weeks in a neonatal care unit approaches that of a term delivery. The benefits from other systemic therapies may not justify the risks associated with them, and experience with adjuvant high-dose interferon-α therapy in pregnancy is minimal.

OTHER MALIGNANT SKIN TUMORS

There is currently no epidemiologic data on the prevalence of nonmelanoma skin cancer in pregnancy. Preliminary evidence suggests that stromal tumors, such as dermatofibrosarcoma protuberans, may grow in pregnancy,[40] and Kaposi sarcoma (KS) may not be adversely affected by pregnancy.[41]

Basal Cell and Squamous Cell Carcinoma

The rarity of reports on basal cell carcinomas (BCCs) occurring in pregnancy indicates that they may not be affected by gestation. Cases of metastatic BCC[42] and multiple BCCs related to human papillomavirus during pregnancy[43] have been reported. There are several case reports of aggressive squamous cell carcinoma (SCC) of the aerodigestive track presenting during pregnancy, which suggests a hormonal stimulation of the growth and/or aggressive behavior of these tumors. In one case, progression from a benign odontogenic cyst to a hybrid verrucous carcinoma/SCC was attributed to the hormonal changes of pregnancy.[44] Also, there are a number of cases of aggressive vulvar SCCs (Fig. 15.10) that developed in pregnancy. All suspicious vulvar lesions should be promptly biopsied, and vulvar symptoms, not secondary to an infectious etiology, should be thoroughly examined. The management of vulvar

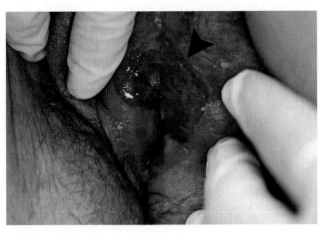

Figure 15.10. Vulvar squamous cell carcinoma (lesion shown with *arrow*). (Courtesy of Dr. Joe Brooks.)

carcinoma in pregnancy is not different than in the non-pregnant state, but the gestational age must be considered.[45]

Kaposi Sarcoma

Spontaneous remissions of KS (see Fig. 15.11) during pregnancy have stimulated investigations into the potential anti-KS activity of human chorionic gonadotropin (hCG). Clinical-grade preparations of hCG have been shown to be toxic to KS cells.[41] However, the mechanism of the anti-KS activity of these preparations remains unclear, and results of studies using commercial hCG preparations in human KS are contradictory due to the fact that pro- and anti-KS components are present in varying proportions in different hCG preparations. Crude urine from first trimester pregnant women, the source for commercial hCG, had a growth stimulatory effect on KS cells, whereas urine from third trimester women, nonpregnant young women, menopausal women, and men exhibited no effect on the growth of KS cells.[46] Given these diverse effects, a cautious use of hCG purified from pregnancy urine for the treatment of KS is recommended.

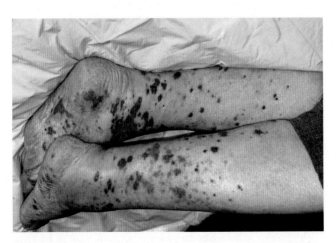

Figure 15.11. Kaposi sarcoma in an HIV-positive female patient presenting with typical violaceous plaques on the lower extremities.

KS in HIV-infected women, which is often misdiagnosed, has an aggressive clinical course, with high rates of visceral involvement and decreased survival. One case of isolated pulmonary KS in pregnancy has been reported.[47] A patient was diagnosed with AIDS after presenting at 25 weeks' gestation with a cough and multiple pulmonary nodules. A thorascopic lung biopsy revealed KS. Despite antiretroviral therapy, KS progressed. Labor was induced at 33.5 weeks' gestation after fetal distress. Postpartum chemotherapy resulted in remission.

Dermatofibrosarcoma Protuberans

There have been several reports of dermatofibrosarcoma protuberans growing rapidly in pregnancy.[40] The tumors showed expression of a progesterone receptor, which may account for their accelerated growth in pregnancy.

Merkel Cell Carcinoma

Whether pregnancy accelerates the progression of Merkel cell carcinoma remains unknown. There are a handful of reports of Merkel cell carcinoma that developed rapidly during pregnancy.[48–50] The outcome was dismal in two of three cases[49–50]; patients died within 2 years of diagnosis.

Mycosis Fungoides

The effect of pregnancy on mycosis fungoides (MF) is unknown. The largest case series is comprised of 12 patients: 9 with MF and 3 with parapsoriasis en plaques (PPP).[51] Of the 12 pregnancies, 11 were uneventful and 1 was associated with abortion. There was no indication that pregnancy changed the course or prognosis of MF or PPP. A patient with advanced (stage IVb) MF presented around the period of conception with a relapse.[52] The relapse responded intrapartum to photon radiotherapy, and the pregnancy was otherwise uneventful. Another patient presented with tumor stage MF in pregnancy was induced at 36 weeks and succumbed to the disease at 3 months' postpartum while being treated with denileukin diftitox.[53]

MATERNAL RISKS

Benign tumors: Symptomatic aggravation
Melanoma: Same as in the nonpregnant patient
Other malignant skin tumors: Same as in the nonpregnant patient

FETAL RISKS

Benign tumors: None
Melanoma: Placental and/or fetal metastasis and death; risks from chemotherapy, radiotherapy, or radiodiagnostic procedures
Other malignant skin tumors: Risks from chemotherapy, radiotherapy, or radiodiagnostic procedures

KEY POINTS

- A wide spectrum of epidermal, fibrous, vascular, neural, and other benign tumors may develop or grow in pregnancy.

- Clinical and dermoscopic changes of benign melanocytic nevi during gestation are mild and often transient; however, dysplastic nevi may develop substantial changes.

- The approach to melanocytic nevi is not different than in the nonpregnant patient; any significantly changing nevi should be biopsied.

- Large population studies indicate that overall survival of melanoma developing in pregnancy is not affected by gestation; however, data are insufficient for stage III/IV disease.

- For stage I/II melanoma, treatment with wide local excision is the standard of care; for stage III/IV disease, a risk benefit analysis should determine whether tailored treatment should be provided before or after delivery.

- The relationship of other malignant skin tumors with pregnancy remains unclear, and the course of most may not be adversely affected by gestation.

REFERENCES

1. Kroumpouzos G, Cohen LM. Dermatoses of pregnancy. *J Am Acad Dermatol*. 2001;45:1–19.
2. Sanchez JL, Figueroa LD, Rodriguez E. Behavior of melanocytic nevi during pregnancy. *Am J Dermapathol*. 1984;6:s84–s89.
3. Ellis DL. Pregnancy and sex steroid hormone effects on nevi of patients with the dysplastic nevus syndrome. *J Am Acad Dermatol*. 1991;2:467–482.
4. Yılmaz E, Kelekci KH, Kelekci S. Skin tag and acanthosis nigricans: do they have a predictive value for gestational diabetes mellitus? *Exp Clin Endocrinol Diabetes*. 2011;119:419–422.
5. Stainforth J, Goodfield MJ. Multiple dermatofibromata developing during pregnancy. *Clin Exp Dermatol*. 1994;19:59–60.
6. McClung AA, Blumberg MA, Huttenbach Y, et al. Development of collagenomas during pregnancy. *J Am Acad Dermatol*. 2005;53:S150–S153.
7. Maldonado Cid P, Sendagorta Cudós E, Noguera Morel L, et al. Bilateral segmental neurofibromatosis diagnosed during pregnancy. *Dermatol Online J*. 2011;17(5):6.
8. Onsun N, Saracoglu S, Demirkesen C, et al. Eruptive widespread Spitz nevi: can pregnancy be a stimulating factor? *J Am Acad Dermatol*. 1999;40:866–867.
9. Nading MA, Nanney LB, Boyd AS, et al. Estrogen receptor beta expression in nevi during pregnancy. *Exp Dermatol*. 2008;17:489–497.
10. Chan MP, Chan MM, Tahan SR. Melanocytic nevi in pregnancy: histologic features and Ki-67 proliferation index. *J Cutan Pathol*. 2010;37:843–851.
11. Foucar E, Bentley TJ, Laube DW, et al. A histopathologic evaluation of nevocellular nevi in pregnancy. *Arch Dermatol*. 1985;121:350–354.
12. Pennoyer JW, Grin CM, Driscoll MS, et al. Changes in size of melanocytic nevi during pregnancy. *J Am Acad Dermatol*. 1997;36:378–382.
13. Zampino MR, Corazza M, Costantino D, et al. Are melanocytic nevi influenced by pregnancy? A dermoscopic evaluation. *Dermatol Surg*. 2006;32:1497–1504.
14. Aktürk AS, Bilen N, Bayrämgürler D, et al. Dermoscopy is a suitable method for the observation of the pregnancy-related changes in melanocytic nevi. *J Eur Acad Dermatol Venereol*. 2007;21:1086–1090.
15. Rubegni P, Sbano P, Burroni M, et al. Melanocytic skin lesions and pregnancy: digital dermoscopy analysis. *Skin Res Technol*. 2007;13:143–147.
16. Wyon Y, Synnerstadt I, Fredrickson M, et al. Spectrophotometric analysis of melanocytic naevi during pregnancy. *Acta Derm Venereol*. 2007;87:231–237.
17. Stensheim H, Møller B, van Dijk T, et al. Cause-specific survival for women diagnosed with cancer during pregnancy or lactation: a registry-based cohort study. *J Clin Oncol*. 2009;27:45–51.
18. O'Meara T, Cress R, Xing G, et al. Malignant melanoma in pregnancy. A population-based evaluation. *Cancer*. 2005;103:1217–1226.
19. Lens M, Bataille V. Melanoma in relation to reproductive and hormonal factors in women: current review on controversial issues. *Cancer Causes Control*. 2008;19:437–442.
20. Di Giorgi V, Gori A, Grazzini M, et al. Estrogens, estrogen receptors and melanoma. *Expert Rev Anticancer Ther*. 2011;11:739–747.
21. Kvaskoff M, Bijon A, Mesrine S, et al. Cutaneous melanoma and endogenous hormonal factors: a large French prospective study. *Am J Epidemiol*. 2011;173:1192–1202.
22. Wong JH, Sterns EE, Kopald KH, et al. Prognostic significance of pregnancy in stage I melanoma. *Arch Surg*. 1989;124:1227–1230.
23. MacKie RM, Bufalino R, Morabito A, et al. Lack of effect of pregnancy on outcome of melanoma. For The World Health Organisation Melanoma Programme. *Lancet*. 1991;337:653–655.
24. Travers RL, Sober AJ, Berwick M, et al. Increased thickness of pregnancy-associated melanoma. *Br J Dermatol*. 1995;132:876–883.
25. Slingluff CL, Reintgen D, Vollmer R, et al. Malignant melanoma arising during pregnancy. A study of 100 patients. *Ann Surg*. 1990;211:552–557.
26. Daryanani D, Plukker JT, De Hullu JA, et al. Pregnancy and early-stage melanoma. *Cancer*. 2003;97:2248–2253.
27. Lens MB, Rosdahl I, Ahlbom A, et al. Effect of pregnancy on survival in women with cutaneous malignant melanoma. *J Clin Oncol*. 2004;22:4369–4375.
28. Trapeznikov NN, Khasanov ShR, Iavorski VV. Melanoma of the skin and pregnancy. *Vopr Onkol*. 1987;33:40–46.
29. Reintgen D, McCarty KS Jr, Vollmer R, et al. Malignant melanoma and pregnancy. *Cancer*. 1985;55:1340–1344.
30. Lens MB, Rosdahl I, Newton-Bishop J. Cutaneous melanoma during pregnancy: is the controversy over? *J Clin Oncol*. 2009;27:e11–e12.
31. Alexander A, Samlowski WE, Grossman D, et al. Metastatic melanoma in pregnancy: risk of transplacental metastases in the infant. *J Clin Oncol*. 2003;21:2179–2186.
32. Altman JF, Altman JF, Lowe L, et al. Placental metastasis of maternal melanoma. *J Am Acad Dermatol*. 2003;49:1150–1154.
33. Schwartz JL, Mozurkewich EL, Johnson TM. Current management of patients with melanoma who are pregnant, want to get pregnant, or do not want to get pregnant. *Cancer*. 2003;97:2130–2133.
34. Leachman SA, Jackson R, Eliason MJ, et al. Management of melanoma during pregnancy. *Dermatol Nurs*. 2007;19:145–152.

35. Gershenwald JE, Thompson W, Mansfield PF, et al. Multi-institutional melanoma lymphatic mapping experience: the prognostic value of sentinel lymph node status in 612 Stage I or II melanoma patients. *J Clin Oncol.* 1999;17:976–983.

36. Cimmino VM, Brown AC, Szocik JF, et al. Allergic reactions to isosulfan blue during sentinel node biopsy—a common event. *Surgery.* 2001;130:439–442.

37. Broer N, Buonocore S, Goldberg C, et al. A proposal for the timing of management of patients with melanoma presenting during pregnancy. *J Surg Oncol.* 2012;106:36–40.

38. Pentheroudakis G, Orecchia R, Hoekstra HJ, et al. Cancer, fertility and pregnancy: ESMO Clinical Practice Guidelines for diagnosis, treatment and follow-up. *Ann Oncol.* 2010;21(suppl 5): v266–v273.

39. Beyeler M, Hafner J, Beinder E, et al. Special considerations for stage IV melanoma during pregnancy. *Arch Dermatol.* 2005;141: 1077–1079.

40. Parlette LE, Smith CK, Germain LM, et al. Accelerated growth of dermatofibrosarcoma protuberans during pregnancy. *J Am Acad Dermatol.* 1999;41:778–783.

41. Simonart T, Van Vooren JP, Meuris S. Treatment of Kaposi's sarcoma with human chorionic gonadotropin. *Dermatology.* 2002;204:330–333.

42. Sass U, Theunis A, Noël JC, et al. Multiple HPV-positive basal cell carcinomas on the abdomen in a young pregnant woman. *Dermatology.* 2002;204:362–364.

43. Larciprete F, De Felice G, Figliolini M. [Metastatic basalioma during pregnancy. (Description of a case)]. *Quad Clin Ostet Ginecol.* 1967;22:433–439.

44. Cudney N, Ochs MW, Johnson J, et al. A unique presentation of a squamous cell carcinoma in a pregnant patient. *Quintessence Int.* 2010;41:581–583.

45. Couvreux-Dif D, Lhommé C, Querleu D, et al. [Cancer of the vulva and pregnancy: two cases and review of the literature]. *J Gynecol Obstet Biol Reprod (Paris).* 2003;32:46–50.

46. Simonart T, Hermans P, Delogne-Desnoeck J, et al. Stimulation of Kaposi's sarcoma cell growth by urine from women in early pregnancy, the current source for clinical-grade human chorionic gonadotropin preparations. *Exp Dermatol.* 2002;11: 365–369.

47. Bryant AE, Genc M, Hurtado RM, et al. Pulmonary Kaposi's sarcoma in pregnancy. *Am J Perinatol.* 2004;21:355–363.

48. Kukko H, Vuola J, Suominen S, et al. Merkel cell carcinoma in a young pregnant woman. *J Plast Reconstr Aesthet Surg.* 2008;61: 1530–1533.

49. Kuppuswami N, Sivarajan KM, Hussein L, et al. Merkel cell tumor in pregnancy. A case report. *J Reprod Med.* 1991;36:613–615.

50. Chao TC, Park JM, Rhee H, et al. Merkel cell tumor of the back detected during pregnancy. *Plast Reconstr Surg.* 1990;86: 347–351.

51. Amitay-Layish I, David M, Kafri B, et al. Early-stage mycosis fungoides, parapsoriasis en plaque, and pregnancy. *Int J Dermatol.* 2007;46:160–165.

52. Castelo-Branco C, Torné A, Cararach V, et al. Mycosis fungoides and pregnancy. *Oncol Rep.* 2001;8:197–199.

53. Dalton SR, Hicks M, Shabanowitz R, et al. Ethical dilemmas in the management of tumor-stage mycosis fungoides in a pregnant patient. *J Am Acad Dermatol.* 2012;66:661–663.

CHAPTER 16

Miscellaneous Skin Disease

Joe Brooks ■ Paulo R. Cunha ■ George Kroumpouzos

INTRODUCTION

A large number of skin diseases, including genodermatoses and neutrophilic dermatoses, can be affected by pregnancy and/or are associated with significant maternal and fetal risks.[1–3] A multidisciplinary approach is often necessary in order to minimize risks and to provide optimal management.[4,5] This chapter highlights the course, management (see Table 16.1), and maternal and fetal risks associated with a variety of skin diseases in pregnancy.

GENODERMATOSES

Ehlers–Danlos Syndrome

Ehlers–Danlos syndrome (EDS) is a heterogeneous group of inherited disorders of collagen metabolism. Dermatologic manifestations include hyperextensible and fragile skin, "cigarette paper" thin scars that stretch excessively after healing (Fig. 16.1A), atrophic scars that become widened over time (Fig. 16.1B), bruising easily, cutaneous hemorrhages, delayed wound healing, and dehiscence.[6] Gingival bleeding after minor trauma and bleeding after surgical procedures are common. Extracutaneous manifestations include, among others, joint hypermobility, other musculoskeletal abnormalities, coronary and cerebral aneurysms, valve prolapse, major vessel dilatation or spontaneous dissections, and ocular and neurologic complications. Women with EDS types I to II (classic EDS), III (hypermobility EDS), and X (fibronectin abnormality) tolerate pregnancy well, and maternal and neonatal outcomes are favorable.[4,6,7] Common complications include pelvic instability, obstetric problems often causing preterm delivery, postpartum hemorrhage, complicated perineal lacerations, and poor wound healing of the episiotomy wound.

Patients with EDS type IV (ecchymotic or arterial) are particularly likely to develop complications during pregnancy. This type of EDS is associated with a pregnancy-related maternal mortality of 20% for each pregnancy and 38.5% for each pregnant woman.[6,8] The risks include premature rupture of the membranes; postpartum bleeding; rupture of major vessels, including the aorta and pulmonary artery; poor wound healing and dehiscence; uterine, vaginal, and perineal lacerations; bladder and uterine prolapse; and abdominal hernias. The rupture of major vessels in pregnancy is more common in type IV. The risks are such that women with EDS type IV should undergo preconception counseling and be advised against pregnancy.[9] Elective termination before 16 weeks has been accomplished, and risks have been manageable in most cases. If the patient chooses to continue pregnancy, serious consideration should be given to cesarean delivery at 32 weeks[8] because the majority of spontaneous deliveries occur between 32 and 35 weeks.[6] A cesarean delivery, however, has its own risks, such as perioperative hemorrhage and wound dehiscence,[6] and consultation with anesthesia is required. Other authors recommended early termination of pregnancy when ultrasonic examination of the aortic root reveals more than 20% enlargement above baseline or a diameter greater than 4 cm.[7]

Fetal risks include prematurity, intrauterine growth restriction (IUGR), and adverse outcome associated with maternal vascular prolapsed or musculoskeletal abnormalities, among others. Other risks include joint luxations; hernias; abnormal fetal presentations (19%), particularly with EDS type III; and floppy infant syndrome (13%). Clinical decisions should be based on knowledge of the specific type of EDS, and the mode of delivery should be tailored to the individual patient's needs. Because the disease is predominantly an autosomal dominant disorder, the risk of transmission to the fetus is 50%. A prenatal diagnosis via chorionic villous sampling or amniocentesis is possible if there is prior knowledge of the disease-causing mutation in the affected patient.[4]

Pseudoxanthoma Elasticum

Pseudoxanthoma elasticum (PXE) is a genetic disorder characterized by calcified dystrophic elastic fibers in the skin, retina, and arteries.[10] The mode of inheritance is autosomal recessive and, less often, autosomal dominant. Clinical manifestations include yellowish papules and plaques, with or without cutaneous laxity, on the neck (Fig. 16.2) and flexural areas, angioid streaks in the eye, and vascular complications including cardiovascular disease and gastrointestinal hemorrhage. Perforating periumbilical PXE (Fig. 16.3) has been reported in multiparous women; however, a clear etiology has not been established. The early literature that was reviewed by Berde, Willis, and Sandberg[11] indicated that pregnancy may worsen the

TABLE 16.1	Summary of Management Options
Condition	**Comment**
EDS, HHT, Marfan syndrome, PXE, Tuberous sclerosis, neurofibromatosis type 1	■ Preconception evaluation and counseling; multidisciplinary approach to prevent serious maternal and fetal complications; monitor blood pressure in PXE and blood transfusion for gastrointestinal bleeding; imaging studies in gestation; u/s scans of brain and heart in fetuses of TS-affected mothers; consider cesarean delivery at 32 weeks in EDS type IV; counsel about the risk of fetal transmission
Hereditary angioedema	■ C1 esterase concentrate[23]; prophylaxis with tranexamic acid or fresh frozen plasma[23]; inspect sites of trauma; regional anesthesia for operative deliveries
Pyoderma gangrenosum	■ High-dose systemic corticosteroids[27]; cyclosporine allows tapering of steroids[27]; azathioprine (one case)[27]; IVIG (one case)[30]; topical/intralesional corticosteroids[27]; local care; rule out underlying disease
Erythema nodosum	■ Rule out underlying disease; supportive Rx (bed rest, paracetamol); removal of culprit drugs; Rx of underlying disease; short course of systemic steroid, if necessary
Vasculitides	■ Conservative approach (i.e., observation or topical steroids, for purely cutaneous disease) ■ Systemic vasculitis[35]: Systemic corticosteroids; azathioprine; cyclophosphamide (severe disease; may use after first trimester); IVIG (second-line Rx)
Sarcoidosis	■ Systemic corticosteroids[42]; other Rx depending on specific organ involvement
Mastocytosis	■ Prophylactic H_1 (chlorpheniramine, cetirizine, loratadine) and H_2 antihistamines (ranitidine)[48]

EDS, Ehlers–Danlos syndrome; HHT, hereditary hemorrhagic telangiectasia; IVIG, intravenous immunoglobulin; PXE, pseudoxanthoma elasticum; Rx, treatment; TS, tuberous sclerosis; u/s, ultrasound.

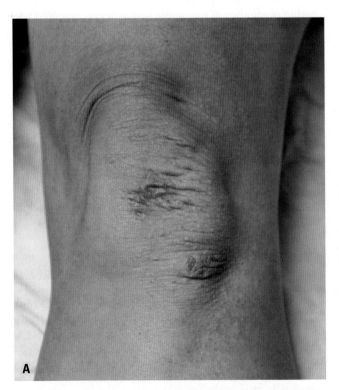

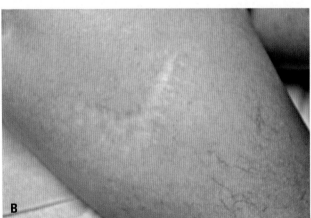

Figure 16.1. Ehlers–Danlos syndrome type II (classic). (**A**) "Cigarette paper" scars on the knee. (**B**) A scar on the thigh developed in pregnancy without prior trauma; scar become widened over time. Patient had two miscarriages and a stillborn at 26 weeks secondary to premature shortening of the cervix. However, three other pregnancies were uncomplicated.

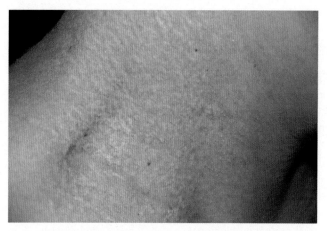

Figure 16.2. Pseudoxanthoma elasticum: Yellow papules coalescing to plaques are typically distributed on the neck. (Courtesy of Dr. Lionel Bercovitch.)

vascular complications of PXE. The main complication is massive hematemesis from gastrointestinal, especially gastric, bleeding, but case reports of repeated epistaxis and congestive heart failure with ventricular arrhythmia have been published.[11] A gastroscopy shows patches of petechiae or a generalized oozing of gastric mucosa[3] and mucosal biopsy degeneration of the elastic fibers in medium-sized arteries with disruption of internal lamellae and formation of microaneurysms.[11] Obstetric complications included hypertension, an increased risk of first-trimester miscarriage, and IUGR secondary to placental insufficiency.

Nevertheless, a retrospective study of 54 pregnancies in 20 South African women with PXE indicated an increased risk of first-trimester abortion (not substantiated by statistical analysis) and cosmetic deterioration of abdominal skin.[12] A subsequent study by Bercovitch and associates[10] showed that PXE was not associated with markedly increased fetal loss or adverse reproductive outcomes. The study reported that the incidence of gastric bleeding and

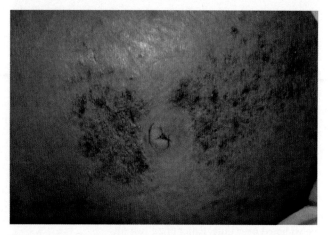

Figure 16.3. Periumbilical perforating pseudoxanthoma elasticum: Yellow to brown plaque composed of coalescing keratotic papules. This presentation is more common in multiparous women of African descent. (Courtesy of Dr. Mayra Ianhez.)

retinal complications is lower than previously reported, although probably higher than in the general population. Worsening of skin manifestation was noted in 12% of patients. It was concluded that most pregnancies are uncomplicated, and there is no basis for advising women with PXE to avoid becoming pregnant. Because of the vascular complications of PXE in pregnancy, vigilant control of the blood pressure to decrease the risk of hemorrhage is crucial.[11] Blood transfusion is required to manage gastrointestinal bleeding.[3] However, a patient who plans a pregnancy should be advised about the possibility of disease exacerbation during pregnancy, fetal complications, and the risk of genetic transmission of the disease to the child.

Tuberous Sclerosis

Tuberous sclerosis (TS) is an autosomal dominant genetic disorder characterized by hamartomas in several organs, including the eyes, brain, kidneys, heart, and lungs, as well as seizures and mental retardation.[13] Mucocutaneous manifestations can be the only sign of the disease and include congenital hypopigmented macules, facial angiofibromas, collagenomas, periungual fibromas (Fig. 16.4), gingival fibromas, and dental enamel pits. The course of TS in pregnancy varies considerably and depends on the maternal expression of the disease.[13] Several successful pregnancies have been reported. Of the six reported cases that were reviewed by Gounden,[14] the diagnosis was made during pregnancy in two; these two patients presented with a retroperitoneal mass antenatally, which turned out to be angiolipoma of the kidney. King and Stamilio[15] reported rates of complications in 23 pregnancies complicated by maternal TS: 43% of patients, including all patients with TS-associated renal disease, had perinatal complications, and rates of preterm and cesarean delivery were 35% and 33%, respectively. Perinatal complications included, among others, polyhydramnios, hemorrhage from ruptured renal tumors, acute renal failure, placental abruption, preeclampsia, IUGR, hydrops fetalis, and fetal demise. Renal involvement was the most important prognostic factor in six pregnancies reviewed by Petrikovsky et al.,[13] and renal evaluation should be included in preconception counseling. Ultrasound scans should be performed to detect any intracranial lesions, cardiac rhabdomyoma, and renal size. Fetal prognosis depends on maternal disease status in pregnancy, as well as the presence of TS lesions in the fetus, such as cardiac rhabdomyomas, which have been associated a mortality rate of 16%.[15] Ultrasound scans of the heart and brain should be performed in fetuses of affected mothers.[15] Delivery is indicated at the earliest sign of fetal compromise.[15]

Neurofibromatosis Type 1

Neurofibromatosis type 1 (NF1) is an autosomal dominant disorder characterized by the presence of pigmented lesions, such as café au lait spots and axillary/inguinal freckling (Fig. 16.5A), cutaneous neurofibromas

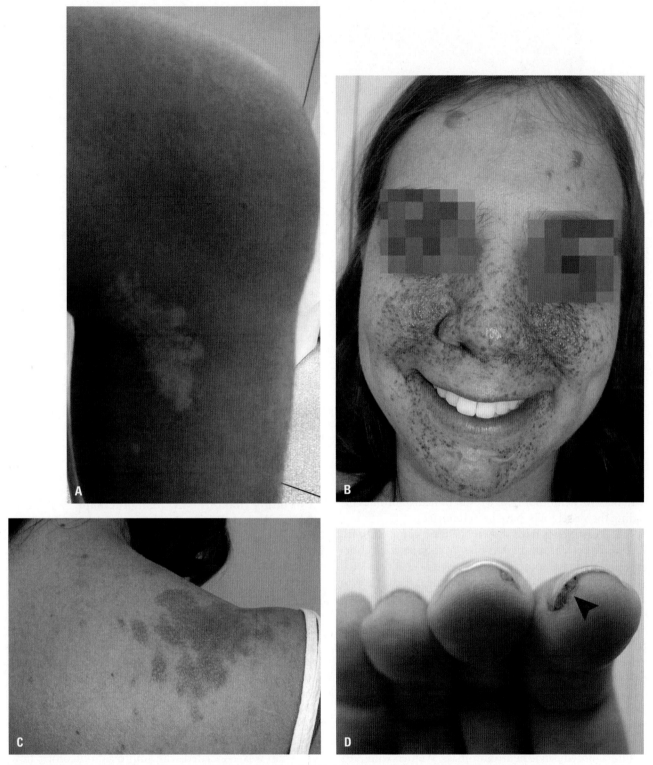

Figure 16.4. Cutaneous manifestations of tuberous sclerosis. **(A)** Ash leaf macule, a congenital hypopigmented lesion. **(B)** Facial angiofibromas are typically noted in the centrofacial area. **(C)** A shagreen ("leather") patch is a connective tissue nevus most commonly located in the lumbosacral area. **(D)** Koenen tumors are periungual fibromas; here, shown in a subungual location *(arrow)*. (Courtesy of Dr. Mayra Ianhez.)

(Fig. 16.5B), Lisch nodules of the iris, and osseous lesions.[5] Tumors of the spinal cord or cranial nerves have a potential of malignant transformation. The most common effect of pregnancy on NF1 is an increase in the growth of new or existing neurofibromas in 55% to 60% of patients.[5]

Neurofibroma size may decrease postpartum in approximately 30% of these patients. Cases of malignant tumor growth in pregnancy, such as a mediastinal malignant peripheral nerve sheath tumor, have been reported. Both renal artery rupture and vessel rupture in the pleural cavity

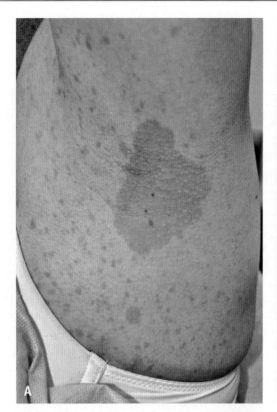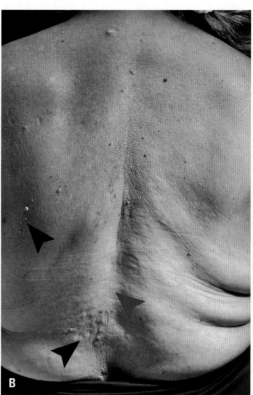

Figure 16.5. Neurofibromatosis type 1. (**A**) Axillary freckling and a café au lait macule. (**B**) Solitary and grouped neurofibromas *(black arrows)* on the back and kyphoscoliosis *(red arrow)*. Kyphoscoliosis caused fetal malpresentation in this patient's pregnancy, which necessitated a cesarean delivery. This is a common obstetric complication of the disease.

with massive hemothorax, as a result of neurofibromas invading the vessel walls, have been reported.

Small case series have shown obstetric complications, such as hypertension, first-trimester spontaneous abortion, and perinatal complications as well as fetal risks such as stillbirth, and IUGR.[16,17] However, the largest study to date did not confirm them and showed only a higher incidence of cesarean delivery (36% of deliveries that resulted in live births), a small part of which related to maternal NF1 complications.[18] The study reported a 17.8% incidence of first-trimester spontaneous abortions but did not report on that of the general population. The most common indication for cesarean delivery was cephalopelvic disproportion or fetal malpresentation (55% of all cesarean deliveries).[18] The authors suggested that this could be related to kyphoscoliosis of the lower spine (see Fig. 16.5B) or undiagnosed pelvic neurofibromas.[5] Women with NF1 should be assessed at their first visit for any history of seizures or visual disturbance, and pulmonary function tests should be performed if kyphoscoliosis is noted.[5] The status of neurofibromas in the pelvic area should be monitored, and fetal growth should be closely assessed, particularly in the cases associated with hypertension. Genetic counseling is mandatory because the risk of fetal transmission is 50%. Identifying the disease-causing mutation enables prenatal diagnosis via chorionic villous sampling or amniocentesis.

Hereditary Hemorrhagic Telangiectasia (Osler–Weber–Rendu Syndrome)

Hereditary hemorrhagic telangiectasia (HHT) is an autosomal dominant disorder characterized by arteriovenous malformations (AVMs), which is associated with susceptibility to rupture and abnormal shunting.[4] Mucocutaneous telangiectasias are noted in the mouth, lips, and nose (Fig. 16.6), and most patients begin having symptoms such as nosebleeds in adolescence. Serious complications can arise from gastrointestinal, pulmonary, and brain AVMs. A large study[19] reported on the outcomes of 262 pregnancies in 111 women with HHT: 3% of women experienced major morbidity in pregnancy, including pulmonary AVM bleeding (1%), stroke (1.2%), and maternal death (1%). Diagnosis of HHT before gestation was associated with improved outcomes; however, 74% of patients did not have an established HHT diagnosis prior to gestation. The likelihood of pregnancy complications and optimal surveillance during pregnancy should be determined in the preconception period, whenever there is an established HHT diagnosis. Important imaging studies include head magnetic resonance imaging (MRI) scan, chest computed tomography (CT), contrast echocardiogram, and ultrasound of right upper quadrant. Pulmonary AVMs should be treated before pregnancy.

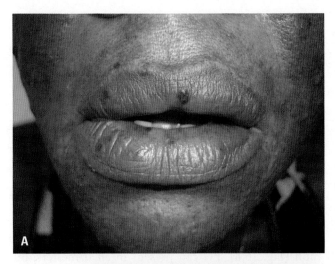

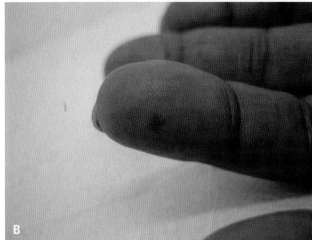

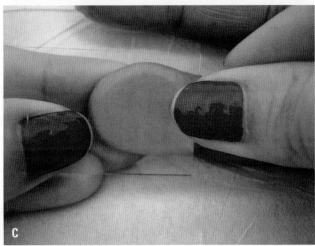

Figure 16.6. Hereditary hemorrhagic telangiectasia: Telangiectasias are shown on the vermilion of (**A**) the lips and (**B**) fingertip. (**C**) Telangiectasia on the fingertip blanches upon pressure with glass. (Courtesy of Dr. Bernard Kawa Kac.)

Patients should be counseled that the offspring has a 50% risk of inheriting the disorder. Prenatal testing is possible if the disease-causing mutation is identified in the family.

Hereditary Angioedema

Attacks of hereditary angioedema (HAE) may increase in pregnancy[20]; however, there has been some inconsistency as to whether attacks are increased[20] or decreased[21] in the second and third trimesters. Some patients experience attacks of HAE only during pregnancy, and it was postulated that they exhibit a unique estrogen-dependent phenotype.[21] Angioedema attacks are rare during delivery despite the injury to the birth canal; however, the trauma of normal labor can precipitate airway difficulties.[22] An increased frequency of postpartum attacks has been reported.[21]

Acute attacks of HAE in pregnancy are treated with concentrates of C1 esterase inhibitor; it is also administered before major procedures and surgery. Tranexamic acid (pregnancy category B) may be used for long-term prophylaxis when C1 esterase inhibitor concentrate is unavailable.[23] Androgens, such as danazol, are contraindicated in pregnancy, and aminocaproic acid (pregnancy

category C) is limited by its serious adverse effects (muscle necrosis, weakness, thrombotic potential).[22] Regional anesthesia is preferable for operative deliveries.[22] No specific precautions are required for vaginal delivery, but sites of local trauma need careful inspection[22]; after vaginal delivery, patients should be carefully checked for any abnormal perineal swelling.[22]

Marfan Syndrome

Marfan syndrome is an autosomal dominant disorder characterized by skeletal, cardiovascular, and ocular manifestations. Significant maternal morbidity in pregnancy is primarily due to cardiovascular complications, especially aortic dissection, which is more likely with an aortic root diameter >40 mm before pregnancy.[4] The serious maternal risks associated to Marfan syndrome should be promptly recognized, and optimal care can be provided through a multidisciplinary approach. Women should be counseled that the risk for having an affected child is 50%. Prenatal diagnosis via chorionic villous sampling is available if the disease-causing allele has been identified in the affected parent.[4]

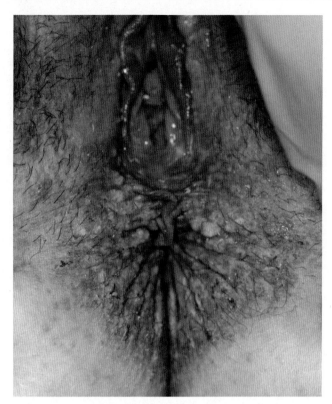

Figure 16.7. Darier disease involving the perianal area: Confluent, erythematous, keratotic papules form malodorous papillomatous plaques. Warty, macerated lesions are typical in this area. Papillomatous lesions are prone to infections that can cause exacerbation of the disease.

Darier Disease

Darier disease is an autosomal dominant genodermatosis with characteristic findings that include moderately pruritic keratotic papules on the upper trunk ("seborrheic" areas) and involvement of the flexures and nails; intertriginous/anogenital areas are affected less commonly (Fig. 16.7). In a study of 163 patients, pregnancy did not affect Darier disease in most women; 22% improved and 11% became worse.[24] Only 14% mentioned perimenstrual exacerbations, and oral contraceptives may help in these cases. In one case, Darier disease flared in each of the six pregnancies of the patient. Other cases showed exacerbation due to herpes or vaccinia virus infection in pregnancy. Localized or segmental Darier disease associated with pregnancy has been reported.[25] Some cases showed verrucous or vegetating lesions in pregnancy.

Other Genodermatoses

Disorders of keratinization, such as ichthyosis vulgaris, are not known to be affected by pregnancy, although sparse reports of exacerbation in pregnancy have been published.[2] A case of exacerbation of erythrokeratoderma variabilis in two female members of the same family has been published.[26] Both experienced exacerbation of the disease during each of their three pregnancies; the flare

was noticed during the last 6 months of gestation and resolved postpartum.

Sparse cases of exacerbation of bullous congenital ichthyosiform erythroderma and epidermolysis bullosa simplex have been reported.

NEUTROPHILIC DERMATOSES

Pyoderma Gangrenosum

Twenty cases of pyoderma gangrenosum (PG) with an onset in pregnancy or in the early postpartum period have been reported, and more than half of these were idiopathic[27–29]; the ulcerative form was the most common (Fig. 16.8). PG can present in all trimesters, but presentation in the immediate postpartum period has been the most common (10 out of 20 cases). Nine cases developed postpartum on the scar of the cesarean section.[27,29] No fetal complications were noted. Most cases respond to high-dose systemic corticosteroids; cyclosporine has been successfully used in order to taper systemic steroids.[27,29] Isolated cases were treated successfully with topical or intralesional corticosteroids[27] and a case with aggravation during pregnancy was treated with intravenous immunoglobulin.[30] One case showed the "pathergic phenomenon" (i.e., localization of PG to sites of trauma

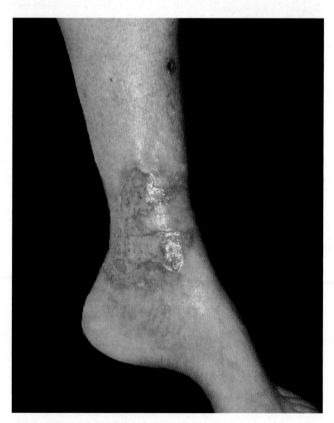

Figure 16.8. Early pyoderma gangrenosum: Shallow ulcerations on an erythematous, indurated base with a tendency to coalesce. The border extends centrifugally and is irregular; it becomes undermined and overhanging in fully developed lesions.

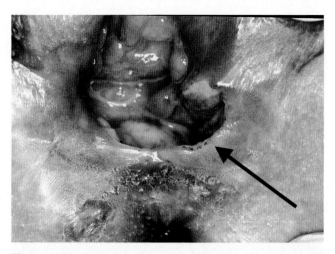

Figure 16.9. Behçet disease: Deep painful ulceration at vaginal introitus *(arrow)*. Compared to oral lesions, anogenital ulcerations are larger, deeper, and with irregular margins.

or surgery), which characterizes the disease. It has been suggested that the immunologic changes of gestation, including a decrease in interleukin-1 and -2, and polymorphonuclear leukocyte function, may predispose one to the development of PG. The diagnosis of PG should always be considered in cases of ulcers with no bacteriologic evidence of infection that do not respond to antibiotic treatment, especially if the ulcers are recurrent or secondary to trauma.[29] Investigations should be carried out to exclude underlying etiologies such as myelodysplasia, inflammatory bowel disease, and connective tissue disease.[28]

Behçet Disease

Behçet disease (BD) is a multisystem disorder characterized by recurrent oral/genital ulcerations (Fig. 16.9), especially aphthous stomatitis, ocular abnormalities, and a variety of other skin lesions. A study indicated that BD may adversely affect pregnancy, as indicated by a higher rate of miscarriage rate, other pregnancy complications, and cesarean delivery.[31] Nevertheless, a large study did not confirm an increased risk of pregnancy complications.[32] Pregnancy did not adversely affect the course of BD and may possibly ameliorate its course[31]; exacerbations were noted only in one-sixth of patients. Exacerbation in other studies was noted in one-third[33] to two-thirds[34] of patients. Patients who improved often showed exacerbations related to menstruation or postpartum.[34] Pregnant women with BD should be closely followed for evidence of IUGR and fetal compromise.[35]

Sweet Syndrome

Sweet syndrome is a neutrophilic dermatosis associated with infections, hematologic malignancies, inflammatory bowel disease, autoimmune disorders, drugs, and pregnancy. A minimum of 12 cases showed an onset in pregnancy, and the first 5 cases were reviewed by Satra

and associates.[36] Most cases resulted in healthy offspring, except for a second-trimester spontaneous abortion. Lesions resolved either spontaneously or after systemic or topical steroid treatment. A search for an underlying etiology is required, although some cases are idiopathic.

OTHER SKIN DISEASES

Erythema Nodosum

Erythema nodosum (EN) is the most common panniculitis, an inflammatory process that involves subcutaneous fat. It typically manifests with painful erythematous nodules on the extensor surfaces of the lower extremities (Fig. 16.10), often with concomitant constitutional symptoms such as fever, malaise, and arthralgias. Etiologies include streptococcal infections, tuberculosis, leprosy, coccidioidomycosis, drugs (e.g., sulfonamides, oral contraceptives), sarcoidosis, inflammatory bowel disease, antiphospholipid syndrome, and BD.[37] Exacerbation or new onset of EN in pregnancy, or with oral contraceptive intake, has been reported.[37] Salvatore and Lynch[38] described five patients that experienced EN episodes both during gestation and with oral contraceptive or other hormonal use. Pregnancy was the cause of 2% of EN cases in a study

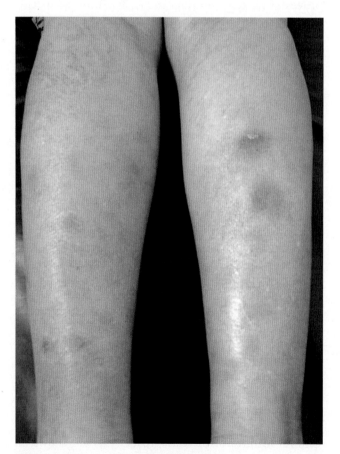

Figure 16.10. Erythema nodosum: Typical presentation of tender erythematous nodules on the legs. (Courtesy of Dr. Mayra Ianhez.)

of 100 cases.[39] EN has been described in all trimesters and resolved spontaneously by delivery. Lesions typically last no more than 6 to 8 weeks. Investigations should be carried out to exclude infectious and other etiologies.[37] Treatment is supportive, and mild analgesics, such as paracetamol, can be helpful. Nonsteroidal anti-inflammatory medications should be avoided in the first and third trimesters. Treatment of the underlying disease and removal of culprit drugs are important. A short course of systemic corticosteroid can also help if it does not adversely interfere with the underlying disease.

Sarcoidosis

Some series have reported that sarcoidosis may improve in pregnancy and relapse in parturition.[40,41] The improvement during gestation may be due to the elevated levels of glucocorticoids.[41] However, in other studies, pregnancy did not predictably influence the course of sarcoidosis. A study did not find any changes during gestation in sarcoidosis that was cured/inactive as of the beginning of pregnancy; the course of active disease varied (three out of five patients were better or stable).[42] Other authors indicated that patients with stage I disease (hilar adenopathy) do better than those with stage II through IV (parenchymal disease).[40,41] Cutaneous lesions of sarcoidosis may improve during gestation (Fig. 16.11). There are no specific fetal risks other than those relevant to severe maternal disease from pulmonary or other organ involvement. The maternal and fetal prognosis is poor in those patients with severe pulmonary involvement. Sarcoid granulomas have been noted in the placenta but not in the fetus.

Vasculitides

The literature is replete with cases of systemic vasculitis diagnosed in pregnancy, although the prevalence of new-onset vasculitis in pregnancy is low.[35] Outcomes in systemic vasculitis are not universally poor and depend on effective preconception planning, the status of the underlying vasculitis, and management during pregnancy. Pregnancy should be planned only after prolonged remission has been achieved. Women who have inactive vasculitis and those with purely cutaneous vasculitis may not be subject to unusual complications during pregnancy. Systemic corticosteroids and azathioprine can be used for systemic vasculitis in pregnancy.[35] Cyclophosphamide can be used in severe disease in the late second or third trimesters.[35] Intravenous immunoglobulin may be used when cyclophosphamide is contraindicated but may not be as effective.[35]

Pityriasis Rosea

Clinical features of pityriasis rosea (PR) are shown in Figure 16.12. A study indicated that PR may occur in pregnancy more often than in the general population (18% versus 6%).[43] Attention has been drawn to possible fetal

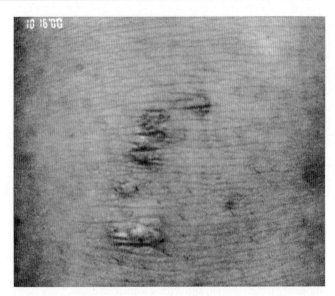

Figure 16.11. Cutaneous sarcoidosis: The patient had extensive disease prior to pregnancy but spontaneously improved in the first two trimesters. Residual granulomatous papules on the knee are shown in the third trimester.

adverse effects from PR with onset in the first 20 weeks of gestation. In a series of 38 patients, 9 had a premature delivery and 5 miscarried; all premature infants thrived.[44] Also, 62% of the women who developed PR within 15 weeks' gestation aborted. Additionally, neonatal hypotonia, weak motility, and hyporeactivity were observed in six cases. Herpes simplex virus-6 was shown in one case; however, other reports[45] did not confirm it, and a recent case report showed herpes simplex virus-2 reactivation. Whether these viruses could be associated with the aforementioned fetal risks remains speculative, and more studies are needed.

Pityriasis Lichenoides et Varioliformis Acuta

Four cases of pityriasis lichenoides et varioliformis acuta in pregnancy have been reported.[46,47] There were no fetal adverse effects. Threatened preterm labor in two of them did not progress after successful treatment of the disease with penicillin[46] or tocolytic agents.[47] Data do not allow concluding that the disease can adversely affect pregnancy.

Mastocytosis

In a recent series of 30 patients,[48] mastocytosis had a heterogeneous behavior during pregnancy: symptoms remained unchanged in half of the cases, whereas they improved or worsened in the other half. Indolent systemic mastocytosis was noted in one patient. These results confirm those of a previous study of eight patients.[49] Prematurity, low birth weight, and respiratory distress were detected in 16% of infants[48] and were all successfully managed with conservative measures. Cutaneous mastocytosis several years after birth was noted in one infant. Patients with nonaggressive forms of mastocytosis should

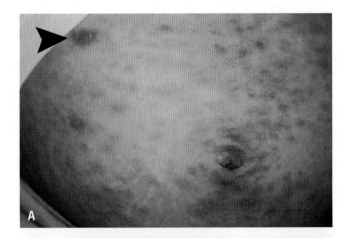

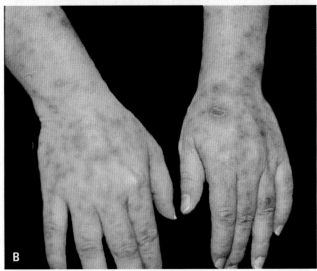

Figure 16.12. Pityriasis rosea in pregnancy: Numerous lesions are shown on (**A**) the abdomen and (**B**) the upper extremities. The "herald patch" *(arrow)* is the first lesion that develops. Lesions typically show central fine scales, and their advancing margin has a larger collarette of scale with the free edge pointing inward. Involvement of the umbilicus and the absence of urticarial lesions helped rule out polymorphic eruption of pregnancy in this case.

not be advised against pregnancy. Prophylactic H₁, such as dexchlorpheniramine, cetirizine, loratadine, and H₂ antihistamines, such as ranitidine, should be systematically administered during pregnancy.[48] Anesthetics and narcotic analgesics used during labor and general anesthetic procedures appear to be safe in these patients.[48,49]

MATERNAL RISKS

EDS type IV, HHT, Marfan syndrome: Vascular complications; EDS associated with PROM, poor wound healing, lacerations, abdominal hernias, bladder and uterine prolapse

Pseudoxanthoma elasticum: Hypertension, gastrointestinal bleeding, retinal complication, worsening of skin disease

Tuberous sclerosis: Renal complications; other risks, including fetal demise, less common

Neurofibromatosis type 1: ↑ rate of cesarean delivery

Hereditary angioedema: Respiratory compromise; severe symptomatic aggravation

Pyoderma gangrenosum: Risks from superinfection, pharmacologic Rx

Sarcoidosis: Risks relevant to severe pulmonary or other organ involvement

Vasculitides: Risks relevant to severe organ involvement

FETAL RISKS

EDS type IV, HHT, Marfan syndrome: Mortality; prematurity, IUGR with EDS; neonatal disease

Pseudoxanthoma elasticum: First-trimester miscarriage and IUGR (not confirmed)

Tuberous sclerosis: Preeclampsia, IUGR, hydrops fetalis, fetal demise, complications related to fetal cardiac rhabdomyomas

Neurofibromatosis type 1: First-trimester miscarriage, IUGR, and stillbirth (not confirmed)

Hereditary angioedema: None when disease is controlled

Pyoderma gangrenosum: Risks from pharmacologic Rx

Behçet disease: ↑ miscarriage, ↑ rate of cesarean delivery (one study)

Sarcoidosis: Risks relevant to maternal pulmonary or other organ involvement

Vasculitides: Risks dependent on the status of maternal organ involvement

Pityriasis rosea: Prematurity, neonatal hypotonia, weak motility, hyporeactivity

EDS, Ehlers–Danlos syndrome; HHT, hereditary hemorrhagic telangiectasia, IUGR, intrauterine growth restriction; PROM, premature rupture of membranes; Rx, treatment; ↑, increased.

KEY POINTS

■ EDS type IV, Marfan syndrome, and HHT have been associated with serious maternal and fetal risks, and preconception counseling is recommended; a multidisciplinary approach is required during pregnancy in order to optimize outcomes.

■ Tuberous sclerosis has been associated with high rates of perinatal complications, and renal involvement adversely affects prognosis; the presence of cardiac rhabdomyoma in the fetus increases fetal mortality.

■ Vascular complications from PXE as well as risks from neurofibromatosis 1 seem milder than previously thought; vigilance and prompt management can minimize complications.

■ Attacks of hereditary angioedema may increase in pregnancy and can be treated with concentrates of C1 esterase inhibitor.

■ Pyoderma gangrenosum and erythema nodosum can develop in pregnancy with no association to the underlying disease; treatment of pyoderma gangrenosum with systemic steroids is typically successful, whereas a conservative approach is recommended for erythema nodosum.

■ Behçet disease, sarcoidosis, and mastocytosis run a variable course in pregnancy and may improve; serious risks are exceptionally noted in sarcoidosis cases with severe pulmonary involvement and aggressive types of mastocytosis.

■ Pityriasis rosea has been associated with fetal risks.

REFERENCES

1. Kroumpouzos G, Cohen LM. Dermatoses of pregnancy. *J Am Acad Dermatol.* 2001;45:1–19.
2. Kumari R, Jaisankar TJ, Thappa DM. A clinical study of skin changes in pregnancy. *Indian J Dermatol Venereol Leprol.* 2007; 73:141.
3. Winton GB. Skin diseases aggravated by pregnancy. *J Am Acad Dermatol.* 1989;20:1–13.
4. Chetty SP, Shaffer BL, Norton ME. Management of pregnancy in women with genetic disorders, Part 1: disorders of the connective tissue, muscle, vascular, and skeletal systems. *Obstet Gynecol Surv.* 2011;66:699–709.
5. Chetty SP, Shaffer BL, Norton ME. Management of pregnancy in women with genetic disorders, Part 2: inborn errors of metabolism, cystic fibrosis, neurofibromatosis type 1, and Turner syndrome in pregnancy. *Obstet Gynecol Surv.* 2011;66:765–776.
6. Volkov N, Nisenblat V, Ohel G, et al. Ehlers-Danlos syndrome: insights on obstetric aspects. *Obstet Gynecol Surv.* 2007;62:51–57.
7. Hammerschmidt DE, Arneson MA, Larson SL, et al. Maternal Ehlers-Danlos syndrome type X. Successful management of pregnancy and parturition. *JAMA.* 1982;248:2487–2488.
8. Lurie S, Manor M, Hagay ZJ. The threat of type IV Ehlers-Danlos syndrome on maternal well-being during pregnancy: early delivery may make the difference. *J Obstet Gynaecol.* 1998; 18:245–248.
9. Pepin M, Schwarze U, Superti-Furga A, et al. Clinical and genetic features of Ehlers-Danlos syndrome type IV, the vascular type. *N Engl J Med.* 2000;342:673–680.
10. Bercovitch L, Leroux T, Terry S, et al. Pregnancy and obstetric outcomes in pseudoxanthoma elasticum. *Br J Dermatol.* 2004;151: 1011–1018.
11. Berde C, Willis DC, Sandberg EC. Pregnancy in women with pseudoxanthoma elasticum. *Obstet Gynecol Surv.* 1983;38:339–344.
12. Viljoen DL, Beatty S, Beighton P. The obstetric and gynaecological implications of pseudoxanthoma elasticum. *Br J Obstet Gynaecol.* 1987;94:884–888.
13. Petrikovsky BM, Vintzileos AM, Cassidy SB, et al. Tuberous sclerosis in pregnancy. *Am J Perinatol.* 1990;7:133–135.
14. Gounden YP. Tuberous sclerosis in pregnancy: a case report and review of the literature. *Aust N Z J Obstet Gynaecol.* 2002;42:551–552.
15. King JA, Stamilio DM. Maternal and fetal tuberous sclerosis complicating pregnancy: a case report and overview of the literature. *Am J Perinatol.* 2005;22:103–108.
16. Swapp GH, Main RA. Neurofibromatosis in pregnancy. *Br J Dermatol.* 1973;88:431–435.
17. Segal D, Holcberg G, Sapir O, et al. Neurofibromatosis in pregnancy: maternal and perinatal outcome. *Eur J Obstet Gynecol Repr Biol.* 1999;84:59–61.
18. Dugoff L, Sujansky E. Neurofibromatosis type 1 and pregnancy. *Am J Med Genet.* 1996;66:7–10.
19. Shovlin CL, Sodhi V, McCarthy A, et al. Estimates of maternal risks of pregnancy for women with hereditary haemorrhagic telangiectasia (Osler-Weber-Rendu syndrome): suggested approach for obstetric services. *BJOG.* 2008;115:1108–1115.
20. Martinez-Saguer I, Rusicke E, Aygören-Pürsün E, et al. Characterization of acute hereditary angioedema attacks during pregnancy and breast-feeding and their treatment with C1 inhibitor concentrate. *Am J Obstet Gynecol.* 2010;203:131.e1–e7.
21. Chinniah N, Katelaris CH. Hereditary angioedema and pregnancy. *Aust N Z J Obstet Gynaecol.* 2009;49:2–5.
22. Duvvur S, Khan F, Powell K. Hereditary angioedema and pregnancy. *J Matern Fetal Neonatal Med.* 2007;20:563–565.
23. Caballero T, Farkas H, Bouillet L, et al. International consensus and practical guidelines on the gynecologic and obstetric management of female patients with hereditary angioedema caused by C1 inhibitor deficiency. *J Allergy Clin Immunol.* 2012; 129:308–320.
24. Burge SM, Wilkinson JD. Darier-White disease: a review of the clinical features in 163 patients. *J Am Acad Dermatol.* 1992;27: 40–50.
25. Telang GH, Atillasoy E, Stierstorfer M. Localized keratosis follicularis associated with menotropin treatment and pregnancy. *J Am Acad Dermatol.* 1994;30:271–272.
26. Gewirtzman GB, Winkler NW, Dobson RL. Erythrokeratodermia variabilis, a family study. *Arch Dermatol.* 1978;114:259–261.
27. Sanz-Muñoz C, Martínez-Morán C, Miranda-Romero A. [Pyoderma gangrenosum following cesarean delivery]. *Actas Dermosifiliogr.* 2008;99:477–480.
28. Sergent F, Joly P, Gravier A, et al. [Pregnancy: A possible etiology of pyoderma gangrenosum. A case report and review of the literature]. *J Gynecol Obstet Biol Reprod (Paris).* 2002;31:506–511.
29. Karim AA, Ahmed N, Salman TA, et al. Pyoderma gangrenosum in pregnancy. *J Obstet Gynaecol.* 2006;26:463–465.
30. Erfurt-Berge C, Herbst C, Schuler G, et al. Successful treatment of pyoderma gangrenosum with intravenous immunoglobulins during pregnancy. *J Cutan Med Surg.* 2012;16:205–207.
31. Jadaon J, Shushan A, Ezra Y, et al. Behçet's disease and pregnancy. *Acta Obstet Gynecol Scand.* 2005;84:939–944.
32. Marsal S, Falgá C, Simeon CP, et al. Behçet's disease and pregnancy relationship study. *Br J Rheumatol.* 1997;36:234–238.
33. Uzun S, Alpsoy E, Durdu M, et al. The clinical course of Behçet's disease in pregnancy: a retrospective analysis and review of the literature. *J Dermatol.* 2003;30:499–502.
34. Bang D, Chun YS, Haam IB, et al. The influence of pregnancy on Behçet's disease. *Yonsei Med J.* 1997;38:437–443.
35. Seo P. Pregnancy and vasculitis. *Rheum Dis Clin North Am.* 2007; 33:299–317.
36. Satra K, Zalka A, Cohen PR, et al. Sweet's syndrome and pregnancy. *J Am Acad Dermatol.* 1994;30:297–300.
37. Bartelsmeyer JA, Petrie RH. Erythema nodosum, estrogens, and pregnancy. *Clin Obstet Gynecol.* 1990;33:777–781.
38. Salvatore MA, Lynch PJ. Erythema nodosum, estrogens, and pregnancy. *Arch Dermatol.* 1980;116:557–578.
39. Mert A, Kumbasar H, Ozaras R, et al. Erythema nodosum: an evaluation of 100 cases. *Clin Exp Rheumatol.* 2007;25:563–570.
40. Agha FP, Vade A, Amendola MA, et al. Effects of pregnancy on sarcoidosis. *Surg Gynecol Obstet.* 1982;155:817–822.
41. Haynes de Regt R. Sarcoidosis and pregnancy. *Obstet Gynecol.* 1987;70:369–372.

42. Chapelon Abric C, Ginsburg C, Biousse V, et al. [Sarcoidosis and pregnancy. A retrospective study of 11 cases]. *Rev Med Interne.* 1998;19:305–312.

43. Corson EF, Luscombe HA. Coincidence of pityriasis rosea with pregnancy. *AMA Arch Derm Syphilol.* 1950;62:562–564.

44. Drago F, Broccolo F, Zaccaria E, et al. Pregnancy outcome in patients with pityriasis rosea. *J Am Acad Dermatol.* 2008;58: S78–S83.

45. Chuh AA, Lee A, Chan PK. Pityriasis rosea in pregnancy— specific diagnostic implications and management considerations. *Aust N Z J Obstet Gynaecol.* 2005;45:252–253.

46. Fukada Y, Okuda Y, Yasumizu T, et al. Pityriasis lichenoides et varioliformis acuta in pregnancy: a case report. *J Obstet Gynaecol Res.* 1998;24:363–366.

47. Eskandar MA. Pityriasis lichenoides et varioliformis acuta in pregnancy. *Saudi Med J.* 2001;22:1127–1129.

48. Matito A, Álvarez-Twose I, Morgado JM, et al. Clinical impact of pregnancy in mastocytosis: a study of the Spanish Network on Mastocytosis (REMA) in 45 cases. *Int Arch Allergy Immunol.* 2011;156:104–111.

49. Worobec AS, Akin C, Scott LM, et al. Mastocytosis complicating pregnancy. *Obstet Gynecol.* 2000;95:391–395.

CHAPTER 17

Pruritus and Obstetric Cholestasis

Victoria Geenes ■ Catherine Williamson

INTRODUCTION

Pruritus is a common symptom of pregnancy reported in 3% to 14% of pregnancies.[1] It commonly affects the abdomen and is often attributed to the stretching of the skin. However, significant pruritus is much less common, affecting only 1.6% of pregnancies.[2] In establishing the cause of pruritus in pregnancy, a broad differential diagnosis needs to be considered (Table 17.1), and clinicians should take into account the constellation of clinical and laboratory findings. Obstetric cholestasis (OC), also known as intrahepatic cholestasis of pregnancy (ICP), is the most common cause of liver dysfunction in pregnancy. It typically presents with maternal pruritus and raised serum bile acids (BAs) in the third trimester and is associated with increased risk of adverse fetal outcomes, including spontaneous preterm delivery, fetal distress during labor, and stillbirth.[3]

EPIDEMIOLOGY

There is a marked variation in the incidence of OC, not only with the geographical location but also with ethnicity.[3] The highest reported rates come from South America, with an overall incidence of 10% in Chile reported in the 1970s.[4] More recently, the incidence has declined to between 1.5% and 4%, but it remains more common in women of Araucanian Indian origin.[5] The reason for this decline is unclear but may reflect more robust diagnostic criteria or changes in environmental factors. In Europe, rates are considerably lower: 1.5% in Sweden and 0.7% in the United Kingdom,[6,7] but similar racial variation is observed, with OC being almost twice as common in women of Asian origin in the United Kingdom.

OC is more common in twin pregnancies (20% to 22%) and following in vitro fertilization treatment (2.7% versus 0.7%). Studies have also suggested that it is more common during the winter months and in women older than the age of 35 years. Hepatitis C infection is associated with OC and may result in earlier onset of the condition. Finally, gallstones are more common in both women with OC and their families.[3]

ETIOLOGY

The etiology of OC is complex and relates to the cholestatic effects of reproductive hormones in genetically susceptible women. Immunologic and environmental/dietary factors may also play a role.

Genetic Factors

Evidence for a genetic component to the etiology of OC comes from the familial clustering, higher prevalence in certain ethnic groups, and mothers of patients with progressive familial intrahepatic cholestasis (PFIC) or benign recurrent intrahepatic cholestasis (BRIC). Several pedigrees, containing small numbers of cases, suggest an autosomal-dominant, sex-limited inheritance pattern.[8,9] Furthermore, a study of Finnish patients with OC showed that OC was experienced in 9% of the parous sisters of patients (odds ratio [OR], 12).[10] In a similar U.K. study, 14% of the sisters of patients developed OC.[11]

PFIC and BRIC are autosomal-recessive syndromes caused by mutations in genes encoding biliary transport proteins and resulting in severe childhood liver disease. A subgroup of the heterozygous mothers of affected children had OC.[11] There are three subtypes of PFIC (types 1 through 3) caused by mutations in *ATP8B1* (FIC1), *ABCB11* (BSEP), and *ABCB4* (MDR3), respectively. The localization of these transporters within the hepatocyte and their substrate specificity is shown in Figure 17.1. The most extensively studied gene in OC is *ABCB4* (encodes the multidrug resistance protein 3 [MDR3]), and mutations of *ABCB4* have been linked to OC. Studies have identified a spectrum of different genetic variants occurring in the majority of the exons of the gene, an *ABCB4* haplotype and four splicing mutations.[11] Although initially thought to be associated specifically with cases of OC with a raised serum gamma glutamyl transpeptidase (GGT) level, a phenotype shared with PFIC type 3, recent studies have demonstrated genetic variation in women with normal GGT levels. Mutations in *ABCB4* have been reported in estrogen-induced cholestasis and low phospholipid cholelithiasis, and women with a history of OC are at increased risk of these disorders.

TABLE 17.1	Differential Diagnosis of Obstetric Cholestasis

Without Jaundice
Atopic dermatitis
Specific dermatoses (P-type atopic eruption, polymorphic eruption, prurigo, pruritic folliculitis)
Pruritus gravidarum
Allergic reaction
Drug eruption
Infestation (i.e., scabies)
Viral or bacterial infection
Striae gravidarum with pruritus
Systemic disease with pruritus (liver, renal, and thyroid disease)

With Jaundice
Viral hepatitis
Hyperbilirubinemic states
Acute fatty liver of pregnancy
Preeclampsia with increased liver enzymes
Hyperemesis gravidarum complicated by cholestasis
Drug-induced hepatitis/icterus
Bile duct obstruction
Other liver disease (i.e., biliary cirrhosis)
Hemolytic and metabolic disease

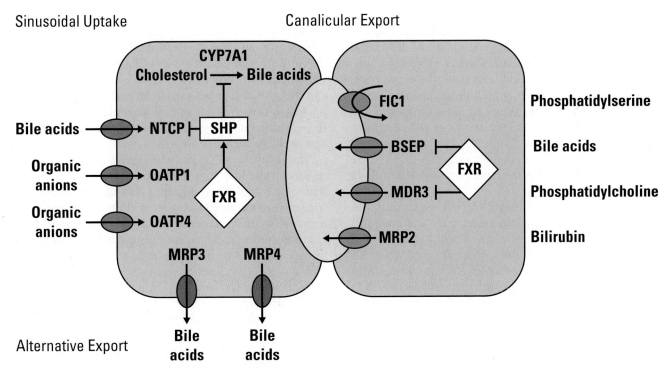

Figure 17.1. A schematic showing the major hepatobiliary uptake and export proteins involved in bile acid homeostasis and their substrate specificities. Bile acids are synthesized from cholesterol in the liver and act as the main route for cholesterol excretion. The synthesis and homeostasis of bile acids is tightly regulated by the nuclear hormone receptor FXR. In response to raised intracellular bile acid levels, FXR downregulates the synthesis, acting via the promoter-specific repressor SHP, and uptakes and upregulates the export. *Green*, canalicular export; *purple*, sinusoidal uptake; *blue*, alternative export. BSEP, bile salt export pump; FIC, familial intrahepatic cholestasis; FXR, farnesoid X receptor; MDR3, multidrug resistance protein 3; MRP, multidrug resistance protein; NTCP, sodium taurocholate cotransporting polypeptide; OATP, organic anion transporting polypeptide; SHP, small heterodimer partner.

Recent studies on *ABCB11* have reported three rare mutations in OC and a single nucleotide polymorphism (SNP) (V444A) that is also associated with estrogen-induced cholestasis. The V444A allele was confirmed as a population susceptibility locus for OC in a white European cohort of 491 cases, in which a heterozygous variation of two of the common PFIC type 2 variants was also identified in a small number of OC cases.[12]

Genetic variation in *FIC 1* has been identified in a small number of OC cases, although its functional significance remains unclear.[11] Of the other biliary transporters, genetic variation has only been reported in *ABCC2*, which encodes the multidrug resistance protein 2 (MRP2). A polymorphism in exon 28 has been found in South American patients with OC.[11] BA homeostasis and transport within the hepatocyte is tightly regulated by a nuclear hormone receptor, the farnesoid X receptor (FXR), which is encoded by *NR1H4*. Four heterozygous variants in *NR1H4* have been described in a white European cohort of OC cases, of which three have demonstrable functional effects.[11] Finally, common polymorphisms of the xenobiotic receptor (pregnane X receptor [*PXR*]), which may contribute to the genetic susceptibility to OC, were found in a South American population but were not confirmed in a white European cohort.

Hormonal Factors

Evidence for a role for reproductive hormones in the etiology of OC comes from the presentation of the disease in the third trimester, at a time when the levels of reproductive hormones peak, and also from the observation that OC is more common in multiple pregnancies where levels of reproductive hormones are naturally higher. This is further supported by the recurrence of OC symptoms with oral contraceptives.[13] Most studies have examined the effects of estrogens rather than progesterone, but there is growing evidence that the latter plays a greater role in the pathogenesis.

Clinical studies have shown that estrogens cause reduced sulfobromophthalein clearance[14] and that this effect is more marked in women with a history of OC and their male relatives. They also increase the total serum BA concentration,[15] and in particular, the concentration of taurine conjugates, which are the principal form of BAs raised in OC. The mechanism by which estrogens induce cholestasis appears to relate to an impairment in the function of the principle BA export pump BSEP, in a manner that is dependent on MRP2, an organic anion transporter at the canalicular membrane.[3] Studies indicate that estrogens may also impair FXR function.

Evidence supporting a role for progesterone in the etiology of OC comes from the observation that the administration of natural progestin to women with threatened preterm labor resulted in the development of OC in more than 90% of those treated.[16] Interestingly, the serum level of progesterone is unchanged in OC compared with normal pregnancy, but the profile of progester-

one metabolites is considerably different, with an excess of mono- and disulfated isomers in the serum and the urine of affected women.[17] Furthermore, there is an increased level of disulfated metabolites in the umbilical cord serum of OC-affected infants.[18] These findings suggest either abnormal synthesis of these compounds or impaired excretion at the canalicular membrane. Supporting the latter, a recent study showed that sulfated progesterone metabolites competitively inhibit both sodium-dependent and -independent uptake of taurocholic acid.[19] These findings suggest that sulfated progesterone metabolites impair the function of the sodium taurocholate cotransporting polypeptide (NTCP) and other uptake transporters. They have also been shown to inhibit taurocholic acid transport by bile salt export pump (BSEP) and the function of FXR in human hepatocyte models and a rodent model of OC.

Immunologic Factors

Increased cell-mediated (Th1-type) reaction and levels of interferon-gamma have been reported along with increased numbers of natural killer cells and natural killer T cells and decreased numbers of T cells in *decidual parietalis*.

Environmental Factors

Dietary intake of selenium is lower in countries with a higher incidence of OC, including Finland and Chile.[3] Selenium levels typically decrease with advancing gestation and are lower in OC patients than pregnant controls. Given that both BAs and estrogens cause oxidative stress and that glutathione peroxidase, an antioxidant that helps protect against this damage, is dependent on selenium, these findings may in part explain the geographical variation in the incidence of OC.

The incidence of OC in Scandinavia and Chile shows seasonal variation, with higher rates observed in winter than in summer. This suggests a possible environmental trigger, such as infection for the condition. Alternatively, it may relate to lower vitamin D levels in winter months because studies of cholestatic animals have reported improved excretion of BAs in animals treated with vitamin D. Along the same lines, a recent study showed decreased 1,25-dihydroxy vitamin D levels in women with OC. The most widely reported infection associated with OC is hepatitis C, which is reported to have a higher incidence in OC pregnancies than normal pregnancies. Furthermore, women with hepatitis C develop OC at earlier gestations. Patients with OC have higher rates of urinary tract infections and pyelonephritis early in pregnancy and increased gut permeability ("leaky gut").[3]

One study has reported higher rates of drug-induced cholestasis in women with OC, in particular, sensitivity to antibiotics.[3] This may reflect an overlap in the etiology of drug sensitivity and OC especially because the V444A variant in BSEP is more commonly found in individuals with drug-induced cholestasis in addition to being a susceptibility factor for OC.[11] Genetic variation in *ABCB4* is also associated with both disorders.

CLINICAL FEATURES

Maternal Disease

OC typically presents with pruritus, raised serum BAs, and deranged liver function in the third trimester.[3] It manifests in 80% of cases at around 30 weeks' gestation, although onset as early as in the first trimester has been reported[20] and may be associated with a more severe phenotype. Pruritus is classically reported to occur on the palms and soles, although any part of the body may be affected. It is frequently worse at night and may be so severe as to cause insomnia. It also tends to worsen as gestation advances and resolves rapidly following delivery, typically within 48 hours. There are no specific dermatologic features, and the presence of a rash other than skin lesions secondary to scratching would make the diagnosis of OC less likely. Excoriations may be the only skin manifestation and are typically seen early in the course of OC (Fig. 17.2). Other skin manifestations, such as prurigo type lesions, also result from the intense desire to scratch and correlate with disease duration (Figs. 17.3 and 17.4). Abrasions and friction blisters can be exceptionally seen. Pruritus may precede or lag behind the liver function abnormalities.[21] Furthermore, the intensity of pruritus does not correlate well with the degree of liver impairment and laboratory parameters.

Equally, the etiology of pruritus is not fully understood. It is classically thought to be caused by the irritant effect of BAs deposited in the skin. Indeed, intradermal injections of BAs and the application of BAs to the blister base provoke a scratch response.[3] However, the concentration of BAs in skin biopsy samples does not correlate well to the sensation of pruritus, and some women with OC report an itch before a rise in serum BA levels is detected. These findings suggest

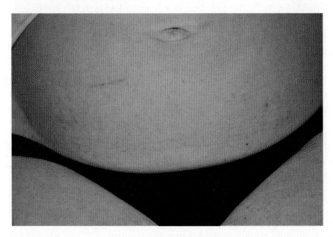

Figure 17.2. Excoriations in a patient with early obstetric cholestasis. Excoriations can be the only skin manifestation of the condition and are typically seen early in the course of the disease and throughout.

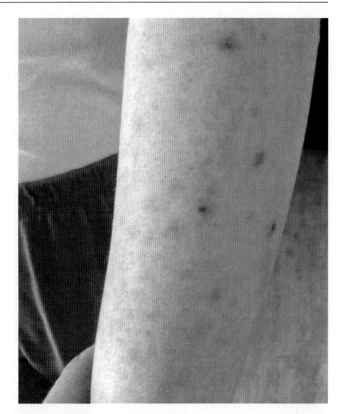

Figure 17.3. Excoriated prurigo type lesions are shown on the arm in a patient with obstetric cholestasis.

that other compounds, such as the reproductive hormones, may be responsible or that a more central mechanism plays a role. Sulfated progesterone metabolites are significantly reduced in the serum of women with OC following treatment with ursodeoxycholic acid (UDCA) and this correlates with a significant reduction in pruritus as recorded on a visual analogue scale.[22] Ondansetron, a 5-hydroxytryptamine 3-receptor antagonist, has also been shown to reduce pruritus in OC, suggesting that serotonin may play a role in the etiology of pruritus.[3] More recently, a study of OC and other cholestatic liver diseases associated with pruritus has implicated lysophosphatidic acid (LPA) as a potent pruritogen in these disorders.[23] LPA is a small phospholipid that plays a role in the development of neuropathic pain and can induce a scratch response when injected in the skin of mice. Serum levels of LPA are significantly higher in women with OC and other cholestatic liver disease associated with pruritus than pregnant controls and patients with other cholestatic liver disease but no pruritus, and the level correlates to the intensity of itch reported by patients.

Jaundice is uncommon, affecting between 10% and 15% of women. The rise in bilirubin rarely exceeds 100 μmol/L. Constitutional symptoms, including anorexia, malaise, and right upper quadrant pain, may be present. In addition, pale stools and dark urine may occur, and some women report steatorrhea. Steatorrhea can result in an increased risk of postpartum hemorrhage secondary to malabsorption of vitamin K. However, this appears to be a rare complication of OC with only very few reports in the literature.[3]

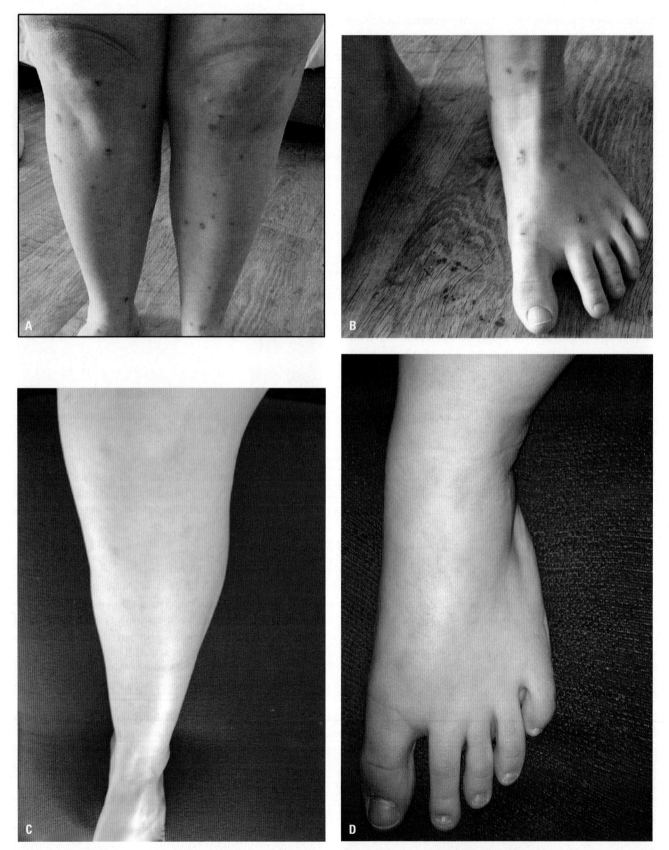

Figure 17.4. (**A, B**) Cutaneous lesions secondary to scratching are shown in a patient with pruritus of several months' duration caused by severe obstetric cholestasis. Extensive, excoriated prurigo type lesions are seen on the shins and dorsa of the feet. (**C, D**) The dermatologic findings and pruritus resolve rapidly following delivery.

Finally, OC may coexist with other pregnancy-related disorders, such as preeclampsia, gestational diabetes, and acute fatty liver of pregnancy.[3] This may reflect a shared underlying etiology. Although there is no evidence to quantify the increased risks in pregnancies affected by OC and another disorder, it is likely that there is an excess of both maternal and fetal morbidity, and, therefore, these subgroups of women require closer monitoring during pregnancy.

Fetal Disease

OC has been consistently associated with an increased risk of adverse fetal outcomes (see box), which has not been accurately quantified.[3] In addition, the etiology of the adverse fetal outcomes is not entirely clear. One study reported an increased risk of adverse events in patients with jaundice.[3] BAs have been repeatedly implicated in all adverse outcomes,[24,25] but the relationship between maternal BA levels and fetal risk is just being established. The largest study to date, a Swedish cohort of 690 women with OC, reported a 1% to 2% increase in the risk of fetal complications (i.e., spontaneous preterm delivery, asphyxia events [operative delivery due to asphyxia; Apgar score <7 at 5 minutes; postpartum pH <7.05 in umbilical arterial blood]; and meconium staining of the amniotic fluid, placenta, and membranes, per additional μmol/L of maternal serum BAs above 40 μmol/L) (Fig. 17.5).[7] Similar findings have been found in small numbers of Hispanic and Turkish patients,[26–28] although there was some variability in the BA level above which the increase in risk occurred. Fetal complications are possibly related to an increased flux of BAs into the fetal circulation, which is evidenced by elevated levels in the umbilical cord serum, the meconium, and amniotic fluid.[3] Vectorial transfer of BAs from the fetus to the mother is impaired in OC, which contributes to the accumulation of BAs in the fetal circulation.[3]

Preterm delivery (i.e., delivery at <38 weeks) is reported in up to 60% of OC pregnancies.[3] Although a significant proportion of these deliveries appear to be iatrogenic, there have been consistent reports of spontaneous preterm labor, with most studies reporting rates of 30% to 40% in the absence of policies of active management.[3] BA levels correlated with rates of preterm delivery in one study

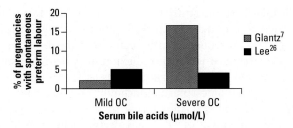

Figure 17.6. A graph demonstrating the incidence of spontaneous preterm labor in studies, examining the association of adverse pregnancy outcomes and maternal serum bile acid levels. Obstetric cholestasis is categorized into two serum bile acid levels: mild (10–40 μmol/L) or severe (>40 μmol/L).

(Fig. 17.6).[7] BAs have been shown to increase myometrial contractility in nonpregnant rat myometrium, and infusions of BAs in sheep resulted in an increased incidence of preterm labor. One study suggested that the myometrium of OC patients may be more responsive to oxytocin.[3]

Meconium staining of the amniotic fluid, a sign of fetal distress, has been reported in approximately 15% of normal term deliveries. In OC, rates between 16% and 58% have been reported.[3] Furthermore, meconium-stained amniotic fluid was reported in 17.9% of OC cases but only 2.9% of controls at 37 weeks.[3] However, meconium staining is seen in virtually all cases of OC that are complicated by intrauterine death.[29] BAs are known to cause an increase in colonic motility, which may account for these findings. Supporting this hypothesis is the finding that 100% of fetal lambs infused with BAs had meconium-stained amniotic fluid at birth.

Both antenatal and intrapartum **cardiotocograph (CTG) abnormalities** have been reported in OC, affecting up to 20% of fetuses during labor.[3] Reported CTG abnormalities include reduced variability in fetal heart rate, tachycardias, and bradycardias. In addition, there have been case reports of fetal atrial flutter and supraventricular tachycardia in association with OC.

Stillbirth was reported in up to 15% of OC pregnancies in older studies and more recently in approximately 1% to 3.5%.[3] The etiology of stillbirth is unclear, but it appears to be a sudden event, and many women report normal fetal movements in the days and hours prior to the fetal loss. This is supported by case reports demonstrating normal CTG traces in the hours prior to stillbirth. Postmortem examinations of the infants typically reveal an appropriately grown infant, with no evidence of chronic uteroplacental insufficiency but signs of acute anoxia.[3] There are several theories about the occurrence of an acute anoxic event. Individual rat neonatal cardiomyocytes lose the ability to beat synchronously following the addition of taurocholic acid, which is the main BA raised in fetal serum in OC, and this in turn results in arrhythmogenic activity. This effect may explain the CTG abnormalities described in OC. Furthermore, meconium has been shown to cause vasoconstriction of the placental chorionic veins, an effect that may be exacerbated by BAs, the level

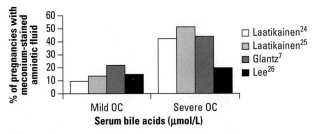

Figure 17.5. A graph demonstrating the incidence of meconium-stained amniotic fluid in studies examining the association of adverse pregnancy outcomes and maternal serum bile acid levels. Obstetric cholestasis is categorized into two serum bile acid levels: mild (10–40 μmol/L) or severe (>40 μmol/L).

of which is significantly higher in meconium from OC pregnancies compared to that from normal pregnancies.[3]

The recent reduction in the rates of stillbirth has been largely attributed to the introduction of policies of active management of OC pregnancies. This term encompasses a wide range of clinical practices including increased antenatal surveillance with CTG monitoring, frequent maternal blood tests, treatment with UDCA and elective delivery at 37 to 38 weeks. The evidence for the practice of early delivery is based on the clustering of OC-associated stillbirths at 37 to 39 weeks.[3] However, stillbirth has been reported as early as 31 weeks.[13] It is likely that the risk of stillbirth increases with increasing levels of serum BAs, but there have been no studies sufficiently powered to conclusively establish a link. However, there are several reports of stillbirths occurring in pregnancies with relatively modest rises in serum BAs (15 to 27 µmol/L).[3] Nevertheless, the BA level may not be representative of the severity of the hypercholanemia in these reports, especially because the serum BA level progressively increases with advancing gestation; therefore, a relatively low BA level from an early gestational week with no subsequent measurement could result in the incorrect conclusion that the serum BA level was not significantly elevated in the context of an adverse pregnancy outcome.

Although there are no specific data relating to the rates of **respiratory distress syndrome** (RDS) following elective preterm delivery in OC, there is some evidence that the incidence of RDS may be increased, affecting up to 25% of OC infants.[3] An analysis of bronchoalveolar fluid from these infants shows that it contains high levels of BAs, suggesting that the RDS is a direct consequence of the disease itself. Several studies have shown that OC is not associated with an increased frequency of small-for-gestational age infants, and although a lower mean birth weight has been described in three studies, it is not associated with intrauterine growth restriction.[3]

DIFFERENTIAL DIAGNOSIS

Before diagnosing OC, other causes of pruritus and/or hepatic impairment should be excluded (see Table 17.1). Diseases listed in Table 17.1 often present with pruritus, and some may coexist with OC. Atopic dermatitis/atopic eruption of pregnancy (AEP) presents with pruritus and primary skin lesions early in pregnancy (75% in the first or second trimester) and shows no liver function test (LFT) abnormalities. Approximately 20% of patients with AEP have a history of atopic dermatitis; the rest have been classified as atopic based on personal and/or family history of atopy and/or elevated serum immunoglobulin E (IgE) levels. Specific dermatoses of pregnancy, such as polymorphic eruption (PEP), prurigo, and pruritic folliculitis of pregnancy, present with primary skin lesions, which are absent in OC. In contrast to OC, there are neither LFT abnormalities nor fetal risks associated with these specific dermatoses. PEP typically affects primigravidas in the third trimester. It usually presents with pruritic lesions on the abdomen that show periumbilical sparing and are often urticarial. Unlike OC, a recurrence of PEP in subsequent pregnancies is uncommon.

Prurigo of pregnancy presents with pruritic papules and nodules on the extensor surfaces of the extremities and occasionally on the abdomen and elsewhere, at about 25 to 30 weeks' gestation and persists until delivery. It may recur in subsequent pregnancies. Serology may show an elevated serum IgE level. Pruritic folliculitis of pregnancy presents during the second or third trimester as follicular and/or acneiform sterile papulopustules on the trunk, thighs, and arms. The eruption may recur in subsequent pregnancies. *Pruritus gravidarum* presents in a manner similar to OC (i.e., pruritus in the third trimester). However, unlike OC, it is not associated with abnormal LFTs, and serum BAs remain within normal limits. Also, *pruritus gravidarum* is not associated with adverse fetal outcomes and resolves in the immediate postpartum period. The etiology of *pruritus gravidarum* is unclear; it may relate to the pruritic effects of reproductive hormones and therefore shares some etiologic factors with OC.

DIAGNOSIS

OC diagnosis is based on the clinical presentation of pruritus in association with raised serum BAs and deranged LFTs in the absence of any other obvious cause. Serum BAs are the most sensitive and specific markers for the diagnosis and monitoring of OC. In normal pregnancy, there is a subtle rise in BA level with advancing gestation, but the level remains within the normal range. BA levels in OC are elevated up to 100 times the upper limit of normal.[3] The rise in serum BAs may precede the onset of pruritus and any other laboratory abnormalities.[21] Although in clinical practice, total BAs are measured, there are reports that the level of individual BAs may be even more sensitive. It has been suggested that the cholic acid (CA) level or the ratio of the primary BAs (cholic:chenodeoxycholic acid [CA:CDCA]) are even more sensitive indicators for the early diagnosis of OC.[3]

Alanine transaminase (ALT) and aspartate transaminase (AST) levels increase in OC, indicating hepatocellular damage. The rise in transaminases may occur prior to or after the rise in serum BAs and, in a small proportion of cases, they remain in the normal range.[3] ALT is reported to be more sensitive than AST, and the increase in ALT tends to be greater than that in AST. Bilirubin levels are elevated in approximately 10% of cases and are therefore of limited value in the diagnosis. If raised, hyperbilirubinemia is typically conjugated.[3] GGT is elevated in a subset of approximately 30% of patients. Increased GGT levels may be associated with a greater level of impairment of the other LFTs.[3] Alkaline phosphatase (ALP) may be elevated, but the production of this enzyme by the placenta renders it largely unhelpful in the diagnosis of OC. In addition, OC has been reported to be associated with deranged lipid profiles, impaired glucose tolerance, and abnormal clotting,[3] although these abnormalities have only been observed in a small number of patients.

MANAGEMENT

The management of OC aims at alleviating maternal symptoms, correcting biochemical abnormalities, and reducing the risk of adverse pregnancy outcomes (Table 17.2). Increased fetal monitoring, by means of fetal movement charts and CTG, is recommended. However, it should be noted that there are several case reports of normal fetal movements and/or CTG recordings in the hours preceding fetal death.[3]

The mainstay of pharmacologic therapy is UDCA. UDCA is a hydrophilic BA, which occurs in trace amounts in normal human bile. It has a direct protective role on the placenta in that it decreases placental apoptosis (Fig. 17.7). UDCA stimulates biliary secretion by posttranscriptional modification of the main export pump, BSEP, and the alternative exporters MRP3 and MRP4 (Fig. 17.8).[30] A recent meta-analysis of nine randomized controlled trials (RCTs) of UDCA in OC reported significant improvements in pruritus and LFT abnormalities, including reductions in serum ALT and BAs.[31] Furthermore, this study also reported an improvement in fetal outcomes with fewer preterm deliveries, fewer admissions to neonatal intensive care units, and less frequent fetal distress and respiratory distress. Of note, this meta-analysis did not consider the single largest RCT of UDCA to date,[32] which includes 125 women, that was simultaneously performed. This trial showed significant reductions in maternal pruritus, ALT, GGT, and bilirubin levels but not in serum BAs.[32] In terms of fetal outcome, this trial showed a significant

TABLE 17.2 Summary of Management Options

Treatment	Comment
Symptomatic treatments	Aqueous cream with 2% menthol, oral antihistamines, cool baths
Ursodeoxycholic acid[a]	First-line Rx; 15 mg/kg/d; relief from pruritus and correction of abnormal LFTs; safe and may improve fetal outcome[22,33,34]
Rifampicin[a]	Second-line Rx; works synergistically with UDCA; no trial data on pruritus or correction of abnormal LFTs[30]
S-adenosyl-L-methionine	Inconsistent effects on pruritus and LFT abnormalities; synergistic effect with UDCA but inferior to UDCA in a comparative study[33]
Dexamethasone	Pruritus relief and correction of LFT abnormalities; promise from initial study[34] not confirmed[35]
Cholestyramine	Up to 18 g/d; only for mild-to-moderate OC; needs to be administered for several days before pruritus relief is achieved and does not improve the LFT abnormalities; vitamin K supplementation required[36]
Phenobarbital	Limited success; mild reduction in pruritus, no effect on BAs[36]
Guar gum	Minimal reduction in pruritus; does not correct the LFT abnormalities[37]
Activated charcoal	Reduction in serum BAs; no effect on pruritus[38]
UVB	Anecdotal; may help with pruritus in mild OC
Epomediol, silymarin	Mild reduction in pruritus, no effect on LFTs (insufficient data)[39]
Vitamin K supplementation[a]	Oral dose 10 mg/d; may protect from postpartum haemorrhage[41]
Obstetric management	■ There is no consensus; however, weighing the risks of elective early delivery against the risk of continuing the pregnancy (stillbirth) may justify the induction of labor after 37 weeks of pregnancy.[42] ■ The Royal College of Obstetricians and Gynecologists advises[43]: ■ Patients should have consultant-led, team-based care and delivery in a hospital unit. ■ Patients should be informed of the increased risks of preterm delivery and meconium staining of the amniotic fluid. ■ There is no specific method of antenatal fetal monitoring to predict stillbirth; the current additional risk of stillbirth has not been accurately quantified. ■ The risks and benefits of delivery after 37 weeks' gestation should be discussed with patients.

[a] Treatments used and recommended by the authors.

BA, bile acid; LFT, liver function test; OC, obstetric cholestasis; Rx, treatment; UDCA, ursodeoxycholic acid; UVB, ultraviolet light B.

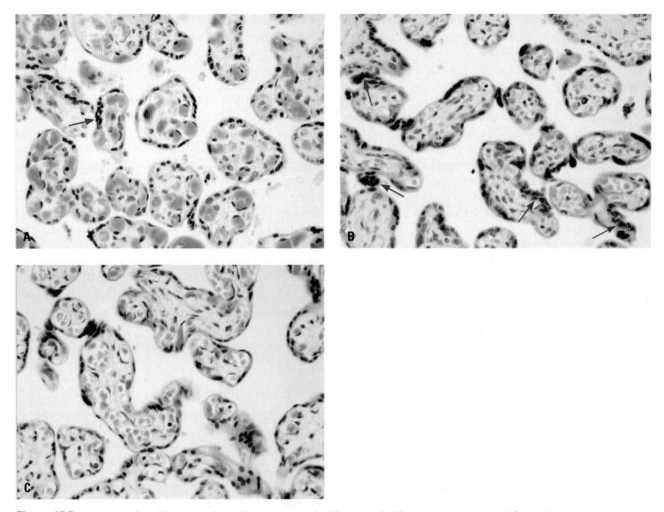

Figure 17.7. Micrographs of hematoxylin and eosin–stained villous trophoblast sections prepared from (**A**) normal and (**B**) obstetric cholestasis pregnancies with untreated obstetric cholestasis; (**C**) after treatment with ursodeoxycholic acid. Morphologic abnormalities identified in the obstetric cholestasis samples include an increased number of syncytial knots *(arrows)*. These represent areas of degenerating nuclei and are associated with other conditions in which there is increased placental apoptosis. The number of syncytial knots is reduced following treatment with ursodeoxycholic acid, suggesting a direct protective role for this drug on the placenta.

reduction in the rate of meconium staining. Therefore, the evidence for an association between UDCA and improved fetal outcomes remains weak. However, the drug is well tolerated by patients. At higher doses, patients may exceptionally complain of diarrhea and gastrointestinal upset.

Rifampicin has been shown to significantly reduce serum transaminases and BAs and to improve pruritus in several liver diseases.[30] There are no studies on the use of rifampicin in OC; however, the authors are aware of several cases that did not respond to UDCA monotherapy but that did subsequently respond to a combination of UDCA and rifampicin. The complementary mechanisms of action of UDCA and rifampicin are shown in Figure 17.8. S-adenosyl-L-methionine has inconsistent effects on pruritus and LFT abnormalities, and its administration as a twice daily and usually intravenous infusion make it a less appealing option. It was shown to have a synergistic effect with UDCA in one study.[33] Dexamethasone was originally reported to improve symptoms,[34] but this finding was not

reproduced.[35] Dexamethasone is now rarely used in OC because of its ability to cross the placenta and its association with fetal risks, such as decreased birth weight and abnormal neurologic development.[3] Other drugs, including cholestyramine,[36] phenobarbital,[36] guar gum,[37] activated charcoal, epomediol, and silymarin[38] have not been subjected to RTCs and have now been largely superseded by UDCA. Antenatal use of oral vitamin K may protect against the risk of postpartum maternal hemorrhage and fetal or neonatal bleeding. There are no RCTs in this area; however, a study showed that postpartum hemorrhage was more common in women who had not received vitamin K compared with those who had (45% versus 12%).[39]

Obstetric Management

There are no clinical and/or laboratory parameters that can predict the risk of intrauterine death. Traditional methods of fetal surveillance, such as regular CTG as early

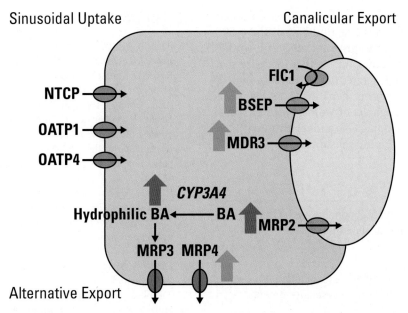

Sinusoidal Uptake

Canalicular Export

Alternative Export

Figure 17.8. A schematic showing the complementary effects of ursodeoxycholic acid *(orange arrows)* and rifampicin *(purple arrows)* in the treatment of cholestatic liver disease. Ursodeoxycholic acid induces the protein expression of BSEP and MDR3, thereby enhancing the canalicular excretion of bile acids and phosphatidylcholine, respectively. It also induces MRP4 at the basolateral membrane, facilitating further excretion of bile acids via alternative export pathways. Rifampicin enhances the excretion of bilirubin via the induction of MRP2 and also facilitates the conversion of hydrophobic bile acids to more hydrophilic species via the induction of CYP3A4. This then promotes bile acid excretion via the basolateral exporter MRP3. *Green,* canalicular export; *purple,* sinusoidal uptake; *blue,* alternative export. BSEP, bile salt export pump; FIC, familial intrahepatic cholestasis; MDR3, multidrug resistance protein 3; MRP, multidrug resistance protein; NTCP, sodium taurocholate cotransporting polypeptide; OATP, organic anion transporting polypeptide.

as the 34th week, are not reliable for predicting the risk of fetal distress or death. Amniocentesis for the presence of meconium has been proposed as a way to predict fetal risks[40] because meconium staining in OC preceded fetal death in 86% of the reported cases.[3] This approach was used in a study that included 206 patients with severe OC and followed a protocol of elective delivery at 37 weeks in the presence of meconium and/or nonreassuring fetal testing and/or severe maternal disease.[40] Of note, no intrauterine deaths were reported with this management strategy and there was no increase in cesarean delivery rate. However, some obstetricians may find this approach too invasive.

There is no consensus about the benefits of an early delivery.[41] Still, a significant body of literature supports delivery between 37 and 38 weeks in women with elevated serum BAs because this may reduce the risk of intrauterine death due to the fact that the majority of stillbirths cluster around the 38th week.[42] Some authors consider delivery around 36 weeks or earlier for severe cases presenting with jaundice, progressive BA elevations, and suspected fetal distress if lung maturity is achieved and the cervix is favorable.[40] Two studies have indicated that rates of cesarean sections are not increased with preterm

elective delivery in OC.[32,40] Along the same lines, many authors consider the iatrogenic risks associated with active management (i.e., greater incidence of failed induction, instrumental delivery) less serious than the risk of intrauterine death posed by spontaneous labor.[42] A study showed iatrogenic risks (i.e., increase in neonatal care admissions, neonates requiring ventilator support) associated with active OC management but no stillbirths or perinatal deaths.[41]

PROGNOSIS

OC resolves rapidly following delivery, typically within 2 to 8 weeks' postpartum. However, there are a few case reports of a more prolonged disease with hepatic impairment lasting up to 82 weeks.[3] Therefore, it is essential to repeat LFTs and serum BA levels at 8 to 12 weeks' postpartum and to consider alternative diagnoses in cases with continued liver dysfunction. There is a high rate of recurrence of OC in subsequent pregnancies, but disease severity and fetal outcomes cannot be predicted by an individual's history.[3] Recurrence is less likely following multiple pregnancies. Women with a history of OC may also experience a recurrence of symptoms with their menstrual cycle (usually in the second half of the cycle) and when taking oral contraceptives.[3] Long-term studies of patients with OC are scanty, but there is evidence that affected women have higher rates of gallstones, nonalcoholic cirrhosis and pancreatitis, hepatitis C, and autoimmune hepatitis.[3] The daughters of women with OC have an increased risk of developing OC, and relatives may have an increased risk of developing gallstones.

MATERNAL RISKS

Recurrence in subsequent pregnancies, with oral contraceptives, or during menstrual cycle

Postpartum hemorrhage

Gallstones

Minor gastrointestinal symptoms (e.g., bloating) in association with ursodeoxycholic acid treatment

FETAL RISKS

Preterm delivery

Fetal distress

Meconium staining of the amniotic fluid

Stillbirth

Neonatal respiratory distress syndrome

Risks from pharmacologic treatment

KEY POINTS

■ Obstetric cholestasis is a common cause of pruritus in pregnancy that can be differentiated from other causes by the absence of primary skin lesions and by the presence of typical laboratory abnormalities.

■ An elevation in the maternal serum bile acid level is mandatory for the diagnosis; once the diagnosis is made, liver function tests should be monitored once a week.

■ Obstetric cholestasis is associated with increased fetal risks, including preterm delivery, fetal distress, meconium staining of the amniotic fluid, and intrauterine death; there is no method of fetal monitoring that can predict fetal risks.

■ Ursodeoxycholic acid is the treatment of choice and improves pruritus and biochemical abnormalities; however, the data to support a beneficial effect of the medication on fetal outcome or on safety are weak.

■ The optimal obstetric management has been debated; benefits and risks from elective delivery by 38 weeks' gestation should be weighed against a risk of stillbirth with expectant management, and a decision should be made on a case-by-case basis and after careful counseling.

REFERENCES

1. Furhoff AK. Itching in pregnancy. A 15-year follow-up study. *Acta Med Scand.* 1974;196:403–410.

2. Roger D, Vaillant L, Fignon A, et al. Specific pruritic diseases of pregnancy. A prospective study of 3192 pregnant women. *Arch Dermatol.* 1994;130:734–739.

3. Geenes V, Williamson C. Intrahepatic cholestasis of pregnancy. *World J Gastroenterol.* 2009;15:2049–2066.

4. Reyes H, Gonzalez MC, Ribalta J, et al. Prevalence of intrahepatic cholestasis of pregnancy in Chile. *Ann Intern Med.* 1978;88: 487–493.

5. Reyes H. Sex hormones and bile acids in intrahepatic cholestasis of pregnancy. *Hepatology.* 2008;47:376–379.

6. Abedin P, Weaver JB, Egginton E. Intrahepatic cholestasis of pregnancy: prevalence and ethnic distribution. *Ethn Health.* 1999;4: 35–37.

7. Glantz A, Marschall HU, Mattsson LA. Intrahepatic cholestasis of pregnancy: relationships between bile acid levels and fetal complication rates. *Hepatology.* 2004;40:467–474.

8. Holzbach RT, Sivak DA, Braun WE. Familial recurrent intrahepatic cholestasis of pregnancy: a genetic study providing evidence for transmission of a sex-limited, dominant trait. *Gastroenterology.* 1983;85:175–179.

9. Reyes H, Ribalta J, Gonzalez-Ceron M. Idiopathic cholestasis of pregnancy in a large kindred. *Gut.* 1976;17:709–713.

10. Eloranta ML, Heinonen S, Mononen T, et al. Risk of obstetric cholestasis in sisters of index patients. *Clin Genet.* 2001;60: 42–45.

11. Dixon PH, Williamson C. The molecular genetics of intrahepatic cholestasis of pregnancy. *Obstet Med.* 2009;1:65–71.

12. Dixon PH, van Mil SW, Chambers J, et al. Contribution of variant alleles of ABCB11 to susceptibility to intrahepatic cholestasis of pregnancy. *Gut.* 2009;58:537–544.

13. Williamson C, Hems LM, Goulis DG, et al. Clinical outcome in a series of cases of obstetric cholestasis identified via a patient support group. *BJOG.* 2004;111:676–681.

14. Reyes H, Ribalta J, Gonzalez MC, et al. Sulfobromophthalein clearance tests before and after ethinyl estradiol administration, in women and men with familial history of intrahepatic cholestasis of pregnancy. *Gastroenterology.* 1981;81:226–231.

15. Barth A, Klinger G, Rost M. Influence of ethinyloestradiol propanolsulphonate on serum bile acids in healthy volunteers. *Exp Toxicol Pathol.* 2003;54:381–386.

16. Bacq Y, Myara A, Brechot MC, et al. Serum conjugated bile acid profile during intrahepatic cholestasis of pregnancy. *J Hepatol.* 1995;22:66–70.

17. Meng LJ, Reyes H, Palma J, et al. Profiles of bile acids and progesterone metabolites in the urine and serum of women with intrahepatic cholestasis of pregnancy. *J Hepatol.* 1997;27: 346–357.

18. Laatikainen TJ, Peltonen JI, Nylander PL. Effect of maternal intrahepatic cholestasis on fetal steroid metabolism. *J Clin Invest.* 1974;53(6):1709–1715.

19. Abu-Hayyeh S, Martinez-Becerra P, Sheikh Abdul Kadir SH, et al. Inhibition of Na+-taurocholate Co-transporting polypeptide-mediated bile acid transport by cholestatic sulfated progesterone metabolites. *J Biol Chem.* 2010;285:16504–16512.

20. Berg B, Helm G, Petersohn L, et al. Cholestasis of pregnancy. Clinical and laboratory studies. *Acta Obstet Gynecol Scand.* 1986; 65:107–113.

21. Kenyon AP, Piercy CN, Girling J, et al. Pruritus may precede abnormal liver function tests in pregnant women with obstetric cholestasis: a longitudinal analysis. *BJOG.* 2001;108:1190–1192.

22. Glantz A, Reilly SJ, Benthin L, et al. Intrahepatic cholestasis of pregnancy: amelioration of pruritus by UDCA is associated with decreased progesterone disulphates in urine. *Hepatology.* 2008;47:544–551.

23. Kremer AE, Martens JJ, Kulik W, et al. Lysophosphatidic acid is a potential mediator of cholestatic pruritu. *Gastroenterology.* 2010;139:1008–1018.

24. Laatikainen T, Ikonen E. Serum bile acids in cholestasis of pregnancy. *Obstet Gynecol.* 1977;50:313–318.

25. Laatikainen T, Tulenheimo A. Maternal serum bile acid levels and fetal distress in cholestasis of pregnancy. *Int J Gynaecol Obstet.* 1984;22:91–94.

26. Lee RH, Kwok KM, Ingles S, et al. Pregnancy outcomes during an era of aggressive management for intrahepatic cholestasis of pregnancy. *Am J Perinatol.* 2008;25:341–345.

27. Oztekin D, Aydal I, Oztekin O, et al. Predicting fetal asphyxia in intrahepatic cholestasis of pregnancy. *Arch Gynecol Obstet.* 2009;280:975–979.

28. Pata O, Vardarelı E, Ozcan A, et al. Intrahepatic cholestasis of pregnancy: correlation of preterm delivery with bile acids. *Turk J Gastroenterol.* 2011;22:602–605.

29. Davies MH, da Silva RC, Jones SR, et al. Fetal mortality associated with cholestasis of pregnancy and the potential benefit of therapy with ursodeoxycholic acid. *Gut.* 1995;37:580–584.

30. Marschall HU, Wagner M, Zollner G, et al. Complementary stimulation of hepatobiliary transport and detoxification systems by rifampicin and ursodeoxycholic acid in humans. *Gastroenterology.* 2005;129:476–485.

31. Bacq Y, Sentilhes L, Reyes HB, et al. Efficacy of ursodeoxycholic acid in treating intrahepatic cholestasis of pregnancy: a meta-analysis. *Gastroenterology.* 2012;143:1492–1501.

32. Chappell LC, Gurung V, Seed PT, et al. Ursodeoxycholic acid versus placebo, and early term delivery versus expectant management, in women with intrahepatic cholestasis of pregnancy: semifactorial randomised clinical trial. *BMJ.* 2012;344:e3799. doi:10.1136/bmj.e3799

33. Nicastri PL, Diaferia A, Tartagni M, et al. A randomised placebo-controlled trial of ursodeoxycholic acid and S-adenosylmethionine in the treatment of intrahepatic cholestasis of pregnancy. *Br J Obstet Gynaecol.* 1998;105:1205–1207.

34. Hirvioja ML, Tuimala R, Vuori J. The treatment of intrahepatic cholestasis of pregnancy by dexamethasone. *Br J Obstet Gynaecol.* 1992;99:109–111.

35. Glantz A, Marschall HU, Lammert F, et al. Intrahepatic cholestasis of pregnancy: a randomized controlled trial comparing dexamethasone and ursodeoxycholic acid. *Hepatology.* 2005;42:1399–1405.

36. Laatikainen T. Effect of cholestyramine and phenobarbital on pruritus and serum bile acid levels in cholestasis of pregnancy. *Am J Obstet Gynecol.* 1978;132:501–506.

37. Riikonen S, Savonius H, Gylling H, et al. Oral guar gum, a gel-forming dietary fiber relieves pruritus in intrahepatic cholestasis of pregnancy. *Acta Obstet Gynecol Scand.* 2000;79:260–264.

38. Kaaja RJ, Kontula KK, Raiha A, et al. Treatment of cholestasis of pregnancy with peroral activated charcoal. A preliminary study. *Scand J Gastroenterol.* 1994;29:178–181.

39. Gonzalez MC, Iglesias J, Tiribelli C, et al. Epomediol ameliorates pruritus in patients with intrahepatic cholestasis of pregnancy. *J Hepatol.* 1992;16:241–242.

40. Roncaglia N, Arreghini A, Locatelli A, et al. Obstetric cholestasis: outcome with active management. *Eur J Obstet Gynecol Reprod Biol.* 2002;100:167–170.

41. Kenyon AP, Piercy CN, Girling J, et al. Obstetric cholestasis, outcome with active management: a series of 70 cases. *BJOG.* 2002;109:282–288.

42. Mays JK. The active management of intrahepatic cholestasis of pregnancy. *Curr Opin Obstet Gynecol.* 2010;22:100–103.

43. Royal College of Obstetricians and Gynaecologists. Obstetric cholestasis. (Green-top 43). http://www.rcog.org.uk/womens-health/clinical-guidance/obstetric-cholestasis-green-top-43. Published May 19, 2011. Accessed June 25, 2013.

Iris K. Aronson ■ George Kroumpouzos

INTRODUCTION

The terminology of specific dermatoses has been confusing and often misleading as a result of poor definition of several of these entities,[1,2] which is mainly due to a poor understanding of their etiopathogenesis. The etiopathogenesis of pemphigoid gestationis (PG) and obstetric cholestasis (OC) has been clarified; however, little is known about the etiopathogenesis of polymorphic eruption (PEP), prurigo (PP), and pruritic folliculitis of pregnancy (PFP). This chapter reviews the history, nomenclature (Table 18.1), and classifications of specific dermatoses and highlights their differentiating features.

HISTORY AND NOMENCLATURE

Herpes gestationis was historically introduced by Milton[3] and is still used in certain countries, including the United States. However, it has been extensively replaced by PG, which is more appropriate because of striking similarities of the disease with the pemphigoid group of disorders. *Cholestasis of pregnancy* and *intrahepatic cholestasis of pregnancy* are synonymous with OC, and they are all appropriate.

Nomenclature of Urticarial Eruptions

PEP has been described under various designations as a result of its variable clinical presentations. It was initially described as *erythema multiforme of pregnancy*,[4] which reflected the presence of targetoid, erythema multiforme-like lesions,[5] and then as *toxemic rash of pregnancy*[6] despite the lack of association with preeclampsia. Nurse[7] reported PEP under the term *late-onset prurigo of pregnancy*, which reflects the onset of the disease in late pregnancy. *Toxic erythema of pregnancy*[8] was then introduced but has not been widely used. The term *pruritic urticarial papules and plaques of pregnancy* (PUPPP), introduced by Lawley, Hertz, and Wade[9] in 1979 is still used, especially in the United States, because the eruption shows predominantly urticarial lesions. PEP, introduced by Holmes and Black,[10] emphasizes on the variable presentations of the eruption and has gained wide support.

Nomenclature of Papular and Prurigo-Type Eruptions

Besnier, Brocq, and Jacquet used the term *prurigo gestationis* to describe all pruritic, pregnancy-related dermatoses other than PG.[11] *Prurigo gestationis of Besnier* was used

by Costello to characterize these dermatoses.[12] *Papular dermatitis of pregnancy* (PDP), an eruption similar to widespread *prurigo gestationis*, was then reported (see the following paragraph).[13] The term *early-onset prurigo of pregnancy*, which was introduced by Nurse, described cases with clinical similarities to PDP.[7] Although Nurse did not report on liver function studies and histopathology and did not exclude the biochemical abnormalities of PDP, most authors concur that early-onset prurigo of pregnancy is not different than PP. The term *PP* was introduced in order to comprise the previous entities.[10] Holmes and Black then suggested that PP can be a result of *pruritus gravidarum* in women with atopic diathesis.[5] The group recently reclassified PP under *atopic eruption of pregnancy* (AEP) based on personal and/or family history of atopy in a significant percentage of PP patients and/or serum immunoglobulin E (IgE) elevations.[14]

Papular dermatitis of pregnancy was described by Spangler et al. in 1962 and estimated its incidence to be approximately 1 in 2,400 pregnancies.[13] The lesions were 3- to 5-mm pruritic papules in a generalized distribution; urticarial lesions have also been described.[15] The eruption occurred throughout pregnancy and cleared after delivery. Histopathology of the skin was nonspecific, and skin immunofluorescence was negative. Significant hormonal abnormalities were found, including an elevated level of urinary chorionic gonadotropin in the third trimester, and low levels of plasma cortisol and urinary estriol. Spangler et al.[13] reported a high fetal mortality rate (27%) and recommended systemic steroids (prednisone or prednisolone, up to 200 mg/d) or diethylstilbestrol. They claimed that these treatments can decrease fetal risks. However, they later discounted the suggestion about diethylstilbestrol because of its association to vaginal carcinoma in female offspring. A high fetal mortality in PDP was not reproduced by other authors, and several authors reported on the efficacy of steroid tapers.[15] Since then, several large series have not found cases of PDP.[16,17] The dismal fetal outcome reported by Spangler et al. may have been biased by the methodology used in data collection.[18] Because of clinical similarities with widespread PP, most authors agree that PDP should be classified under PP.

Linear immunoglobulin M (IgM) dermatosis of pregnancy (LMDP) was described in a patient who presented at the 37th week of gestation with intensely pruritic, erythematous, follicular papulopustules on the abdomen,

TABLE 18.1	Nomenclature of Specific Dermatoses

Disease	Synonyms
Pemphigoid gestationis	■ Herpes gestationis ■ Gestational pemphigoid
Polymorphic eruption of pregnancy	■ Pruritic urticarial papules and plaques of pregnancy ■ Late-onset prurigo of pregnancy ■ Toxemic rash of pregnancy ■ Toxemic erythema
Prurigo of pregnancy	■ Prurigo gestationis (of Besnier) ■ Early-onset prurigo of pregnancy ■ Papular dermatitis of pregnancy ■ Linear IgM disease of pregnancy
Pruritic folliculitis of pregnancy	■ Acneiform eruption of pregnancy[a] ■ Atopic eruption of pregnancy
Atopic eruption of pregnancy	■ Eczema in pregnancy ■ Prurigo gestationis (of Besnier) ■ Early-onset prurigo of pregnancy ■ Papular dermatitis of pregnancy ■ Pruritic folliculitis of pregnancy (papular type)
Obstetric cholestasis	■ Cholestasis of pregnancy ■ Intrahepatic cholestasis of pregnancy ■ Jaundice of pregnancy ■ Prurigo gravidarum

[a] Suggested denomination for nonpapular morphology of pruritic folliculitis of pregnancy.[18]

IgM, immunoglobulin M.

forearms, thighs, and legs.[19] The histologic features were those of folliculitis, and direct immunofluorescence of the skin showed bright, dense, linear IgM deposits at the basement membrane zone (BMZ). The eruption resolved within 6 weeks of delivery, and immunofluorescence became negative after resolution. A similar case was triggered by nifedipine.[20] Nevertheless, the specificity of IgM antibodies at the BMZ is low.[20] Some authors categorized LMDP under PEP and others under PP.[21]

CLASSIFICATION

Holmes and Black[5] attempted to rationalize the historic nomenclature by proposing a classification of specific dermatoses into PG, PEP, PP, and PFP (Table 18.2). They suggested that PP encompasses entities such as Besnier PG, early-onset PP, and PDP, whereas PEP includes the entities toxemic rash of pregnancy, toxic erythema of pregnancy, late-onset PP, and PUPPP.[5] Impetigo herpetiformis was excluded from specific dermatoses because it is a flare of pustular psoriasis in pregnancy rather than a specific dermatosis.

A working classification of pruritic entities was subsequently proposed by Shornick.[2] He suggested that PG and PUPPP are distinct specific dermatoses and that PFP should be classified under PP based on clinical similarities between PFP and PDP in the original PFP report.[22] Also, he suggested classifying OC under pruritic dermatoses for working purposes because the entity needs to be routinely differentiated from pruritic dermatoses. However, he indicated that OC is not a dermatosis. Roger et al.[17] suggested classifying PP, PDP, and PFP under PEP, while keeping PG and OC as separate entities; however, this classification has not gained support.

A reclassification was proposed by Black's group (see Table 18.2). The authors introduced the concept of AEP

TABLE 18.2	Classifications of Specific Dermatoses of Pregnancy	

Historic Classification[10]	Established Classification[5]	Recent Reclassification[14]
Herpes gestationis	Pemphigoid gestationis	Pemphigoid gestationis
Toxemic rash of pregnancy Late-onset prurigo of pregnancy Pruritic urticarial papules and plaques of pregnancy	Polymorphic eruption of pregnancy	Polymorphic eruption of pregnancy
Late-onset prurigo of pregnancy Prurigo gestationis of Besnier Papular dermatitis of pregnancy	Prurigo of pregnancy	Atopic eruption of pregnancy[a]
	Pruritic folliculitis of pregnancy	
		Intrahepatic cholestasis of pregnancy

[a] An atopic eruption of pregnancy includes atopic dermatitis in pregnancy, prurigo of pregnancy, and pruritic folliculitis of pregnancy.

(Modified from Kroumpouzos G. Specific dermatoses of pregnancy: advances and controversies. *Expert Rev Dermatol.* 2010;5:633–648.)

TABLE 18.3	**Overview of Specific Dermatoses of Pregnancy**			
Disease	**Prevalence**	**Clinical Data**	**Lesion Morphology and Distribution**	**Important Laboratory Findings**
Obstetric cholestasis[a]	0.7%–4%; ethnic/ geographic variation	■ Onset in late second or third trimester ■ Resolution post-partum ■ +++ recurrence in future pregnancies[b]	■ No primary skin lesions[b]; excoriations and/or prurigo papules from scratching; jaundice (10%–15%)	■ Abnormal liver function tests, most characteristically elevated serum bile acids
Pemphigoid gestationis	1:7,000 to 1:50,000	■ After first trimester or postpartum ■ Flare at delivery (75%), resolution postpartum ■ + recurrence in future pregnancies	■ Abdominal[c] urticarial lesions, involving the umbilicus (>50%), can progress into a generalized bullous eruption	■ Bx: Subepidermal vesicle, infiltrate with eosinophils ■ DIF: Linear C3 ± IgG along basement membrane zone
Polymorphic eruption	1:120 to 1:240	■ Usually third trimester or postpartum ■ Resolution post-partum ■ Primigravidas[b]; assoc multiple gestation pregnancy[b] ■ Rare recurrence in future pregnancies	■ Polymorphous eruption, most often urticarial, starts in the abdominal[d] striae and shows periumbilical sparing; often becomes generalized	■ None
Prurigo[d]	1:300 to 1:450	■ Usually after first trimester ■ Resolution post-partum ■ ++ recurrence in future pregnancies	■ Grouped excoriated papules and/or prurigo nodules over the extremities and occasionally abdomen	■ Serum IgE elevations
Pruritic folliculitis[d]	?	■ Usually after first trimester ■ Resolution post-partum ■ ± recurrence in future pregnancies	■ Follicular[b] papules and pustules on the trunk, less often on extremities	■ Bx: Sterile folliculitis
Atopic eruption	>50% of pruritic dermatoses	■ 75% of cases before 3rd trimester[b] ■ Personal and/or family h/o atopy ■ No h/o AD (80%) ■ ++ recurrence in future pregnancies	■ Patchy eczematous lesions (67%) and papular/prurigo-like lesions (33%); flex-ural distribution is common	■ Serum IgE elevations (20%–70%)

[a] Not a specific dermatosis but included in several working classifications.[2,14]

[b] A clinical diagnostic characteristic that helps differentiate the disease from other specific dermatoses.

[c] Abdominal involvement is more common in pemphigoid gestationis and polymorphic eruption than in other specific dermatoses (P < .001).[14]

[d] Prurigo and papular morphology of pruritic folliculitis of pregnancy included under atopic eruption in a reclassification (see Table 18.2).[14]

AD, atopic dermatitis; assoc, associated with; Bx, biopsy; DIF, direct immunofluorescence of the skin; h/o, history of; IgE, immunoglobulin E.

that encompasses atopic dermatitis (AD), PFP, and PP (see Ch. 21).[14] Lumping these entities together was based on possible atopic diathesis in patients with PP and PFP. The authors also showed an impressive percentage of new AD (AD developing for the first time in gestation), which includes almost 80% of all cases of AD in pregnancy.[14] The study indicated that AEP starts earlier in gestation than PEP and PG, which may facilitate the differentiation among these entities. Nevertheless, it has been challenged whether PP and PFP are always associated with atopy (see Ch. 21).[23] Using low IgE elevations as a diagnostic criterion of AEP[14] needs to be confirmed. The need for further epidemiologic investigations into the relation between the biologic changes of pregnancy and IgE immunoregulation has been stressed by several authors.[23,24]

DIFFERENTIATING FEATURES

The features that differentiate the specific dermatoses are shown in Table 18.3. The differentiation is often a clinical one because with the exception of PG and OC, these entities do not show specific laboratory findings. Some of the specific clinical features, such as distribution of urticarial lesions in abdominal striae in PEP and involvement of the umbilicus in PG, are helpful. The authors who introduced the concept of AEP proposed an algorithm that helps in the differentiation of pruritic skin diseases in pregnancy.[14] The algorithm was mainly based on earlier onset of AEP (before the third trimester) compared to the late onset (third trimester or postpartum) of PEP and PG, and additionally, distribution differences (i.e., AEP is more likely to involve the trunk and limbs, whereas PEP and PG show predominantly abdominal involvement).

The differentiation among specific dermatoses can be challenging. One-third of AEP patients develop the eruption later in gestation, making the clinical differentiation from other entities, such as PEP, difficult. As indicated elsewhere (see Chs. 9 and 21), the criteria for atopy used in the studies (see Table 9.1) may not reliably distinguish between AEP in an atypical (nonflexural) distribution and dermatoses with eczematous or nonspecific features such as PEP. Furthermore, PEP may not be easily distinguished from AEP when it presents with nonurticarial morphology earlier in pregnancy or postpartum. Further studies are required in order to better differentiate among these entities.

REFERENCES

1. Kroumpouzos G, Cohen LM. Specific dermatoses of pregnancy: an evidence-based systematic review. *Am J Obstet Gynecol.* 2003; 188:1083–1092.
2. Shornick JK. Dermatoses of pregnancy. *Semin Cutan Med Surg.* 1998;17:172–181.
3. Milton JL. *The Pathology and Treatment of Disease of the Skin.* London, England: Robert Hardwicke; 1872:205.
4. Gross P. Erythema multiforme gestationis. *Arch Dermatol Syphilol.* 1931;23:567.
5. Holmes RC, Black M. The specific dermatoses of pregnancy. *J Am Acad Dermatol.* 1983;8:405–412.
6. Bourne G. Toxemic rash of pregnancy. *Proc R Soc Med.* 1962; 55:462–464.
7. Nurse D. Prurigo of pregnancy. *Australas J Dermatol.* 1968;9: 258–267.
8. Holmes RC, Black MM, Dann J, et al. A comparative study of toxic erythema of pregnancy and herpes gestationis. *Br J Dermatol.* 1982;106:499–510.
9. Lawley TJ, Hertz KC, Wade TR, et al. Pruritic urticarial papules and plaques of pregnancy. *JAMA.* 1979;241:1696–1699.
10. Holmes RC, Black M. The specific dermatoses of pregnancy: a reappraisal with special emphasis on a proposed simplified clinical classification. *Clin Exp Dermatol.* 1982;7:65–73.
11. Besnier E, Brocq L, Jacquet L. *La Pratique Dermatologique,* Vol. 1. Paris, France: Masson; 1904:75.
12. Costello MJ. Eruptions of pregnancy. *N Y State J Med.* 1941; 41:849–855.
13. Spangler AS, Reddy W, Bardawill WA, et al. Papular dermatitis of pregnancy. *JAMA.* 1962;181:577–581.
14. Ambros-Rudolph CM, Müllegger RR, Vaughan-Jones SA, et al. The specific dermatoses of pregnancy revisited and reclassified: results of a retrospective two-center study on 505 pregnant patients. *J Am Acad Dermatol.* 2006;54:395–404.
15. Rahbari H. Pruritic papules of pregnancy. *J Cutan Pathol.* 1978; 5:347–352.
16. Vaughan Jones SA, Hern S, Nelson-Piercy C, et al. A prospective study of 200 women with dermatoses of pregnancy correlating the clinical findings with hormonal and immunopathological profiles. *Br J Dermatol.* 1999;141:71–81.
17. Roger D, Vaillant L, Fignon A, et al. Specific pruritic dermatoses of pregnancy. A prospective study of 3192 women. *Arch Dermatol.* 1994;130:734–739.
18. Ambros-Rudolph CM, Black MM, Vaughan Jones S. The papular and pruritic dermatoses of pregnancy. In: Black MM, Ambros-Rudolph C, Edwards L, et al., eds. *Obstetric and Gynecologic Dermatology.* 3rd ed. London, England: Mosby Elsevier; 2008:73–77.
19. Alcalay J, Ingber A, Hazaz B, et al. Linear IgM dermatosis of pregnancy. *J Am Acad Dermatol.* 1988;18(2 pt 2):412–415.
20. Ingber A. Linear IgM dermatosis of pregnancy. In: Ingber A, ed. *Obstetric Dermatology.* Berlin, Germany: Springer-Verlag; 2009:147–150.
21. Kroumpouzos G, Cohen LM. Dermatoses of pregnancy. *J Am Acad Dermatol.* 2001;45:1–19.
22. Zoberman E, Farmer ER. Pruritic folliculitis of pregnancy. *Arch Dermatol.* 1981;117:20–22.
23. Koutroulis I, Papoutsis J, Kroumpouzos G. Atopic dermatitis in pregnancy: current status and challenges. *Obstet Gynecol Surv.* 2011;66:654–663.
24. Bos JD. Reappraisal of dermatoses of pregnancy. *Lancet.* 1999; 354:1140.

CHAPTER 19

Pemphigoid Gestationis

George Kroumpouzos ■ Detlef Zillikens

INTRODUCTION

Pemphigoid gestationis (PG) has been historically known by many names, including *herpes gestationis*, which was coined by Milton in 1972. The disease is not related to the herpes virus, and the term PG that was coined by Holmes and Black is more appropriate because of striking similarities between PG and the pemphigoid group of disorders.

EPIDEMIOLOGY

The prevalence of PG ranges from 1 in 7,000 to 1 in 50,000 pregnancies.[1,2] A recent study in a central region of Germany showed PG to be the second most common autoimmune bullous disease, with an incidence of two new patients per million residents per year.[3] The incidence of mucous membrane pemphigoid was the same as that of bullous pemphigoid (BP): 13.4 new patients. Although the number of neonates is decreasing in central Europe and Germany, the rising overall incidence of PG compared to an epidemiologic study of the same region 15 years earlier[4] may be due to increasing awareness that the disease often presents without blisters and due to the availability of more sensitive and easy-to-use detection systems, such as enzyme-linked immunosorbent assays (ELISA). Small series of PG in African Americans does not show clinical and immunopathogenetic differences with Caucasians[5]; however, there is a lack of epidemiologic data in other ethnic groups. PG may exceptionally present itself as a paraneoplastic syndrome of a trophoblastic tumor, such choriocarcinoma or molar pregnancy, and in these cases, the course of the cutaneous disease parallels that of the tumor.[6]

ETIOLOGY

PG is a rare autoimmune subepidermal blistering disease that belongs to the spectrum of the pemphigoid group of diseases.[7,8] The major pathogenic antigen is the BP antigen 2 (collagen XVII), a 180-kd hemidesmosomal transmembrane glycoprotein (BP180).[9,10] Reactivity against both BP180 and BP antigen 1 (230-kd) has been detected in 10% of patients. Genetic susceptibility and hormonal factors may be implicated in the etiopathogenesis of PG. The former are evidenced by human leukocyte antigen (HLA) predisposition and the detection of a nonfunctioning C4 null allele in most patients.[11] The formation of the antibody inciting the disease may be modulated by hormonal factors such as pregnancy, parturition, oral contraceptives, and certain neoplasias.[7] It has been proposed that aberrant expression of Major Histocompatibility Complex (MHC) class II molecules of paternal origin in the placenta can start an allogeneic response to placental basement membrane zone (BMZ) molecules such as BP180; the antibody subsequently cross-reacts with the homologous maternal antigen in the BMZ of the skin.[12]

CLINICAL FEATURES

Onset and Skin Manifestations

PG starts typically in the second or third trimester (mean onset at 21 to 28 weeks' gestation) or the immediate postpartum period (14% to 25% of cases).[11] The onset of PG has been reported as early as 5 weeks after conception and as late as 35 days' postpartum.[8] When PG starts postpartum, its onset typically occurs within hours or 2 to 3 days of delivery and only exceptionally after postpartum day 3. PG starts in more than half of the cases on the abdomen, within the umbilicus and/or periumbilically, with severely pruritic, urticarial papules and plaques (Fig. 19.1) that may become targetoid or polycyclic (Fig. 19.2) and that spread onto other areas of the trunk (Fig. 19.3), buttocks, and extremities, often involving palms and soles (Fig. 19.4).[13] A generalized bullous eruption may follow within days to weeks of the initial presentation of pruritus (Fig. 19.5), but the disease often runs a nonbullous course. If bullae appear, they may develop in urticarial lesions or appear de novo in clinically uninvolved skin. The urticarial lesions enlarge peripherally and are rimmed by vesicles and tense bullae (Fig. 19.6). Involvement of the face (Fig. 19.7) and mucous membranes (Fig. 19.8) is rare, as are pustular lesions. Patients most often present with urticarial or even eczematous lesions; cases without bullae throughout the course of the disease are not uncommon (see

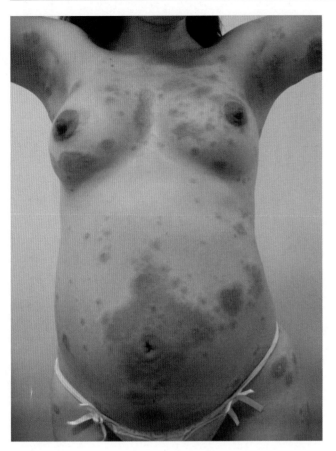

Figure 19.1. Urticarial lesions start within the umbilicus and/or periumbilically in more than half of the cases and often take on a targetoid appearance. (Courtesy of Dr. Paulo R. Cunha.)

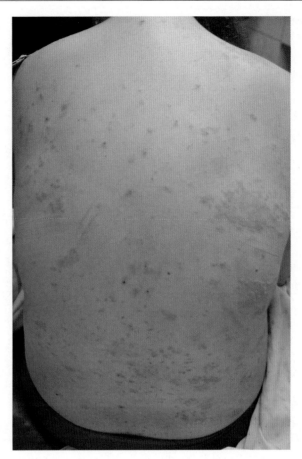

Figure 19.3. Urticarial lesions typically spread on the trunk, may become confluent, and are associated with excoriations as they are usually very pruritic.

Fig. 19.4).[2,14] Lesions heal without scarring unless superinfection occurs. PG should be considered in every pregnant patient with a longer standing history of pruritus. In many of these cases, the pregnancy is too short to take the disease into the blistering stage. This can be compared to the premonitory, nonblistering, pruritic phase of BP that may precede the bullous phase for months and even years.

Natural Course

PG runs an extremely variable clinical course. There is often a period of relative remission in the last few weeks of pregnancy followed by an abrupt relapse at the time of delivery or in the immediate postpartum period in

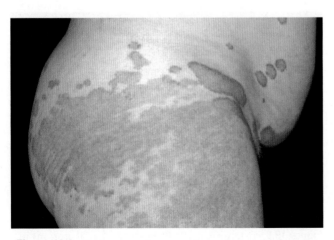

Figure 19.2. Lesions can show annular or polycyclic features.

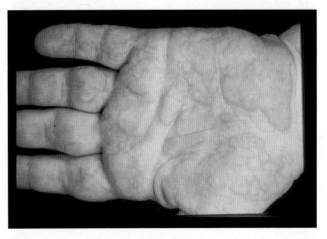

Figure 19.4. Urticarial lesions are shown on the palm of a patient with nonblistering, pemphigoid gestationis.

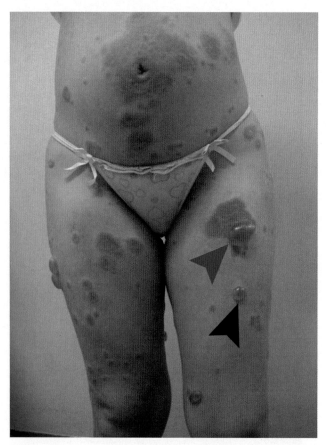

Figure 19.5. A generalized bullous eruption may follow the urticarial phase. Tense bullae develop in both involved (urticarial plaques) *(blue arrow)* and uninvolved, or minimally involved, skin *(black arrow)*. (Courtesy of Dr. Paulo R. Cunha.)

75% of the cases. PG usually subsides spontaneously even without treatment through the weeks to months after parturition, but a protracted course has been exceptionally reported; the medium duration of postpartum flares is 28 weeks[8] but may increase with the number of involved

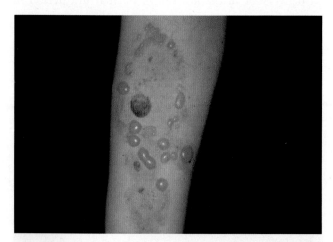

Figure 19.6. The urticarial lesions enlarge peripherally and are rimmed by vesicles and tense bullae. Breakage of some bullae with resulting crusting is shown. (Reprinted from Kroumpouzos G, Cohen LM. Dermatoses of pregnancy. *J Am Acad Dermatol.* 2001;45:1–19, with permission from Elsevier.)

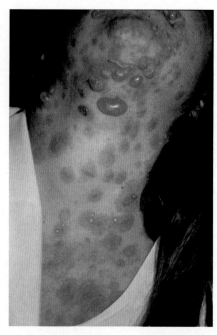

Figure 19.7. Involvement of the face is unusual. (From Kroumpouzos G, Cohen LM. Diseases of pregnancy and their treatment. In: Krieg T, Bickers D, Miyachi Y, eds. *Therapy of Skin Diseases: A Worldwide Perspective on Therapeutic Approaches and their Molecular Basis.* Berlin, Germany: Springer-Verlag; 2010: 677–691. [Courtesy of Dr. Jeffrey Callen.])

pregnancies.[15] A "conversion" to BP has been reported.[16,17] Chronic PG, defined as lasting more than 6 months' postpartum, has been reported in more than 20 cases.[15,18–21] In a case series,[20] chronic PG was more likely in older patients, multigravidas, and in those with a history of PG in previous pregnancies, a widespread eruption, and mucosal involvement.

PG often recurs in subsequent pregnancies, usually appearing more severe and earlier in gestation, and lasting longer postpartum.[2] Unaffected ("skip") pregnancies, however, have been reported (8%)[8,22] and were attributed

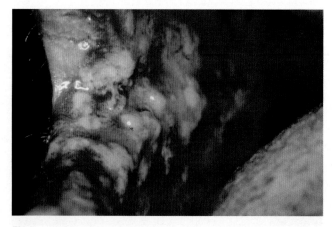

Figure 19.8. Extensive, partly fibrin-covered, oral erosions in a patient with immunoglobulin A (IgA) autoantibodies targeting the C-terminus of BP180.

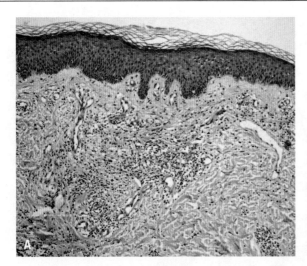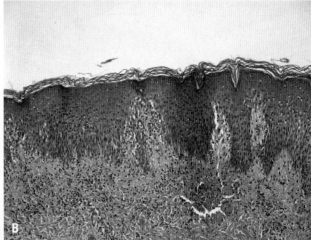

Figure 19.9. Urticarial lesions show papillary dermal edema and a mixed perivascular infiltrate with eosinophils. (**A**) Infiltrate may extend beyond the papillary dermis (hematoxylin-eosin, ×10). (**B**) Spongiosis, intracellular, and papillary dermal edema with conspicuous eosinophils. Eosinophils and neutrophils can be seen along the dermal–epidermal junction that shows vacuolar degeneration (hematoxylin-eosin, ×10). (Courtesy of Drs. Paulo R. Cunha and Lisa M. Cohen, respectively.)

to a male consort change or the expression of full compatibility at the HLA-D locus by the mother and fetus.[22] Nevertheless, skip pregnancies despite constant paternity, and nonidentical HLA-DR alleles have been reported.[8,23] Premenstrual exacerbations are common and may last for months to years. Recurrence with oral contraceptives has been reported in 20% to 50% of patients with a history of PG in small series.[2,22] It typically starts within days to weeks after the initiation of oral contraceptive use and disappears after its withdrawal. The effects of breastfeeding and prolactin on the postpartum duration of PG have not been adequately clarified, although it has been suggested that breastfeeding may reduce the duration of the disease.[15,22]

PATHOLOGY

Histopathology

The histopathologic features correlate with the morphologic characteristics of skin lesions. Urticarial lesions show a marked papillary dermal edema, which results in teardrop-shaped dermal papillae and a mixed perivascular lymphohistiocytic infiltrate with numerous eosinophils that may extend beyond the papillary dermis (Figs. 19.9 and 19.10). Spongiosis and intracellular edema may be seen (see Figs. 19.9B and 19.10A). A subepidermal blister with a large number of eosinophils in the blister cavity (Fig. 19.11) develops during the bullous phase of PG. The

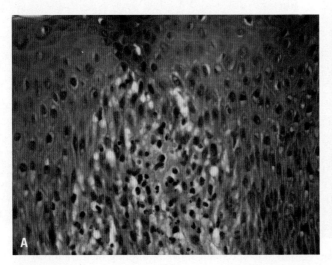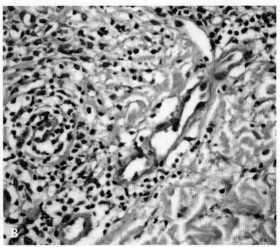

Figure 19.10. (**A**) Conspicuous eosinophils in edematous, teardrop-shaped dermal papillae (hematoxylin-eosin, ×20). (**B**) Numerous eosinophils in a dense dermal infiltrate, also seen in perivascular locations (hematoxylin-eosin, ×20). (Courtesy of Drs. Lisa M. Cohen and Paulo R. Cunha, respectively.)

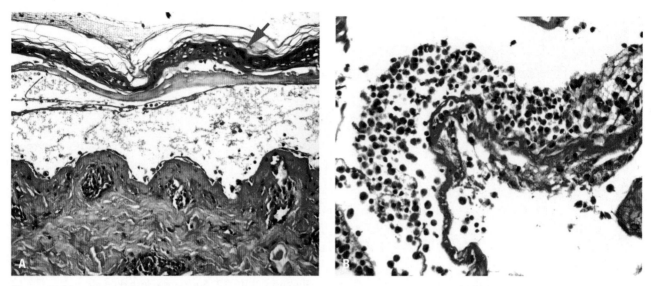

Figure 19.11. (**A**) A subepidermal blister develops secondarily to basal keratinocyte necrosis. The epidermis above the bulla is flattened and necrotic *(arrow)* (hematoxylin-eosin, ×10). (**B**) The blister contains plasma, fibrin, and inflammatory cells; numerous eosinophils can be seen (hematoxylin-eosin, ×20). (Courtesy of Dr. Paulo R. Cunha.)

presence of eosinophils is the most constant feature of PG, whereas the degree of edema or vesiculation varies.[2] PG cannot be differentiated from other subepidermal bullous diseases by a histopathologic evaluation alone.

Immunopathology

Direct immunofluorescence (DIF) microscopy of perilesional skin shows a linear third component of complement (C3) deposition, with or without immunoglobulin G (IgG), along the cutaneous BMZ in all patients (Fig. 19.12).[7] IgG deposition is detected in 25% to 30% of cases with DIF but is more commonly detected in salt-split skin specimens showing separation at the level of lamina lucida. In salt-split skin testing, the antibody binds to the roof (epidermal side) of the vesicle (Fig. 19.13). DIF may remain positive for 6 months to 4 years after clinical remission.[22] Indirect immunofluorescence (IIF) microscopy using normal human skin as substrate detects circulating serum IgG in less than 25% of cases. However, IgG is positive in all patients' sera when a three-step complement-binding IIF technique is used (Fig. 19.14).[7] Figure 19.15 shows a BIOCHIP mosaic

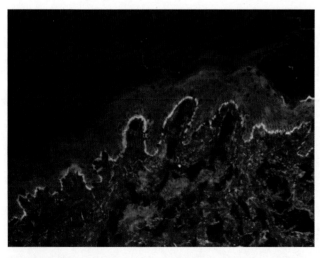

Figure 19.12. Direct immunofluorescence microscopy showing the linear deposition of immunoglobulin G (IgG) along the dermal–epidermal junction of perilesional skin.

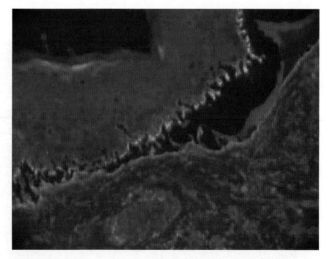

Figure 19.13. Direct immunofluorescence microscopy: Salt-split skin specimen showing binding of the antibody to the roof (epidermal side) of the vesicle. (Courtesy of Dr. Carlos H. Nousari.)

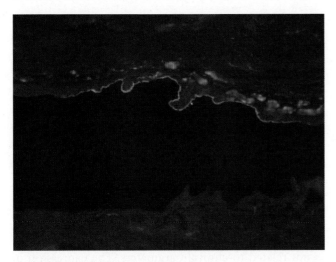

Figure 19.14. The detection of the third component of complement (C3) by an immunofluorescence complement–fixation test. The serum of a patient tested for complement-fixing immunoglobulin G (IgG) antibodies by indirect immunofluorescence microscopy using fresh complement. C3 is fixed at the epidermal side of human salt-split skin specimen.

IIF test for screening and differentiation of skin-specific autoantibodies. The historic term *herpes gestationis* factor was used for an IgG1 autoantibody against the BMZ. Similar linear deposition of C3 and IgG has been observed in the skin of neonates of affected mothers and along the BMZ of the amniotic epithelium (Fig. 19.16).[2,7] Immunoelectron microscopy shows that the deposits of C3 and IgG are localized to the upper lamina lucida beneath the plasma membrane. Table 19.1 summarizes the immunofluorescence findings in PG and autoimmune vesiculobullous diseases that need to be differentiated from PG.

DIAGNOSIS

The diagnosis is based on the constellation of clinical and histopathologic features and immunopathologic testing, especially DIF and serologic analysis (complement-binding test, ELISA), as outlined previously. PG should be considered in a pregnant patient with longer standing

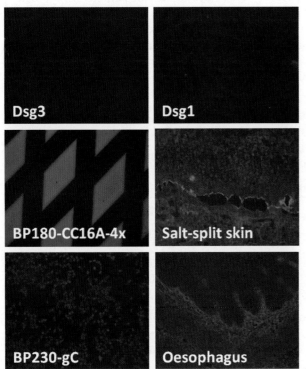

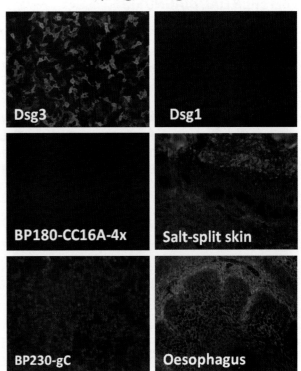

Figure 19.15. A BIOCHIP mosaic indirect immunofluorescence test for screening and differentiation of skin-specific autoantibodies in a single incubation step. Stainings after incubation with a pemphigoid gestations (PG, *left*), and pemphigus vulgaris (PV, *right*) serum. Desmoglein (Dsg) 1, Dsg 3, and BP230gC (C-terminal globular domain of BP230) are expressed in human HEK293 cells. BP180 NC16A is directly coated on the BIOCHIP. Further substrates are primate esophagus and salt-split human skin. For the PG serum, staining of recombinant NC16A and the epidermal side of the salt-split skin is observed, whereas the PV autoantibodies recognize recombinant Dsg 3 and stain monkey esophagus with an intercellular epithelial pattern.

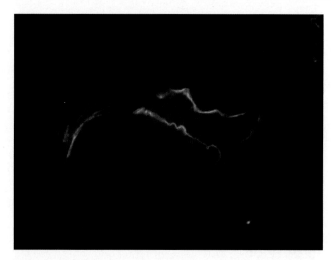

Figure 19.16. Direct immunofluorescence analysis of gestational pemphigoid placenta showed a linear third component of complement (C3) positivity in the trophoblastic villous basement membrane. (Courtesy of Dr. Kaisa Tasanen.)

pruritus. In these cases, at least a serum sample should be analyzed by ELISA and IIF (complement-binding test).

DIFFERENTIAL DIAGNOSIS

The differential diagnosis is summarized in Table 19.2. In the nonbullous phase of PG, differentiation from other inflammatory diseases may be clinically difficult. In particular, polymorphic eruption of pregnancy (PEP) (see Ch. 20) can manifest itself with urticarial lesions that are indistinguishable from those of early stage, prebullous PG. However, DIF (negative in PEP and other inflammatory diseases) can differentiate between these entities.

PATHOGENESIS

Immunogenetics

The expression of MHC class II HLA antigens DR3 (61% to 85%), DR4 (52%), or both (43% to 45%) has been reported (the combination is reported in 3% of healthy controls).[24] HLA-DRB1*0301 (DR3) and DRB1*0401/0340X (DR4) have been associated with PG. Yet, the HLA type is not related to clinical parameters. The expression of HLA-DR2 was reported in 50% of spouses, especially those of patients with the DR3/DR4 combination. The nonfunctioning C4 null allele is present in virtually all patients. The C4A null allele (C4*QO) is detected in 90% of patients and may impair immune complex degradation.[25] Because of close proximity between C4 and DR alleles, there is strong disequilibrium between C4 null alleles and DR3, making it difficult to determine the primary genetic link in PG. Antibodies against paternal HLA molecules were found in 85% of patients with a history of PG as compared to 25% in a control group of healthy multiparous women.[11] However, it remains uncertain whether the high prevalence of anti-HLA antibodies supports the theory of "paternal factor" or is simply an epiphenomenon.

TABLE 19.1	Immunofluorescence Findings That Aid in Differentiating Pemphigoid Gestationis From Other Autoimmune Vesiculobullous Disorders		
Disease	**DIF**	**Salt-Split Test (DIF)**	**IIF**
Pemphigoid gestationis	Linear C3 (100%) and IgG (25%–30%) along BMZ	Roof[a]	Circulating IgG against BMZ (20%); 100% with complement-binding technique
Bullous pemphigoid	Linear C3 (80%–100%) and IgG (50%–90%) along BMZ	Roof > roof + base[b]	Circulating IgG against BMZ (60%–80%), less commonly IgA, IgE
Linear IgA dermatosis	Linear IgA (90%) along BMZ	Roof > roof + base > base	Circulating IgA against BMZ (adults 50%, children 75%)
Bullous lupus erythematosus	Linear or granular IgG (100%), IgA, IgM, C3 (50%–60%) along BMZ	Floor > roof or absent	Circulating IgG against BMZ, rare IgA
Dermatitis herpetiformis	Granular IgA in dermal papillae (85%) or along BMZ (25%)	Not required	Circulating IgA antiendomysial antibody (100%)
Pemphigus vulgaris	Intercellular IgG (100%), IgA, rarely C3 (50%)	Not required	Circulating intercellular IgG (95%)

[a] Roof: Epidermal side of salt-split separation.

[b] Base: Dermal side of salt-split separation.

BMZ, basement membrane zone; C3, third component of complement; DIF, direct immunofluorescence; Ig, immunoglobulin; IIF, indirect immunofluorescence.

TABLE 19.2	Differential Diagnosis of Pemphigoid Gestationis
Disease	**Differentiating Features**
Polymorphic eruption	■ Primiparas (80%) vs. 50% in PG ■ Periumbilical sparing, bullae uncommon ■ Prominent striae, lesions on striae ■ Halo around urticarial lesions ■ Flare around delivery less common ■ DIF and IIF for C3 negative ■ Recurrence in subsequent pregnancies exceptional
Atopic eruption[a]	■ Starts earlier in pregnancy (first through second trimesters) ■ Urticarial and bullous lesions uncommon ■ H/o atopy in patient and/or family
Erythema multiforme[a]	■ H/o HSV or offending drug ■ Urticarial stage missing, mucosae affected ■ Course of disease does not stimulate pemphigoid gestationis
Urticaria[a]	■ No bullae, no predilection for umbilicus ■ No flare around delivery
Drug eruption[a]	■ Hx suggestive of drug-induced rash ■ Bullae less common, no predilection for umbilicus ■ Improvement with discontinuation of offending drug, no flare around delivery
Bullous pemphigoid[b]	■ Age typically >60 years ■ No predilection for umbilicus ■ No hormonal modulation ■ No association with trophoblastic tumors
Linear IgA dermatosis[b]	■ Herpetiform grouping of lesions, "cluster of jewels" sign, mucosal involvement (50%) ■ Pathology: Primarily neutrophilic infiltrate ■ DIF and IIF: Linear IgA along BMZ
Dermatitis herpetiformis[b]	■ Bullae unusual, herpetiform grouping of papulovesicles ■ Pathology: Primarily neutrophilic infiltrate ■ DIF: Granular IgA in papillary dermis (85%) ■ IIF: IgA antiendomysial antibodies
Bullous lupus[b]	■ H/o systemic lupus ■ Urticarial stage missing, no predilection for umbilicus, no flare around delivery ■ Pathology: Primarily neutrophilic infiltrate ■ DIF: Granular and/or linear IgG along BMZ
Pemphigus vulgaris[b]	■ Superficial erosions and flaccid blisters ■ Mucosal involvement ■ DIF and IIF: IgG stain of intercellular spaces

[a] DIF and IIF negative but not typically required for the differentiation.

[b] Immunofluorescence findings are shown in Table 19.1.

BMZ, basement membrane zone; C3, third component of complement; DIF, direct immunofluorescence; Ig, immunoglobulin; IIF, indirect immunofluorescence; HSV, herpes simplex virus; h/o, history of; Hx, history.

Immunopathogenesis

The target epitope in PG is located in the noncollagenous domain (NC16A) of the transmembrane BP180 antigen,[10,26] especially the N-terminal portion of this domain,[27] which is adjacent to the plasma membrane of the hemidesmosomes (Fig. 19.17). However, other epitopes of BP180 may occasionally be targeted.[28,29] Epitopes within the NC16A domain that are relevant for blister induction have been identified.[30] A case with predominantly oral lesions and IgA autoantibodies targeting the C-terminus of BP180 was reported (see Fig. 19.8).[29] Autoantibodies targeting the NC16A domain mainly belong to the complement-activating subclasses IgG1 and

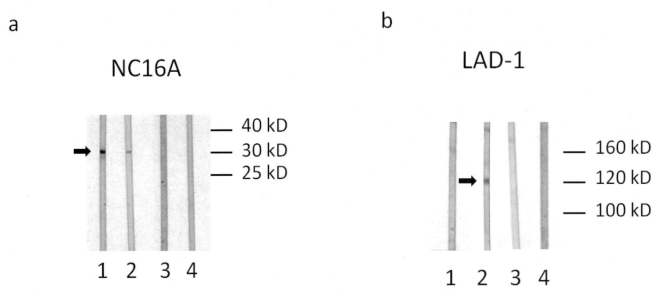

Figure 19.17. The serum from a patient recognizes recombinant NC16A, but not the linear immunoglobulin A (IgA) disease antigen-1 (LAD-1), by immunoblot analysis. **(A)** Representative immunoblot analysis using recombinant NC16A and sera of patients with pemphigoid gestationis (PG, *lane 1*), bullous pemphigoid (BP, *lane 2*), pemphigus vulgaris (PV, *lane 3*), and serum of a healthy volunteer (HV, *lane 4*). PG and BP sera recognize the recombinant protein *(arrow)*, whereas serum of the PV patient and HV do not show any reactivity with NC16A. **(B)** Representative immunoblot analysis using LAD-1, the 120-kDa cell-derived soluble ectodomain of BP180 *(arrow)*, which is the major target antigen of patients with LAD. This antigen does not contain the N-terminal half of the NC16A domain of BP180 LAD-1 is only recognized by serum of the BP patient *(lane 2)*. None of the other sera (same like in label **A**) showed reactivity with this protein.

IgG3.[31] Complement activation results in the attraction of eosinophils, and their subsequent degranulation may release proteolytic enzymes that dissolve the bond between the epidermis and dermis. One study, however, showed a predominance of IgG4 subclass in lesional skin, a finding that mimics classic BP.[32] The pathogenic relevance of autoantibodies to BP180 NC16A could be demonstrated in an ex vivo assay. IgG from PG patients, purified against a recombinant form of the BP180NC16A, induced dermal–epidermal separation in cryosections of human skin when coincubated with neutrophils from healthy volunteers. Antigen-specific T lymphocytes in the peripheral blood were shown to express a Th1 cytokine profile,[33] while a predominance of Th2-type cells was found in the inflammatory infiltrate of lesional skin.[34] Further studies will have to elucidate the role of different T-lymphocyte subsets in the pathogenesis of PG.

Serum antibody levels with conventional (not complement-fixing) IIF do not correlate well with the course of disease and may remain low-positive even after the eruption resolves. Serum antibody levels, however, correlated with disease activity when BP180 NC16A-ELISA was used.[35] ELISA has shown higher sensitivity than IIF[36,37] and can differentiate PG from PEP with a specificity and sensitivity of 96%.[38] It remains a useful diagnostic tool and a monitor marker that can guide management decisions. Two commercially ELISAs for the detection of autoantibodies to BP180 NC16A are available (MBL, Japan; EUROIMMUN, Germany).

Placental antigens may play an important role in the production of autoantibodies to BP180. Because all patients have anti-HLA antibodies against paternal class I antigens and the only source of disparate antigens is the placenta, an immunologic insult during gestation has been postulated. An increased expression of MHC class II antigens within the amniochorionic stroma and focally on the trophoblast epithelium has been shown in PG.[12] Also, the PG autoantibody can bind amniotic membrane, an ectodermal structure antigenically similar to the skin. Based on this, it has been suggested that placental BP180 is presented to the maternal immune system in the context of foreign (placental) MHC, thus triggering the production of autoantibodies that cross-react with the skin.[12] Alternatively, an allogeneic reaction of placental stromal cells to BP180 in the context of paternal MHC molecules may occur, which can bypass the need for antigen-specific helper responses.[7,12] In support of this, a study showed that BP180 is expressed by syncytial and cytotrophoblastic cells of human placenta and epithelial cells of the amniotic membrane during the first trimester, and the clinical symptoms of PG occur after the expression of autoantigen in the placenta.[39] The authors suggested that the earlier onset of PG in subsequent pregnancies could be explained by the presence of autoantigen already in the placenta during the first trimester.

MATERNAL AND FETAL RISKS

The mother is at increased risk for Graves disease (10% to 11% of patients compared to 0.4% in controls), which does not develop simultaneously with PG.[40] An increased frequency of other autoantibodies has been reported in patients with PG and, in family members, an increased frequency of autoimmune disorders, particularly Graves disease, Hashimoto thyroiditis, and pernicious anemia.[40] Despite controversy about fetal risks in PG, most recent studies indicate that these risks are manageable and the fetal/neonatal prognosis remains good.[41] Associations with small-for-gestational age weight at birth and preterm delivery have been reported. In a series of 74 cases, 16% of deliveries occurred before 36 weeks and 32% before 38 weeks' gestation versus 2% and 11%, respectively, in the control group.[42] There was no evidence that systemic steroid treatment could decrease these risks. A borderline increase in spontaneous abortions was reported[8] but is not supported by a previous study.[42] Cases of intrauterine fetal death have been reported as well as two cases of neonates that developed neurologic symptomatology, one of which was associated with convulsions.[43] An increased frequency of other autoimmune diseases has not been reported in neonates born to affected mothers. The onset of PG in the first or second trimester and presence of blisters have been associated with adverse pregnancy outcomes.[44] Because of the rarity of PG, a stratification of pregnancies to low or high risk for fetal complications has not been possible.

The fetal risks are thought to be due to low-grade placental dysfunction induced by PG autoantibodies[41,42] and may not decrease with treatment.[42] Huilaja et al.[39] suggested that BP180 autoantibodies may induce epithelial–stromal microseparation in the placenta, which may lead to minor functional failure and explain the mild fetal risks seen in PG. A recent study by the authors[45] showed an abnormal placental-to-birth weight ratio in half of pregnancies (12 studied), a detachment of basement membranes, and undeveloped hemidesmosomes. Nevertheless, umbilical artery Doppler evaluations of placental function were normal in all but one pregnancy. Although a high rate of prematurity was observed, neonatal outcome was uneventful.

Neonatal PG is a transient eruption that occurs in 5% to 10% of cases.[46] It develops as a result of passive transplacental transfer of the PG antibody, which can be demonstrated in cord blood and neonatal skin. Urticarial or vesiculobullous lesions can be seen (Fig. 19.18) and resolve spontaneously in the course of days to 3 weeks after onset, even before the maternal antibodies clear from the neonate's blood. Interestingly, the titer of the antibody transferred to the neonate is similar to that detected in the mother.[47] DIF of fetal skin is often positive despite the lack of lesions, indicating the presence of subclinical disease. DIF and the circulating IgG autoantibody become negative by the end of the first month of life.

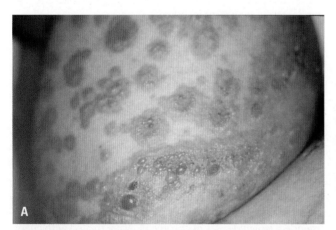

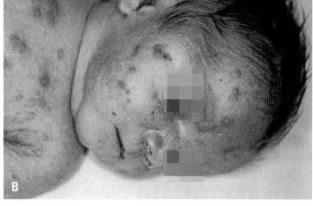

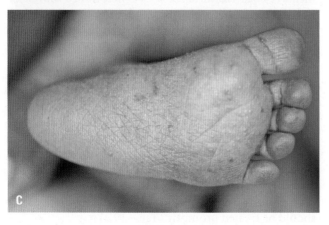

Figure 19.18. Neonatal pemphigoid gestationis. (**A**) Vesicles and bullae developing on urticarial plaques on the trunk. (**B**) Extensive involvement of the face and frontal scalp. (**C**) Minute vesicles on the sole.

MANAGEMENT

Specific Goals

Management should provide symptomatic relief and counseling in order to alleviate patient anxiety. PG is usually very pruritic, and a systemic H_1 antihistamine that is safe in gestation, such as diphenhydramine or chlorpheniramine, can be helpful. Cool compresses may provide symptomatic relief. Local care should focus on promoting healing and preventing superinfection, and the patient should be advised to use a sterile nonadherent dressing on the blisters and eroded areas. The physician may drain large tender bullae to reduce discomfort. If superinfection occurs, it should be treated promptly with an appropriate antibiotic. The patient should be counseled that there is no evidence that any treatment can prevent the fetal risks associated with PG, which can be minimized with fetal surveillance. The patient should be advised that PG may recur in subsequent pregnancies.

Systemic Corticosteroids

Potent topical corticosteroids combined with oral antihistamines are helpful for nonbullous lesions, single vesicles, periods of mild activity, or flares with menstruation. Systemic corticosteroids, in addition to topical corticosteroids, remain the mainstay of therapy for more extensive bullous disease (see Table 19.1), and the overwhelming majority of patients respond within a few days (Fig. 19.19). Most patients are started at low doses of prednisone or prednisolone (0.3 to 0.5 mg per kilogram), and the dosage is then titrated according to the clinical response. Prednisone doses higher than 1 mg per kilogram are not typically required but have been used. High doses of systemic steroids represent a risk factor for maternal and fetal adverse effects (see Ch. 23). Prednisone and prednisolone are relatively safe during gestation, but other systemic steroids such as betamethasone and dexamethasone demonstrate fetal toxicity and should be avoided.[11] Once new blister formation has been suppressed, prednisone should be maintained at the same dose for 1 to 2 weeks and then tapered to lower doses (5 to 10 mg per day) or even discontinued. The dosage may be increased or steroid therapy resumed shortly after delivery to control the anticipated flare of the disease. Postpartum prednisone at daily doses 10 to 20 mg allows for safe breastfeeding.

Nonsteroidal Treatment Options

First-line treatments for steroid-resistant cases include adjuvant immunoapheresis (IA) (immunoadsorption),[48,49] plasmapheresis,[17,50] and intravenous immunoglobulin (IVIG).[18,19,51] All have been used successfully in pregnancy and the postpartum period, and their safety profile is acceptable. A reduction of serum autoantibody levels with IA parallels the clinical response (Fig. 19.20). However, in most cases, a lower dose of systemic steroid is required to block later production of new autoantibody. IVIG has been used alone or in combination with cyclosporine[18] or other immunosuppressant medications[19,51] with some success.

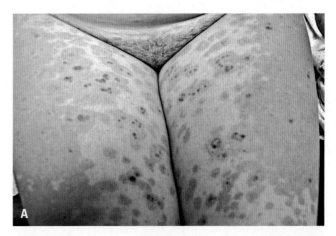

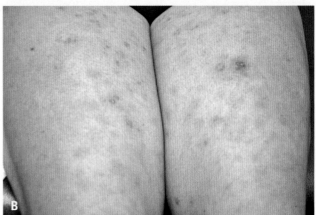

Figure 19.19. Response to systemic steroids can be dramatic. (**A**) Prior to steroid treatment. (**B**) Remission 2 weeks after systemic steroid treatment is shown.

Steroid-sparing agents should also be considered in postpartum recalcitrant or chronic PG. Minocycline or doxycycline, in combination with nicotinamide, has been successfully used in nonbreastfeeding mothers with recalcitrant PG.[52,53] Refractory cases have been treated with azathioprine in conjunction with systemic corticosteroids.[19,51,54] Immunosuppressive and anti-inflammatory agents, such as cyclophosphamide,[21] pyridoxine,[8] sulfapyridine,[8] or dapsone,[8,17,55] have been used postpartum in recalcitrant cases in nonnursing patients, often as an adjunct to systemic steroids. However, they have been inconsistently effective and therefore are not recommended. Isolated cases of chronic PG were treated with chemical oophorectomy with goserelin[16] and rituximab.[55] Early delivery is not indicated because the fetal risks seem to be mild.

Fetal Surveillance and Neonatal Care

Fetal surveillance should include monitoring for growth retardation with periodic ultrasounds, and if growth restriction is confirmed, obstetric management and decisions on early delivery should follow the guidelines for small-for-gestational age neonates.[4] Infants of patients treated with systemic corticosteroids should be evaluated for adrenal insufficiency. Lesions in infants require only simple wound care, but if a superinfection occurs, it should be treated promptly (Table 19.3).

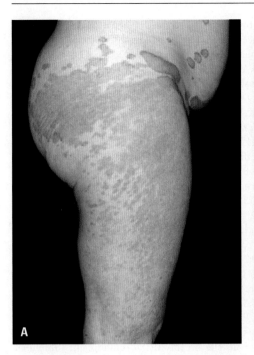
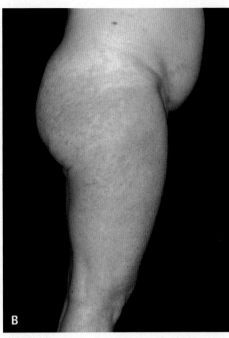

Figure 19.20. Response to immunoapheresis (IA). (**A**) Prior to treatment. (**B**) After ten IA treatments over 4 weeks, in four cycles of two or three procedures on consecutive days. IA resulted in rapid clinical remission and allowed for the tapering of prednisolone dose from 60 mg/d to 7.5 mg/d and safe breast-feeding. (Courtesy of Dr. Enno Schmidt.)

TABLE 19.3	Summary of Management Options

Treatment	Comment
Pregnant/Lactating Patient	
High-potency topical corticosteroids	First-line Rx; helpful especially in the early urticarial stage or menstrual flares and can be combined with systemic corticosteroids if needed[7,11]
Oral H$_1$ antihistamines	First-line Rx; coadministered with topical steroids, may be used in all stages[7]
Systemic corticosteroids	Second-line Rx, first-line Rx for generalized bullous disease; prednisone/prednisolone dose starting at 0.3–0.5 mg/kg,[7] titrate according to clinical response
Plasmapheresis	Second-line Rx for generalized bullous disease; a few cases treated[17,50]; typically combined with adjuvant immunosuppressive Rx, which is required to block later production of autoantibodies; logistics and cost are limiting factors
Immunoapheresis	Second-line Rx for generalized bullous disease; several cases treated[48,49]; safety profile acceptable; clinical response parallels autoantibody level reduction; allows for a low systemic steroid dose and safe breastfeeding; logistics and cost are limiting factors
IVIG	Second-line Rx for generalized bullous disease; alone or in combo with cyclosporine[18] or other immunosuppressive agents[19,51]; no adverse effects reported; cost may limit its use
Termination of pregnancy	Has resulted in resolution of recalcitrant PG[8]
Fetal monitoring/neonatal care	Periodic ultrasounds; if IUGR, obstetric management should follow guidelines for small-for-gestational age neonates; evaluate for adrenal insufficiency neonates born to patients treated with systemic steroids; simple wound care for neonatal PG and prompt Rx of any superinfection
Additional Options Postpartum in Nonlactating Patient	
Minocycline or doxycycline	Alone or in combination with nicotinamide[52,53]
Immunosuppressive medications	Cyclosporine combined with IVIG (case report)[18]; cyclophosphamide (case report)[21]; azathioprine as adjunct in recalcitrant cases[19,51,54]
Anti-CD20 antibody	Rituximab 375 mg/m^2 weekly for 4 weeks (case report)[55]
Dapsone	Used as adjunct with variable efficacy[8,17,55]; suboptimal safety profile in pregnancy/lactation
Chemical oophorectomy	Goserelin used in chronic recalcitrant PG (case report)[16]

IUGR, intrauterine growth restriction; IVIG, intravenous immunoglobulin; PG, pemphigoid gestationis; Rx, treatment.

MATERNAL RISKS

Risk of Graves disease
Risks from pharmacologic treatment

FETAL/NEONATAL RISKS

Small-for-gestational age weight at birth
Premature delivery
Neonatal pemphigoid gestationis
Fetal cerebral hemorrhage (one case)
Convulsions with neonatal pemphigoid gestationis
  (one case)
Risks from pharmacologic treatment

KEY POINTS

- Pemphigoid gestationis is a rare autoimmune disease of pregnancy or the puerperium that is closely related to the pemphigoid group of bullous disorders; it can also occur as a paraneoplastic syndrome of trophoblastic tumors.

- The disease is usually very pruritic and starts with an urticarial eruption that involves the umbilicus/periumbilical area in more than half of the cases; a generalized bullous eruption may follow, which can affect the palms and soles, and exceptionally, the face, neck, and mucous membranes.

- Pemphigoid gestationis typically remits in the last few weeks of pregnancy and relapses at the time of delivery or in the immediate postpartum period; in most cases, it spontaneously resolves through several weeks to months after parturition.

- The antibody that incites the pathology targets the noncollagenous domain of the transmembrane BP180 antigen; DIF microscopy of perilesional skin shows a linear C3 deposition, with or without IgG, along the basement membrane zone.

- Fetal risks include fetal growth restriction and premature delivery; neonatal pemphigoid gestationis is a rare transient bullous eruption.

- The response to topical and systemic corticosteroids can be dramatic; plasmapheresis/immunoapheresis and intravenous immunoglobulin are second-line treatment options.

REFERENCES

1. Zurn A, Celebi CR, Bernard P, et al. A prospective immunofluorescence study of 111 cases of pruritic dermatoses of pregnancy: IgM anti-basement membrane zone antibodies as a novel finding. *Br J Dermatol.* 1992;126:474–478.
2. Shornick JK, Bangert JL, Freeman RG, et al. Herpes gestationis: clinical and histologic features of twenty-eight cases. *J Am Acad Dermatol.* 1983;8:214–224.
3. Bertram F, Bröcker EB, Zillikens D, et al. Prospective analysis of the incidence of autoimmune bullous disorders in Lower Franconia, Germany. *J Dtsch Dermatol Ges.* 2009;7:434–440.
4. Zillikens D, Wever S, Roth A, et al. Incidence of autoimmune subepidermal blistering dermatoses in a region of central Germany. *Arch Dermatol.* 1995;131:957–958.
5. Shornick JK, Meek TJ, Nesbitt LT Jr, et al. Herpes gestationis in blacks. *Arch Dermatol.* 1984;120:511–513.
6. Sinemus K, Zillikens D, Lehmann P. [Pemphigoid gestationis—first sign of metastatic choriocarcinoma]. *J Dtsch Dermatol Ges.* 2004;2:851–854.
7. Shimanovich I, Bröcker EB, Zillikens D. Pemphigoid gestationis: new insights into the pathogenesis lead to novel diagnostic tools. *BJOG.* 2002;109:970–976.
8. Jenkins RE, Hern S, Black MM. Clinical features and management of 87 patients with pemphigoid gestationis. *Clin Exp Dermatol.* 1999;24:255–259.
9. Morrison LH, Labib RS, Zone JJ, et al. Herpes gestationis autoantibodies recognize a 180-kd human epidermal antigen. *J Clin Invest.* 1988;81:2023–2026.
10. Giudice GJ, Emery DJ, Zelickson BD, et al. Bullous pemphigoid and herpes gestationis autoantibodies recognize a common non-collagenous site on the BP180 ectodomain. *J Immunol.* 1993;151:5742–5750.
11. Semkova K, Black M. Pemphigoid gestationis: current insights into pathogenesis and treatment. *Eur J Obst Gynecol Reprod Biol.* 2009;145:138–144.
12. Kelly SE, Black MM, Fleming S. Antigen-presenting cells in the skin and placenta in pemphigoid gestationis. *Br J Dermatol.* 1990;122:593–599.
13. Castro LA, Lundell RB, Krause PK, et al. Clinical experience in pemphigoid gestationis: report of 10 cases. *J Am Acad Dermatol.* 2006;55:823–828.
14. Ogilvie P, Trautmann A, Dummer W, et al. [Pemphigoid gestationis without blisters]. *Hautarzt.* 2000;51:25–30.
15. Holmes RC, Williamson DM, Black MM. Herpes gestationis persisting for 12 years postpartum. *Arch Dermatol.* 1986;122:375–376.
16. Jenkins RE, Vaughan Jones SA, Black MM. Conversion of pemphigoid gestationis to bullous pemphigoid—two refractory cases highlighting this association. *Br J Dermatol.* 1995;135:595–598.
17. Amato L, Mei S, Gallerani I, et al. A case of chronic herpes gestationis: persistent disease or conversion to bullous pemphigoid? *J Am Acad Dermatol.* 2003;49:302–307.
18. Hern S, Harman K, Bhogal BS, et al. A severe persistent case of pemphigoid gestationis treated with intravenous immunoglobulins and cyclosporin. *Clin Exp Dermatol.* 1998;23:185–188.
19. Rodrigues Cdos S, Filipe P, Solana Mdel M, et al. Persistent herpes gestationis treated with high-dose intravenous immunoglobulin. *Acta Derm Venereol.* 2007;87:184–186.
20. Boulinguez S, Bedane C, Prost C, et al. Chronic pemphigoid gestationis: comparative clinical and immunopathological study of 10 patients. *Dermatology.* 2003;206:113–119.
21. Castle SP, Mather-Mondrey M, Bennion S. Chronic herpes gestationis and antiphospholipid syndrome successfully treated with cyclophosphamide. *J Am Acad Dermatol.* 1996;34:333–336.
22. Holmes RC, Black MM, Jurecka W, et al. Clues to the etiology and pathogenesis of herpes gestationis. *Br J Dermatol.* 1983;109:131–139.
23. Black MM, Najem NM. Remarkable follow-up experiences of a severe persistent case of pemphigoid gestationis. *Clin Exp Dermatol.* 2005;30:593–594.

24. Shornick JK, Stastny P, Gilliam JN. High frequency of histocompatibility antigens HLA-DR3 and DR4 in herpes gestationis. *J Clin Invest.* 1981;68:553–555.

25. Shornick JK, Artlett CM, Jenkins RE, et al. Complement polymorphism in herpes gestationis: association with C4 null allele. *J Am Acad Dermatol.* 1993;29:545–549.

26. Lin M-S, Gharia M, Fu CL, et al. Molecular mapping of the major epitopes of BP180 recognized by herpes gestationis autoantibodies. *Clin Immunol.* 1999;92:285–292.

27. Kromminga A, Sitaru C, Meyer J, et al. Cicatricial pemphigoid differs from bullous pemphigoid and pemphigoid gestationis regarding the fine specificity of autoantibodies to the BP180 NC16A domain. *J Dermatol Sci.* 2002;28:68–75.

28. Di Zenzo G, Calabresi V, Grosso F, et al. The intracellular and extracellular domains of BP180 antigen comprise novel epitopes targeted by pemphigoid gestationis autoantibodies. *J Invest Dermatol.* 2007;127:864–873.

29. Shimanovich I, Skrobek C, Rose C, et al. Pemphigoid gestationis with predominant involvement of oral mucous membranes and IgA autoantibodies targeting the C-terminus of BP180. *J Am Acad Dermatol.* 2002;47:780–784.

30. Herrero-Gonzalez JE, Brauns O, Egner R, et al. Immunoadsorption against two distinct epitopes on human type XVII collagen abolishes dermal-epidermal separation induced in vitro by autoantibodies from pemphigoid gestationis patients. *Eur J Immunol.* 2006;36:1039–1048.

31. Chimanovitch I, Schmidt E, Messer G, et al. IgG1 and IgG3 are the major immunoglobulin subclasses targeting epitopes within the NC16A domain of BP180 in pemphigoid gestationis. *J Invest Dermatol.* 1999;113:140–142.

32. Patton T, Plunkett RW, Beutner EH, et al. IgG4 as the predominant IgG subclass in pemphigoides gestationis. *J Cutan Pathol.* 2006;33:299–302.

33. Lin M-S, Gharia MA, Swartz SJ, et al. Identification and characterization of epitopes recognized by T lymphocytes and autoantibodies from patients with herpes gestationis. *J Immunol.* 1999;162:4991–4997.

34. Fabbri P, Caproni M, Berti S, et al. The role of T lymphocytes and cytokines in the pathogenesis of pemphigoid gestationis. *Br J Dermatol.* 2003;148:1141–1148.

35. Sitaru C, Powell J, Messer G, et al. Immunoblotting and enzyme-linked immunosorbent assay for the diagnosis of pemphigoid gestationis. *Obstet Gynecol.* 2004;103:757–763.

36. Barnadas MA, Rubiales MV, González MJ, et al. Enzyme-linked immunosorbent assay (ELISA) and indirect immunofluorescence testing in a bullous pemphigoid and pemphigoid gestationis. *Int J Dermatol.* 2008;47:1245–1249.

37. Sitaru C, Dähnrich C, Probst C, et al. Enzyme-linked immunosorbent assay using multimers of the 16th non-collagenous domain of the BP180 antigen for sensitive and specific detection of pemphigoid autoantibodies. *Exp Dermatol.* 2007;16:770–777.

38. Powell AM, Sakuma-Oyama Y, Oyama N, et al. Usefulness of BP180 NC16a enzyme-linked immunosorbent assay in the serodiagnosis of pemphigoid gestationis and in differentiating between pemphigoid gestationis and pruritic urticarial papules and plaques of pregnancy. *Arch Dermatol.* 2005;141:705–710.

39. Huilaja L, Hurskainen T, Autio-Harmainen H, et al. Pemphigoid gestationis autoantigen, transmembrane collagen XVII, promotes the migration of cytotrophoblastic cells of placenta and is a structural component of fetal membranes. *Matrix Biol.* 2008;27:190–200.

40. Shornick JK, Black MM. Secondary autoimmune diseases in herpes gestationis (pemphigoid gestationis). *J Am Acad Dermatol.* 1992;26:563–566.

41. Mascaró JM Jr, Lecha M, Mascaró JM. Fetal morbidity in herpes gestationis. *Arch Dermatol.* 1995;131:1209–1210.

42. Shornick JK, Black MM. Fetal risks in herpes gestationis. *J Am Acad Dermatol.* 1992;26:63–68.

43. Okumus N, Önal EE, Turkuılmaz C, et al. A case report of neonatal convulsions due to maternal herpes gestationis. *J Child Neurol.* 2007;22:488–491.

44. Chi C-C, Wang S-H, Charles-Holmes R, et al. Pemphigoid gestationis: early onset and blister formation are associated with adverse pregnancy outcomes. *Br J Dermatol.* 2009;160:1222–1228.

45. Huilaja L, Mäkikallio T, Sormunen R, et al. Pemphigoid gestationis: placental morphology and function. *Acta Derm Venereol.* 2013;93:33–38.

46. Karna P, Broecker AH. Neonatal herpes gestationis. *J Pediatr.* 1991;119:299–301.

47. Aoyama Y, Asai K, Hioki K, et al. Herpes gestationis in a mother and newborn. *Arch Dermatol.* 2007;143:1168–1172.

48. Wohrl S, Geusau A, Karlhofer F, et al. Pemphigoid gestationis: treatment with immunoapheresis. *J Dtsch Dermatol Ges.* 2003;1:126–130.

49. Westermann L, Hügel R, Meier M, et al. Glucocorticosteroid-resistant pemphigoid gestationis: successful treatment with adjuvant immunoadsorption. *J Dermatol.* 2012;39:168–171.

50. Van de Wiel A, Hart CH, Flinterman J, et al. Plasma exchange in herpes gestationis. *Br Med J.* 1980;281:1041–1042.

51. Kreuter A, Harati I, Breuckmann F, et al. Intravenous immune globulin in the treatment of persistent pemphigoid gestationis. *J Am Acad Dermatol.* 2004;51:1027–1028.

52. Loo WJ, Dean D, Wojnarowska F. A severe case of recurrent pemphigoid gestationis successfully treated with minocycline and nicotinamide. *Clin Exp Dermatol.* 2001;26:726–727.

53. Amato L, Coronella G, Berti S, et al. Successful treatment with doxycycline and nicotinamide of two cases of persistent pemphigoid gestationis. *J Dermatolog Treat.* 2002;13:143–146.

54. Cobo MF, Santi CG, Maruta CW, et al. Pemphigoid gestationis: clinical and laboratory evaluation. *Clinics (Sao Paulo).* 2009;64:1043–1047.

55. Cianchini G, Masini C, Lupi F, et al. Severe persistent pemphigoid gestationis: long-term remission with rituximab. *Br J Dermatol.* 2007;157:388–431.

CHAPTER 20

Polymorphic Eruption of Pregnancy

Lisa M. Cohen ■ George Kroumpouzos

INTRODUCTION

Polymorphic eruption of pregnancy (PEP) is the most common specific dermatosis of pregnancy. The term *pruritic urticarial papules and plaques of pregnancy* (PUPPP), coined by Lawley et al.,[1] is used synonymously. Historic terms, such as *toxemic rash of pregnancy*, *late-onset prurigo of pregnancy*, and *toxemic rash of pregnancy*, have been replaced by PUPPP or PEP. This distinct eruption shows consistent clinical features, has not been associated with substantial fetal risks, and does not typically recur in subsequent pregnancies.

EPIDEMIOLOGY

The prevalence of PEP has been historically reported between 1 in 120[2] and 1 in 240 pregnancies (0.4% to 0.8%).[3] Roger et al.[4] reported an incidence of 1 in 130 pregnancies (0.7%). Prevalence was much lower in an Israeli study (0.03%)[5] and higher than expected in an Indian study (2.3%).[6] Still, comparisons between various populations cannot easily be made because the magnitude of confounding variables, such as the utilization of medical services and recruitment of patients, may differ in previous studies. The prevalence of PEP in other non-Caucasian ethnic groups has not been well studied. PEP was diagnosed in 26% of pregnant patients that presented with pruritic dermatoses.[7] Most studies indicate that PEP is more common than other specific dermatoses such as pemphigoid gestationis, prurigo of pregnancy, and pruritic folliculitis of pregnancy.

The eruption occurs primarily in primigravidas (70%),[8] with the percentage of nulliparous women being even higher (81%), because a third of multigravidas had not completed the course of their previous pregnancies.[8] The respective rates in the study by Aronson et al.[9] were 42% and 68%. However, an even lower prevalence (40%) in primigravidas[10] and primiparous women (28% to 57%)[4,5,10,11] has been reported in other studies. PEP has been associated with multiple gestation pregnancy.[12] In a meta-analysis of 282 cases,[13] the prevalence of multiple gestation was 11.7% (10% twin and 1.7% triplet pregnancies), whereas in the largest PEP study to date, the prevalence of multiple gestation was 12.7% (11.6% twin and 1.1% triplet pregnancies).[8] There is a predominance of male fetuses (59% to 64%).[5,8,10]

ETIOLOGY

The etiology of PEP remains obscure. There is typically no previous or family history of the eruption, and human leukocyte antigen (HLA) studies have been noncontributory. An abnormal maternal immune reactivity to stretched skin is evidenced by the location of lesions in or adjacent to the abdominal striae in women during the third trimester. Excessive maternal weight gain or fetal birth weight and an association with multiple gestation pregnancy may be contributing factors.[12] Hormonal factors have also been implicated, as well as microchimerism (i.e., a reaction to fetal DNA in maternal skin).

CLINICAL FEATURES

PEP occurs in the third trimester in 83% of patients[8] (range, 75% to 97% in various studies).[7,8,11,14] It occurs less often in the first trimester (range, 0% to 10.5%) and second trimester (range, 0% to 10.5%) or postpartum (range, 0% to 15%).[8,9,11,14] A study suggested that cases with purely urticarial features throughout the course of the eruption may start more often in the third trimester (91%) than those with nonurticarial or polymorphous features (70%).[9] Mean onset is at 32 to 36 weeks in most large studies. The most frequent week of onset has been the 39th week.[14] The eruption tends to be short-lived, with a mean duration of 6 weeks[15]; however, it is rarely severe for more than 1 week. Familial occurrence and recurrence in subsequent pregnancies, with menses, or oral contraceptive use are uncommon.[16]

Pruritus is the most common symptom and is typically contemporaneous with the eruption. It can be severe enough to cause disturbed sleep patterns and difficulty with daily activities.[14] Other symptoms, such as burning or pain can occasionally be encountered. Although pruritus is severe, excoriations are relatively uncommon,[14] which is an important finding that can help differentiate PEP from other pruritic conditions, such as obstetric cholestasis, which commonly present with extensive

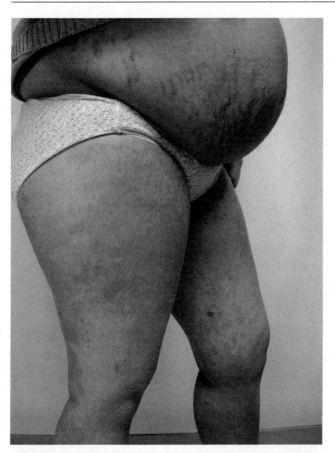

Figure 20.1. Urticarial lesions start on the abdomen and/or proximal thighs in the vast majority of cases. (Courtesy of Bellevue Dermatology Department Collection, New York University.)

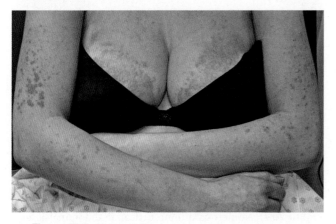

Figure 20.2. Urticarial lesions on the breasts and arms.

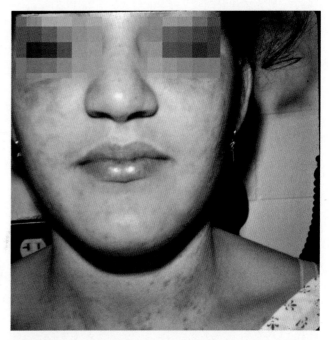

Figure 20.3. Urticarial lesions of polymorphic eruption on the face and neck. (Courtesy of Dr. Iris Aronson.)

excoriations. This intensely pruritic eruption starts on the lower abdomen and/or proximal thighs in up to 91% of cases (Fig. 20.1), and 80% of patients subsequently develop lesions on other areas of the trunk and upper extremities (Fig. 20.2).[8] The largest study shows that 97% of patients had abdominal involvement at some point

through the course of the disease.[8] Nevertheless, exclusive involvement of the extremities has been reported.[8,17] There is sparing of the mucous membranes, and involvement of the face and neck (Fig. 20.3), palm (Fig. 20.4), and soles is uncommon.

The lesions characteristically start within or adjacent to the abdominal striae distensae in up to two-thirds of the cases and demonstrate periumbilical sparing (see Figs. 20.4C and 20.5).[13,18] The prominence of abdominal striae has been reported in 55% of cases (see Figs. 20.5 and 20.6).[8] Periumbilical sparing may be seen in the absence of striae distensae (Fig. 20.7). The lesions are usually urticarial (49%) (see Figs. 20.2 and 20.7), but the eruption often becomes polymorphous throughout the course of the disease, showing eczematous (22%) (Fig. 20.8), vesicular (17%) (see Figs. 20.4 and 20.9), targetoid (6%) (Fig. 20.10), annular/polycyclic (6%), or purpuric lesions. Lesions may show a nonurticarial morphology (Figs. 20.11 and 20.12).[8] Aronson et al. subcategorized PUPPP into three groups[9]: type I, showing predominantly urticarial lesions (40%); type II, showing erythema and nonurticarial papules or vesicles (44%); and type III, showing combinations of features of types I and II (16%). In their study, cases with purely urticarial lesions (type I) were less likely to affect the face, palms, and soles than cases from types II and III[9]; however, there have been sparse reports of purely urticarial cases with facial involvement. Papular lesions blanch upon pressure and demonstrate perilesional pallor (halo) in two-thirds of the cases (Fig. 20.13).[4,14] The presence of perilesional halos is a helpful clinical finding that, along with the distribution within abdominal striae,

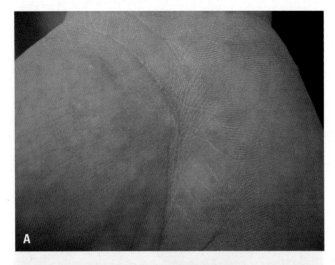

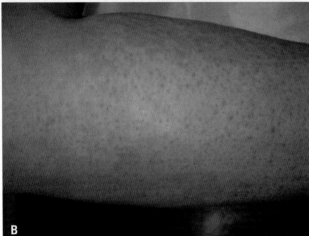

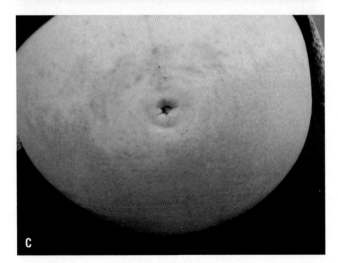

Figure 20.4. (**A**) Minute papulovesicular lesions on the palm. (**B**) Acral vesicular lesions healing with crusting. (**C**) In the same patient, typical abdominal lesions show periumbilical sparing. (Courtesy of Dr. Ossama Abbas.)

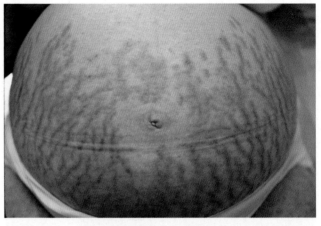

Figure 20.5. Urticarial lesions distributed along abdominal striae distensae, which is a typical distribution of polymorphic eruption. The prominence of the striae distensae is seen. (Courtesy of Dr. Thomas L. Rosenfeld.)

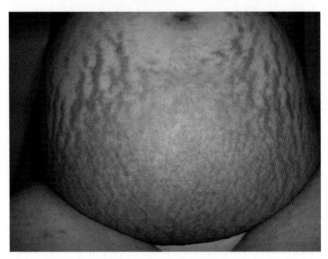

Figure 20.6. The prominence of striae distensae is shown and is reported in approximately 55% of cases of polymorphic eruption. (Courtesy of Dr. Patricia Cristodor.)

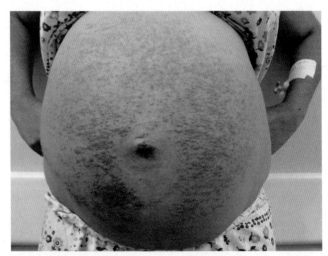

Figure 20.7. Numerous minute urticarial abdominal lesions show periumbilical sparing. There are no *striae distensae* in this patient. (Courtesy of Dr. Mayra Ianhez.)

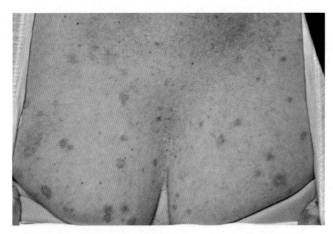

Figure 20.8. Eczematous lesions on the chest.

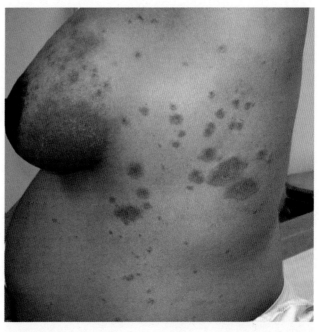

Figure 20.10. Several large targetoid lesions in a polymorphic eruption. (Courtesy of Dr. Iris Aronson.)

periumbilical sparing, and absence of excoriations, can help in the diagnosis.

Sterile pustules and follicular lesions are exceptionally seen (Fig. 20.14).[11] Similarly rare are bullae (Fig. 20.15). Dyshidrosis-like palmoplantar lesions, the predominance of confluent acral vesicular lesions that can form bullae, koebnerization, and photodistribution have been rarely reported.[19–21] Vesicular lesions with necrotic features were reported in a case associated with acquired hemophilia A.[22] Generalized PEP may resolve with extensive desquamation and thus may resemble a toxic erythema

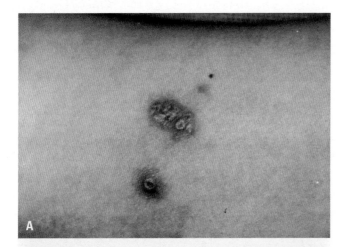

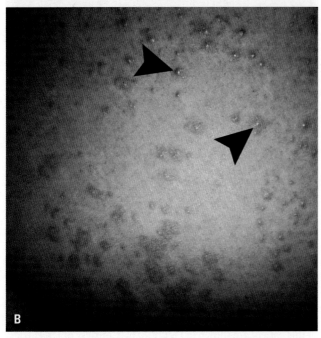

Figure 20.9. (**A**) Minute vesicular lesions on the forearm in polymorphic eruption that developed in the third trimester in a primigravida. (**B**) Numerous microvesicles on the abdomen; many vesicles are superimposed on typical urticarial lesions. (Courtesy of Dr. Iris Aronson.)

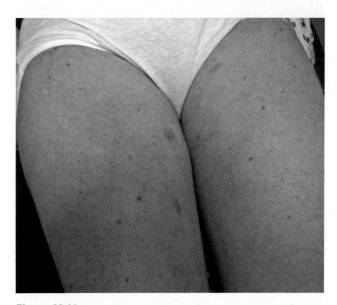

Figure 20.11. Lesions may at times show a nonurticarial, nonspecific morphology, making the diagnosis challenging.

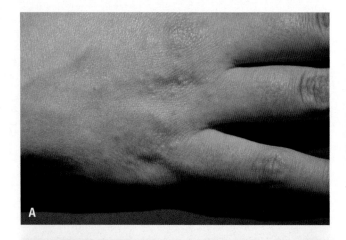

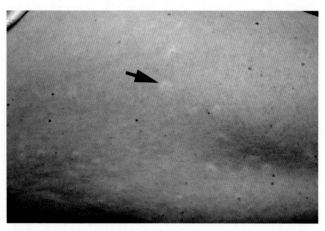

Figure 20.13. Pruritic urticarial papules, most with perilesional halos *(arrow)*, on the thigh.

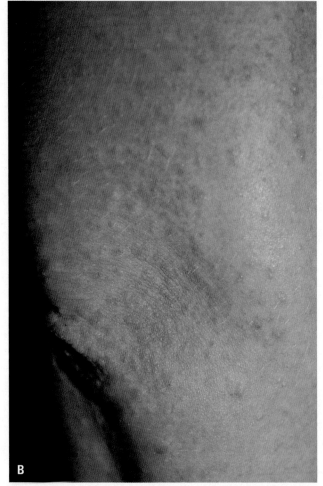

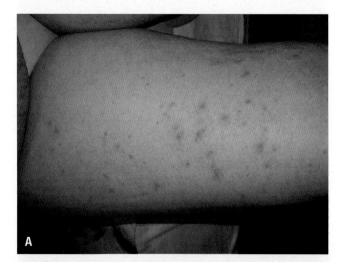

Figure 20.12. Minute pruritic papules (**A**) on the dorsum of the hand and (**B**) on the knee. The urticarial morphology is subtle, but some of the lesions on the knee show perilesional halos.

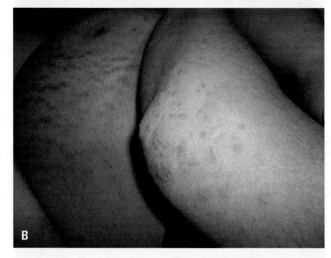

Figure 20.14. (**A**) Minute follicular papulopustules on the thigh. (**B**) Similar lesions on the elbow. The abdominal lesions of this patient are shown in Figure 20.6. (Courtesy of Dr. Patricia Cristodor.)

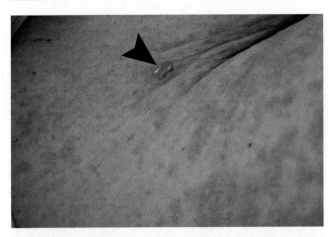

Figure 20.15. Bulla *(arrow)* developed on a urticarial lesion of the polymorphic eruption. This primigravida patient had a twin pregnancy, and her eruption was associated with preeclampsia.

(Fig. 20.16). The presence of polymorphous lesions correlates with disease duration, and an association between nonurticarial morphology and disease duration of more than 6 weeks has been reported.[8] The eruption resolves spontaneously intrapartum, at delivery, or within 6 weeks of delivery; most cases resolve by 3 weeks' postpartum. Nevertheless, postpartum exacerbation[4] and cases with a prolonged course after delivery have been exceptionally reported.[23,24]

PATHOLOGY

Histopathology

Skin histopathology typically shows nonspecific findings, including epidermal changes, upper dermal edema, and a superficial and mid-dermal perivascular lymphohistiocytic

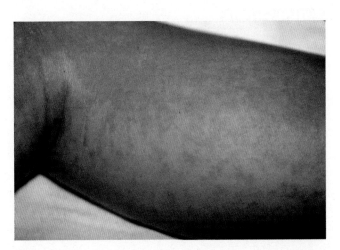

Figure 20.16. Widespread lesions resolving with desquamation, a picture reminiscent of toxic erythema. (Courtesy of Dr. Helen Raynham.)

infiltrate with variable numbers of eosinophils (Figs. 20.17A to 20.17C).[18] Epidermal changes are encountered in almost half of the biopsies and include spongiosis, hyperkeratosis, and/or parakeratosis, acanthosis, and exocytosis (Fig. 20.17D). They are more conspicuous in older lesions or in those with polymorphous morphology. The intensity of the infiltrate and severity of PEP correlated with the presence of epidermal changes in another study.[25] Foci of spongiosis may coalesce into minute vesicles. The infiltrate is primarily composed of T-helper (Th) lymphocytes. Eosinophil infiltration is seen in 60% of cases[8] and is prominent in one-third of them (see Fig. 20.17C) and may rarely be associated with eosinophilic spongiosis. Eosinophil infiltration and granule protein deposition is less prominent in PEP than in pemphigoid gestationis[26,27]; however, a comparison should be done only for urticarial lesions because eosinophils are mainly present in the early urticarial stage of both dermatoses.[28]

Immunopathology

Direct and indirect immunofluorescence has been negative, although some studies have shown the third component of complement (C3) and/or immunoglobulins in blood vessels or at the dermal–epidermal junction in lesional skin.[9,14,29] Most authors concur that these immune reactants may reflect circulating immune complexes and in most cases represent nonspecific immune reactants often found in various inflammatory dermatoses.[9] Serum immunoglobulin E (IgE) elevations were reported in 28% of patients (uncontrolled).[8]

SEROLOGY

Serologic screenings for circulating autoantibodies and hormonal abnormalities have been invariably negative, and a decrease in serum cortisol[11] has not been confirmed.

DIAGNOSIS

PEP remains a clinical diagnosis because histopathology is nonspecific and laboratory tests are noncontributory. A typical presentation of papulourticarial lesions within the abdominal striae, often followed by polymorphous lesions, is highly suggestive of the diagnosis. Nevertheless, the diagnosis may be challenging in patients who present with polymorphous lesions or lesions in atypical distributions.

DIFFERENTIAL DIAGNOSIS

In addition to other specific dermatoses (such as pemphigoid gestationis or obstetric cholestasis), atopic or contact dermatitis, urticaria, viral exanthems, drug eruptions,

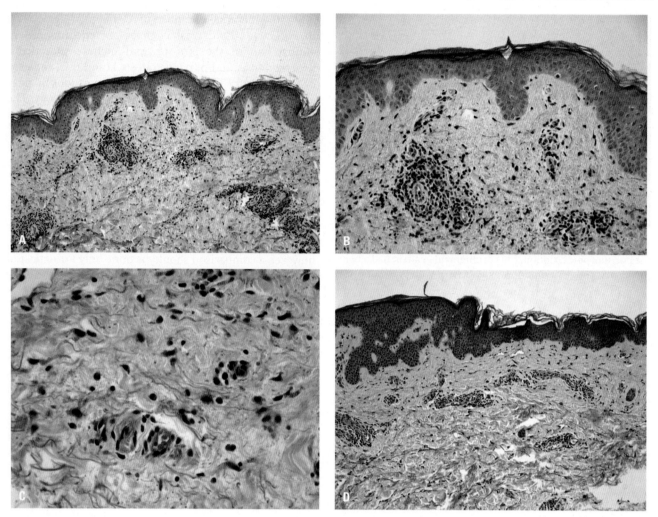

Figure 20.17. (**A**) Superficial and mid-dermal perivascular lymphohistiocytic infiltrate and upper dermal edema (hematoxylin-eosin, ×10). (**B**) Superficial perivascular lymphohistiocytic infiltrate with sparse eosinophils, upper dermal edema, and focal exocytosis (hematoxylin-eosin, ×20). (**C**) Eosinophils can be conspicuous (hematoxylin-eosin, ×40). (**D**) Epidermal changes (i.e., acanthosis, parakeratosis, mild spongiosis, and, occasionally, exocytosis) are shown. They are more common in older lesions and those with polymorphous morphology.

hypersensitivity reactions, insect bites, and infections such as scabies need to be differentiated from PEP (Table 20.1). A detailed history and physical examination are crucial for a diagnosis. Differentiating PEP from early, prebullous pemphigoid gestationis may be challenging, and a skin biopsy of perilesional skin for direct immunofluorescence is required. Prurigo of pregnancy typically begins earlier, persists throughout pregnancy, and shows papulonodular lesions and an absence of urticarial lesions. Pruritic folliculitis of pregnancy is differentiated from PEP by the presence of follicular papulopustules and histopathology of folliculitis. Obstetric cholestasis shows only secondary skin lesions and typical liver function abnormalities. Atopic dermatitis in pregnancy typically presents on flexural areas in patients with a personal and/or a family history of atopy, but the differentiation from atypical presentations of PEP can be challenging.

PATHOGENESIS

The pathogenesis of PEP remains elusive despite the relative frequency of this dermatosis. Genetic predisposition does not seem to be a contributing factor. A role for paternal factors has been suggested by sparse observations[16,30] but not corroborated. Autoimmune mechanisms, such as those encountered in pemphigoid gestationis, are not involved in PEP. Etiologic theories have mainly focused on abdominal distention, hormonal and immunologic factors, and fetal microchimerism, and these will be presented in the following sections.

Abdominal Distention

Several authors postulated that rapid abdominal wall distention in primigravidas in late pregnancy with subsequent damage to the connective tissue may trigger

TABLE 20.1	Differential Diagnosis of Polymorphic Eruption
Disease	**Differentiating Features**
Pemphigoid gestationis	■ No periumbilical sparing, no predilection for striae, no halo around urticarial lesions ■ Bullous stage may develop ■ Flare around delivery ■ DIF positive for linear C3 at the basement membrane zone
Prurigo of pregnancy	■ Starts earlier (first through second trimesters) and persists throughout pregnancy ■ Papulonodular lesions, no urticarial lesions ■ Occasional h/o atopy in patient and/or family
Pruritic folliculitis of pregnancy	■ Follicular papulopustules, no predilection for abdominal striae ■ Histopathology of sterile folliculitis
Atopic dermatitis/atopic eruption of pregnancy	■ Starts earlier in pregnancy (first through second trimesters) ■ Typically flexural distribution, urticarial lesions uncommon ■ Often h/o atopy in patient and/or family
Obstetric cholestasis	■ No primary skin lesions ■ Liver function test abnormalities ■ Recurrence in subsequent pregnancies is common
Urticaria	■ Typical PEP distribution is absent ■ Hx suggestive of underlying etiology
Drug/hypersensitivity eruption	■ Hx suggestive of drug- or allergen-induced rash ■ No predilection for abdominal striae ■ Improvement with discontinuation of offending drug/allergen
Viral exanthem	■ Typically exanthematous, less pruritic ■ Different distribution, often with oral and palmoplantar lesions
Infestations (i.e., scabies)	■ Different distribution (intertriginous areas, genitalia, webs) ■ Hx suggestive ■ Positive scabies preparation
Insect bites	■ Hx suggestive of exposure ■ Grouping of lesions, no typical PEP distribution

C3, third component of complement; DIF, direct immunofluorescence; h/o, history of; Hx, history; PEP, polymorphic eruption of pregnancy.

PEP. This theory is supported by the striking localization of lesions in or adjacent to abdominal striae and associations with multiple gestation pregnancy,[13,31] excessive weight gain in the mother and increased fetal weight,[12] and maternal obesity.[5] A meta-analysis revealed a 10-fold higher prevalence of multiple gestation pregnancy in patients with PEP,[13] which is also supported by several studies,[7,8,31] and lends further support to the theory of abdominal overdistention. Nevertheless, the association with excessive maternal weight gain has been debated,[10,32] and an increased fetal weight has been discounted.[32,33]

As per the previous theory, damage of connective tissue within striae secondary to excessive stretching can trigger an inflammatory reaction.[12,31] Exposure of antigens within collagen that are otherwise hidden from the maternal immune system could possibly elicit an allergic reaction, resulting in the initial distribution of the lesions in or adjacent to the abdominal striae.[15] Alternatively, an altered maternal immune reactivity, which might be exaggerated in multiple pregnancies, could cause an abnormal reaction to stressed skin in the abdominal striae. Along the same lines, multiple gestation pregnancy, the rate of which is increased in PEP, is associated with high progesterone levels, which can aggravate inflammation at the tissue level. Progesterone-triggered tissue inflammation is supported by a study that showed progesterone receptor immunoreactivity only in the lesional skin in PEP.[34] How PEP becomes generalized remains unknown, but cross-reactivity to collagen in otherwise normal skin may play a role.[15]

Hormonal Factors

No consistent hormonal abnormality has been identified, and a reduction in maternal serum cortisol[11] has not been corroborated. As aforementioned, increased progesterone receptor reactivity in skin lesions of PEP has been reported,[34] and the authors suggested that suprabasilar keratinocytes can act as targets of progesterone action by expressing progesterone receptor. This finding indicates a possible role for progesterone in the inflammatory process in PEP. Other authors suggested that a hormonal substance may be released by the aging placenta in the third trimester, which could induce fibroblast proliferation in maternal skin, but factual evidence is scarce.[35]

Immunologic Factors

Immunohistochemical studies have indicated the activation of the maternal immune system[36] and suggested that a graft-versus-host mechanism may be involved.[28] The lymphohistiocytic infiltrate in PEP is composed mainly of Th lymphocytes, activated T cells (HLA DR+, CD25+, LFA-1+), dermal dendritic cells, and epidermal Langerhans cells.[36] This immunohistologic profile that characteristically includes a strong HLA-DR expression indicates activation of the skin immune system secondary to an antigenic stimulus. Caproni et al. showed a predominance of Th1-oriented CD8+ lymphocytes in PEP compared to the Th2 profile (CD4 cells) in pemphigoid gestationis,[28,37] and the authors suggested that the Th1-like cytokine pattern in PEP may indicate a graft-versus-host–like reaction. They also showed a stronger expression of HLA-DR by a wider spectrum of cells and a higher expression of Th1-like cytokines such as interferon-γ and interleukin-2 in PEP as compared to pemphigoid gestationis.[37]

A high prevalence (55%) of personal and/or family history of atopy and/or elevated serum IgE levels in a recent study[8] needs to be confirmed. In this study, IgE elevation was shown in 28% of PEP cases (uncontrolled), but it has been challenged whether mild IgE elevations in pregnancy can serve as an indicator of atopy.[38] Allergic asthma was present in 11% of 57 PUPPP patients by Aronson et al.[9] Whether an atopic background can influence the course of PEP needs to be addressed in prospective studies.[8]

Microchimerism

An increased rate of male infants among the offspring of PEP patients has been reported.[5,8,10] Interestingly, a study demonstrated male fetal DNA in skin lesions of a small number of PEP patients,[39] possibly resulting from fetal cell migration to maternal skin secondary to peripheral blood chimerism. Chimerism is known to start early in gestation and increases as pregnancy progresses. The presence of fetal DNA in maternal skin could elicit an allergic or immune reaction, which could lead to the development of PEP.[15] Immune tolerance or an absence of fetal DNA in maternal skin[15] in subsequent pregnancies may explain why PEP does not typically recur. Along the same lines, case reports have shown the presence of male fetal progenitor cells in maternal circulation for up

to 27 years' postpartum,[40] which may explain recurrent PEP-like lesions in a patient 28 years after her last pregnancy.[24] Furthermore, an immunohistochemical study showed a predominance of CD8+ T cells in lesions of PEP, and the authors suggested that these could be chimeric and serve as an initiator factor with Th1-like molecules and eosinophils as effector mechanisms in the inflammatory process.[28]

MATERNAL AND FETAL RISKS

The perinatal outcome has been favorable, with fetal deaths being uncommon and possibly coincidental,[11,41] or related to other obstetric risk factors such as multiple gestation pregnancy.[8,14] PEP has not been associated with preterm delivery or intrauterine growth restriction.[5] A case of transient neonatal PEP has been described; however, other neonatal eruptions were not entirely ruled out in this case.[42] Maternal risks are related to obstetric risk factors (multiple gestation, cesarean section) rather than the disease itself. The study by Ohel et al. reported high rates of labor induction (50%) and cesarean delivery (28.6%) in PEP patients.[5] Labor induction and cesarean section were independent factors associated with PEP in a multiple logistic regression model, but PEP was not an independent risk factor for cesarean delivery in a multivariate analysis. A high rate of cesarean delivery (40%) in PEP was also shown in another study, with cesarean delivery being independently associated with PEP.[10] A higher rate of cesarean delivery (56%) was also reported in a recent smaller study,[17] with the rate of cesarean delivery in the general population being 25% (O. Abbas, MD, electronic communication, November 2012). However, the higher rate of cesarean delivery in the study correlated with a high rate (50%) of multiple gestation pregnancy. The association between PEP and cesarean delivery needs to be clarified in prospective studies. An association with hypertensive disorders and mild preeclampsia[5] was not statistically significant (P = 0.06) in a subsequent study[10]; however, it is supported by some reports (see Fig. 20.15).[4,41] An association with increased number of hospitalizations[10] needs to be validated.

MANAGEMENT

Mild-to-moderate PEP can be treated symptomatically with general measures (cooling baths, emollients, wet soaks), antipruritic topical medications, mid-potency topical steroids, and oral H_1 antihistamines that are safe in gestation (diphenhydramine, chlorpheniramine, cetirizine) (Table 20.2). Because the eruption usually resolves within 7 to 10 days of delivery, most authors recommend a conservative approach. In cases of severe pruritus and/or when the eruption becomes generalized, a short course of oral steroid, such as prednisone or prednisolone at a

TABLE 20.2	Summary of Management Options
Treatment	**Comment**
General measures	Frequent cooling showers/baths, emollients, wet soaks, topical antipruritic medications such as aqueous cream with 1%–2% menthol[11]
Topical corticosteroids	Required in most patients; mid-potency steroids are effective in mild-to-moderate cases[18]; taper gradually over 1–2 wks after improvement[25]
Oral antihistamines	H_1 antihistamines, such as diphenhydramine, chlorpheniramine, cetirizine, all safe in gestation, can help in pruritus control[8]
Systemic corticosteroids	For very symptomatic or extensive disease; oral prednisone or prednisolone at dose 20–40 mg/d is typically effective[1,14]; safe for the neonate if needed to be administered postpartum
Ultraviolet light B therapy	Anecdotal[18]
Obstetric evaluation	An objective evaluation of labor induction is required in order to minimize unnecessary cesarean delivery[5]
Patient counseling	Minimizes patient anxiety; advise patient that there are no maternal or fetal/neonatal risks with this skin disease; inform patient of associations with multiple gestation pregnancy and cesarean delivery as well as risks associated with these

dose of 20 to 40 mg per day, may be necessary and appears to be safe in late gestation. Response to low-dose prednisone (10 mg per day) may be less prompt.[14] The oral steroid needs to be tapered promptly after the clinical response is noted. The risk of fetal adrenal suppression secondary to systemic steroid treatment is low, especially for prednisolone, because the maternal–fetal gradient of prednisolone is 10:1.[43] Ultraviolet light B (UVB) has been used successfully by the authors but is rarely used during gestation because the eruption is short-lived.[13] Recalcitrant PEP has improved dramatically after delivery with cesarean section.[44] Nevertheless, early delivery has not gained support, and most authors recommend expectant management.

An objective evaluation of labor induction should arise when dealing with patients with PEP in order to minimize unnecessary cesarean delivery.[5] The pregnant female should be counseled that PEP is self-limited, does not typically recur in subsequent pregnancies, and is not associated with substantial maternal or fetal risks. Patients should be made aware of the associations with multiple gestation pregnancy and cesarean delivery, and the maternal and fetal risks that accompany them.

MATERNAL RISKS

No risks from the disease
Theoretical risks associated with multiple gestation pregnancy and cesarean delivery
Risks from pharmacologic treatment

FETAL RISKS

None

KEY POINTS

■ The prevalence of polymorphic eruption is between 1 in 120 and 1 in 240 pregnancies; the eruption occurs predominantly in primigravidas in the third trimester and has been associated with multiple gestation pregnancy.

■ There are variable clinical presentations, the most common being urticarial lesions that start within or adjacent to the abdominal striae and show periumbilical sparing.

■ The histopathology is nonspecific; immunofluorescence is negative (which helps the differentiation from prebullous pemphigoid gestationis); and serologic tests are noncontributory.

■ The etiology is unclear, but the abdominal wall distention, hormonal and immunologic factors, and microchimerism have been implicated.

■ There are no maternal or neonatal/fetal risks.

■ Treatment is with mid-potency topical steroids and oral antihistamines; a conservative approach to a short course of systemic steroid is recommended.

REFERENCES

1. Lawley TJ, Hertz KC, Wade TR, et al. Pruritic urticarial papules and plaques of pregnancy. *JAMA*. 1979;241:1696–1699.
2. Bourne G. Toxaemic rash of pregnancy. *Proc R Soc Med*. 1962;55:462–464.
3. Holmes RC, Black MM, Dann J, et al. A comparative study of toxic erythema of pregnancy and herpes gestationis. *Br J Dermatol*. 1982;106:499–510.

4. Roger D, Vaillant L, Fignon A, et al. Specific pruritic diseases of pregnancy: a prospective study of 3192 pregnancy women. *Arch Dermatol.* 1994;130:734–739.

5. Ohel I, Levy A, Silverstein T, et al. Pregnancy outcome of patients with pruritic urticarial papules and plaques of pregnancy. *J Matern Fetal Neonatal Med.* 2006;19:305–308.

6. Kumari R, Jaisankar TJ, Thappa DM. A clinical study of skin changes in pregnancy. *Indian J Dermatol Venereol Leprol.* 2007; 73:141.

7. Ambros-Rundolph CM, Mullegger RR, Vaughan-Jones SA, et al. The specific dermatoses of pregnancy revisited and reclassified: results of a retrospective two-center study on 505 pregnant patients. *J Am Acad Dermatol.* 2006;54:395–404.

8. Rudolph CM, Al-Fares S, Vaughan-Jones SA, et al. Polymorphic eruption of pregnancy: clinicopathology and potential risk factors in 181 patients. *Br J Dermatol.* 2006;154:54–60.

9. Aronson IK, Bond S, Fiedler VC, et al. Pruritic urticarial papules and plaques of pregnancy: clinical and immunopathologic observations in 57 patients. *J Am Acad Dermatol.* 1998;39:933–939.

10. Regnier S, Fermand V, Levy P, et al. A case-control study of polymorphic eruption of pregnancy. *J Am Acad Dermatol.* 2008;58: 63–67.

11. Vaughan Jones SA, Hern S, Nelson-Piercy C, et al. A prospective study of 200 women with dermatoses of pregnancy correlating the clinical findings with hormonal and immunopathological profiles. *Br J Dermatol.* 1999;141:71–81.

12. Cohen LM, Capeless EL, Krusinski PA, et al. Pruritic urticarial papules and plaques of pregnancy and its relationship to maternal-fetal weight gain and twin pregnancy. *Arch Dermatol.* 1989;125:1534–1536.

13. Kroumpouzos G, Cohen LM. Specific dermatoses of pregnancy: an evidence-based systematic review. *Am J Obstet Gynecol.* 2003; 188:1083–1092.

14. Yancey KB, Hall RP, Lawley TJ. Pruritic urticarial papules and plaques of pregnancy. Clinical experience in twenty-five patients. *J Am Acad Dermatol.* 1984;10:473–480.

15. Ahmadi S, Powel FC. Pruritic urticarial papules and plaques of pregnancy: current status. *Australas J Dermatol.* 2005;46:53–58.

16. Weiss R, Hull P. Familial occurrence of pruritic urticarial papules and plaques of pregnancy. *J Am Acad Dermatol.* 1992;26:715–717.

17. Ghazeeri G, Kibbi AG, Abbas O. Pruritic urticarial papules and plaques of pregnancy: epidemiological, clinical, and histopathological study of 18 cases from Lebanon. *Int J Dermatol.* 2012;51: 1047–1053.

18. Kroumpouzos G, Cohen LM. Dermatoses of pregnancy. *J Am Acad Dermatol.* 2001;45:1–19.

19. Normand F, Armingaud P, Estève E. [Dyshidrosis and acral purpura during polymorphic eruption of pregnancy]. *Ann Dermatol Venereol.* 2001;128:531–533.

20. Sherley-Dale AC, Carr RA, Charles-Holmes R. Polymorphic eruption of pregnancy with bullous lesions: a previously unreported association. *Br J Dermatol.* 2009;162:208–234.

21. Goolamali SI, Salisbury JR, Higgins EM. Polymorphic eruption of pregnancy in a photodistribution: a potentially new association? *Clin Exp Dermatol.* 2009;34:e381–e382.

22. Journet-Tollhupp J, Tchen T, Remy-Leroux V, et al. [Polymorphic eruption of pregnancy and acquired hemophilia A]. *Ann Dermatol Venereol.* 2010;137:713–717.

23. Terai M, Oka M, Tsujimoto M, et al. Recalcitrant pruritic urticarial papules and plaques of pregnancy with a prolonged course after delivery. *Eur J Dermatol.* 2012;22:136–137.

24. Saraswat A, Rai R, Kumar B. Lesions resembling polymorphic eruption of pregnancy several years after pregnancy. *Dermatology.* 2001;202:82.

25. Moreno A, Noguera J, de Moragas JM. Polymorphic eruption of pregnancy: histopathologic study. *Acta Derm Venereol.* 1985;65:313–318.

26. Holmes RC, Jurecka W, Black MM. A comparative histopathologic study of polymorphic eruption of pregnancy and herpes gestationis. *Clin Exp Dermatol.* 1983;8:523–529.

27. Borrego L, Peterson EA, Diez LI, et al. Polymorphic eruption of pregnancy and herpes gestationis: comparison of granulated cell proteins in tissue and serum. *Clin Exp Dermatol.* 1999;24: 213–225.

28. Caproni M, Giomi B, Berti S, et al. Relevance of cellular infiltrate and cytokines in polymorphic eruption of pregnancy (PEP). *J Dermatol Sci.* 2006;43:67–69.

29. Zurn A, Celebi CR, Bernard P, et al. A prospective immunofluorescence study of 111 cases of pruritic dermatoses of pregnancy: IgM anti-basement membrane zone antibodies as a novel finding. *Br J Dermatol.* 1992;126:474–478.

30. Powell FC. Parity, polypregnancy, paternity and PUPPP. *Arch Dermatol.* 1992;128:1551.

31. Elling SV, McKenna P, Powell FC. Pruritic urticarial papules and plaques of pregnancy in twin and triplet pregnancies. *J Eur Acad Dermatol Venereol.* 2000;14:378–381.

32. Roger D, Vaillant L, Lorette G. Pruritic urticarial papules and plaques of pregnancy are not related to maternal or fetal weight gain. *Arch Dermatol.* 1990;126:1517.

33. Pauwels C, Bucaille-Fleury L, Recanati G. Pruritic urticarial papules and plaques of pregnancy: relationship to maternal weight gain and twin or triplet pregnancies. *Arch Dermatol.* 1994;130: 801–802.

34. Im S, Lee ES, Kim W, et al. Expression of progesterone receptor in human keratinocytes. *J. Korean Med Sci.* 2000;15:647–654.

35. Ingber A, Alcalay J, Sandbank M. Multiple dermal fibroblasts in patients with pruritic urticarial papules and plaques of pregnancy. A clue to the etiology? *Med Hypotheses.* 1988;26:11–12.

36. Carli P, Tarocchi S, Mello G, et al. Skin immune system activation in pruritic urticarial papules and plaques of pregnancy. *Int J Dermatol.* 1994;33:884–885.

37. Fabbri P, Caproni M, Berti S, et al. The role of T lymphocytes and cytokines in the pathogenesis of pemphigoid gestationis. *Br J Dermatol.* 2003;148:1141–1148.

38. Cohen LM, Kroumpouzos G. Pruritic dermatoses of pregnancy: to lump or to split? *J Am Acad Dermatol.* 2007;56:708–709.

39. Aractingi S, Berkane N, Bertheau P, et al. Fetal DNA in skin of polymorphic eruptions of pregnancy. *Lancet.* 1998;352:1898–1901.

40. Bianchi DW, Zickwolf GK, Weil GJ, et al. Male fetal progenitor cells persist in maternal blood for as long as 27 years postpartum. *Proc Natl Acad Sci USA.* 1996;93:705–708.

41. Lowenstein L, Solt I, Peleg A, et al. [Is there an association between PUPPP and preeclampsia, abruptio placentae and fetal death?] *Harefuah.* 2004;143:861–862.

42. Uhlin SR. Pruritic urticarial papules and plaques of pregnancy. Involvement in mother and infant. *Arch Dermatol.* 1981;117: 238–239.

43. Gabbe SG. Drug therapy in autoimmune disease. *Clin Obstet Gynecol.* 1987;26:635–641.

44. Beltrani VP, Beltrani VS. Pruritic urticarial papules and plaques of pregnancy: a severe case requiring early delivery for relief of symptoms. *J Am Acad Dermatol.* 1992;26:266–267.

CHAPTER 21

Prurigo, Pruritic Folliculitis, and Atopic Eruption of Pregnancy

George Kroumpouzos ■ Lisa M. Cohen

INTRODUCTION

Prurigo (PP) and pruritic folliculitis (PFP) are the least well characterized specific dermatoses of pregnancy.[1] PP and PFP are less common than polymorphic eruption, with PFP being the least prevalent.[2,3] PP encompasses entities that have been historically reported as Besnier's *prurigo gestationis*,[4] Nurse's *early onset prurigo*,[5] and Spangler's *papular dermatitis of pregnancy*.[6] A traditional classification of specific dermatoses has included PP and PFP as separate entities,[7] but this status has been recently challenged (see Ch. 18).[2] Atopic eruption of pregnancy (AEP) is a concept introduced to include atopic dermatitis (AD), which can worsen or present for the first time in pregnancy as well as specific dermatoses that may be associated with atopy such as PP and PFP. This chapter outlines the historical background, features, pathogenesis, and management options of these entities.

PRURIGO OF PREGNANCY

Epidemiology

PP affects approximately 1 in 300 to 1 in 450 pregnancies.[3,5] The incidence of PP in non-Caucasian patients is unknown.

Clinical Features

Although PP has been reported in all trimesters, it usually starts in midpregnancy, at about 25 to 30 weeks' gestation, and persists throughout gestation. It manifests itself with grouped, extremely pruritic, discrete papules and nodules over the extensor surfaces of the extremities (Figs. 21.1 and 21.2), dorsa of hands and feet, and occasionally on the abdomen and elsewhere; with disease progression, trunk and extremities are equally involved (Fig. 21.3).[2] The lesions are typically smaller than 1 cm in diameter,[8] with the vast majority being no larger than 0.5 cm; lesions can occasionally coalesce into crusted plaques. Marked excoriations and crusting secondary to scratching are invariably seen (see Figs. 21.3 and 21.4), and the lesions may look eczematous (see Fig. 21.1).[3] Nodular lesions similar to those of prurigo nodularis in nonpregnant females can be seen (Fig. 21.5), but the nodules in PP are smaller and of lighter color than those in prurigo nodularis.[8] Pustules secondary to superinfection of lesions may be seen, but vesicles are absent.

Most authors agree that the cases labeled as *papular dermatitis of pregnancy* by Spangler represent severe, widespread PP.[9] Scarring can be seen in lesions that have persisted and have been manipulated (see Fig. 21.4). The disease usually abates in the immediate postpartum period but may occasionally last up to 3 months' postpartum. Mild postinflammatory hyperpigmentation can be seen in active lesions and upon resolution,[10] especially in dark-skinned patients (see Figs. 21.4 and 21.5).[8] The recurrence of PP with subsequent pregnancies varies.

Pathology

Most dermatologists do not perform a skin biopsy because PP is a clinical diagnosis. Histopathologic features are nonspecific and include acanthosis, hyperkeratosis, parakeratosis, and a perivascular lymphohistiocytic infiltrate (Fig. 21.6), containing occasionally eosinophils and neutrophils. Full-thickness excoriation with serum crust is frequently seen (Fig. 21.7).[7] Evidence of scarring can be demonstrated (see Fig. 21.6), often a result of manipulation of the lesions. Direct immunofluorescence (DIF) is negative.

Laboratory Tests

In a retrospective study, an elevated immunoglobulin E (IgE) level was detected in 5 out of 12 patients with PP.[11] There have been no other abnormalities in serologic tests. The hormonal abnormalities (elevated beta-human chorionic gonadotropin, and decreased cortisol and estrogen levels) that were reported by Spangler et al.[6] have not been confirmed.

Diagnosis

PP remains a clinical diagnosis because it lacks specific histopathologic features, and DIF is negative.

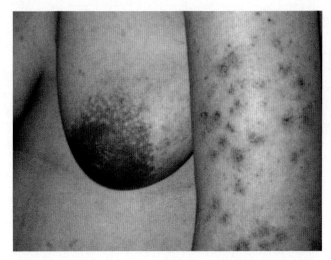

Figure 21.1. Prurigo at 26 weeks' gestation showing excoriated pruritic erythematous papules and crusted, eczematous-looking lesions on the extensor aspect of the arm. The patient had no history of atopy. The lesions responded to oral antihistamines and topical steroids but resolved only postpartum. (Courtesy of Dr. Magdalena Roth.)

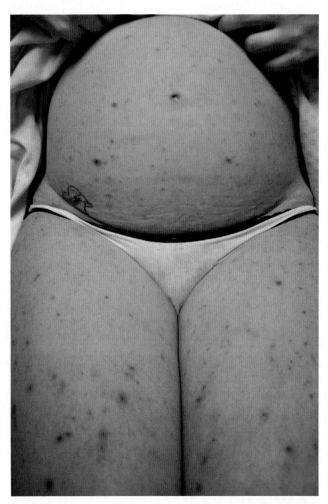

Figure 21.3. A severe, generalized atopic eruption in the third trimester: Numerous excoriated lesions are noticed on the abdomen and lower extremities. The patient had no personal or family history of atopy, and serum immunoglobulin E (IgE) level was 68 kU/L (normal, <114 kU/L).

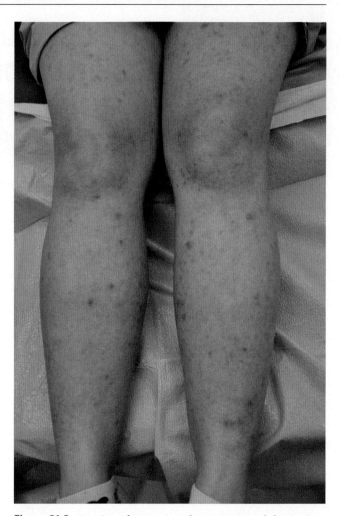

Figure 21.2. Prurigo of pregnancy shown at 26 weeks' gestation: Excoriated pruritic erythematous papules and minute nodules on the extensor surfaces of the lower extremities.

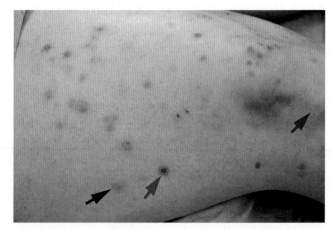

Figure 21.4. Prurigo of pregnancy resolving with hyperpigmentation in an Asian female. A crusted hyperpigmented papule secondary to scratching *(blue arrow)*, atrophic scarring with dyspigmentation *(black arrow)*, and linear scarring secondary to excoriation *(red arrow)*.

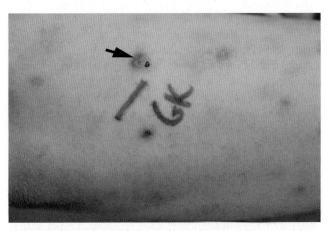

Figure 21.5. Prurigo of pregnancy: Active lesions and mild postinflammatory hyperpigmentation are shown on the forearm. The *arrow* shows a crusted, excoriated nodule that released serosanguinous fluid secondary to repeated scratching. Nodular lesions are typically smaller than the ones encountered in prurigo nodularis of nonpregnant patients.

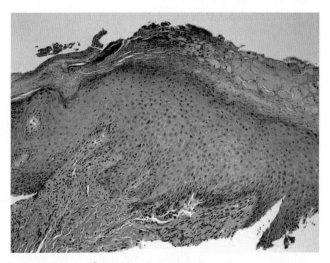

Figure 21.7. Histopathologic examination of the lesion shown with *arrow* in Figure 21.5 demonstrates excoriation with serous crusting and irregular acanthosis (hematoxylin and eosin stain, ×40).

Differential Diagnosis

PP should be differentiated from other specific dermatoses, AD/atopic eruption, obstetric cholestasis, arthropod bites, scabies, and drug eruptions (Table 21.1). Pemphigoid gestationis often starts on the abdomen and typically progresses to bullous lesions. A polymorphic eruption often involves the abdominal striae and shows predominantly urticarial lesions that are absent in PP. PFP lesions are follicular and demonstrate a sterile folliculitis on biopsy, features that are absent in PP. Differentiation from AD/AEP is challenging because these entities show a clinical overlap (see Atopic Eruption of Pregnancy). Scabies, arthropod bites, and drug eruptions can be ruled out by a history and thorough clinical examination.

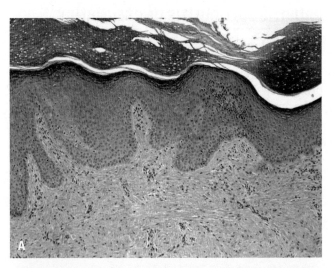

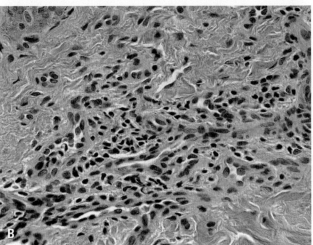

Figure 21.6. **(A)** Histopathologic examination of a nodular lesion demonstrates acanthosis, hyperkeratosis with focal parakeratosis, and dermal fibrosis (hematoxylin and eosin stain, ×10). **(B)** A higher magnification shows a perivascular lymphohistiocytic infiltrate (hematoxylin and eosin stain, ×40).

Pathogenesis

The etiology of PP is unclear, but it is likely that scratching in response to pruritus may play a role.[8] PP has been associated with obstetric cholestasis[12] and/or a family history of obstetric cholestasis[12] or *pruritus gravidarum*.[3] Bos suggested that PP and obstetric cholestasis are closely related disorders and may represent different levels of severity of the same disease.[13] In fact, the absence of primary lesions in obstetric cholestasis is often the only feature that differentiates these entities. Holmes and Black were the first to suggest that PP may result from *pruritus gravidarum* in women with an atopic predisposition.[7] Subsequently, Black and associates reported an association with personal or a family history of AD (4 out of 12 patients) and the elevation of serum IgE (5 out of 12 patients; uncontrolled).[11] The group then suggested that PP be classified under AEP,[2] although 4 out of 49 PP patients in the study fulfilled only minor criteria of atopy. Nevertheless, there has been no history of AD or an established atopic background in some PP patients[2,3];

TABLE 21.1	Differential Diagnosis of Prurigo, Pruritic Folliculitis, and Atopic Eruption of Pregnancy
Disease	**Differential Diagnosis**
Prurigo	■ Pemphigoid gestationis ■ Polymorphic eruption ■ Pruritic folliculitis ■ Atopic eruption[a] ■ Obstetric cholestasis ■ Arthropod bites ■ Infestations (i.e., scabies) ■ Drug eruptions
Pruritic folliculitis	■ Microbial folliculitis ■ Polymorphic eruption ■ Prurigo ■ Atopic eruption[b] ■ Obstetric cholestasis ■ Arthropod bites
Atopic eruption	■ Polymorphic eruption ■ Obstetric cholestasis ■ Prurigo ■ Pruritic folliculitis ■ Contact dermatitis ■ Drug eruptions ■ Infestations (i.e., scabies)

[a] Suggested overlap.

[b] Suggested overlap between papular, nonacneiform morphology of pruritic folliculitis, and atopic eruption.

this has also been these authors' experience (see cases in Figs. 21.1 and 21.3).[1] The association with atopy was not confirmed in a large prospective study of 1,392 patients, and the use of mild, uncontrolled serum IgE elevations in pregnancy as an indicator of atopy has been challenged[14]; only very high IgE levels were included in the criteria for atopy by Hanifin and Rajka.[15] Ingber indicates that the clinical presentation of pruritic papules on the extensor aspects of the extremities in PP is not the distribution of widespread and papular types of AD.[16] PP may be a heterogeneous group and several pathways can be involved.[8] The etiology and clinical associations with atopy and obstetric cholestasis can be clarified only with prospective large-scale clinical studies.

Maternal and Fetal Risks

The disease has not been associated with any maternal risks, and pharmacologic risks are minimal. Fetal outcome is excellent, and the birth weight has been normal. The dismal fetal outcome reported by Spangler[6] has not been reproduced and seems to have been biased by the methodology used in data collection.[9]

Management

Treatment is symptomatic, and lesions respond to moderately or highly potent topical steroids. Intralesional steroids can be helpful for a small number of lesions, as can topical steroids under occlusion, such as flurendrenolone tape.[17] Oral antihistamines, such as diphenhydramine or chlorpheniramine, are safe in gestation.[8,17] Cooling baths and antipruritic topical medications, such as aqueous cream with 1% to 2% menthol,[11] can be helpful. A short course of oral corticosteroid (20 to 30 mg per day) may be necessary in cases of recalcitrant pruritus[10]; higher steroid doses (up to 60 mg per day) have been historically reported in *papular dermatitis of pregnancy* but are not typically required. A taper of oral steroid is usually effective, but a rebound can occur upon discontinuation.[10] Ingber has successfully treated many PP patients with 20 to 30 treatments of narrowband ultraviolet light B (UVB).[8] The pregnant patient should be counseled that PP is not associated with fetal risks.

PRURITIC FOLLICULITIS OF PREGNANCY

Epidemiology

PFP is a rare, benign, and self-limiting condition of pregnancy. Since the original description of 6 cases by Zoberman and Farmer,[18] approximately 25 cases have been reported. The incidence of PFP was approximately 1 in 3,000 pregnancies in a large prospective study.[3] Because of its rarity, its incidence in various ethnic groups remains unknown. The condition is probably underdiagnosed because it is minimally symptomatic and may be misdiagnosed as steroid acne or microbial folliculitis because of clinical similarities with these entities.[19,20] A predominance of male fetuses (male to female ratio, 2:1) in the largest series[11] has not been confirmed.

Clinical Features

PFP has been reported as early as the ninth week of gestation,[21] with the vast majority of cases starting in the second or third trimester. It manifests with sparse, follicular, erythematous, or tan papules and sterile pustules that mainly involve the upper abdomen, chest, and back but can spread to the legs and arms (Figs. 21.8 to 21.10).[18,19] The lesions can be excoriated, but the eruption is usually only mildly pruritic or asymptomatic. The initial report by Zoberman and Farmer described the eruption as papular (see Fig. 21.8)[18]; however, several cases showing acneiform papulopustules have been subsequently reported (see Fig. 21.10).[19,22,23] The acneiform presentations cannot be clinically distinguished from other acneiform eruptions, such as steroid acne or microbial folliculitis (Fig. 21.11). Florid presentations with extensive acneiform lesions have been reported (Fig. 21.12). The eruption resolves spontaneously by delivery or within 1 month postpartum and may recur in subsequent pregnancies.[18]

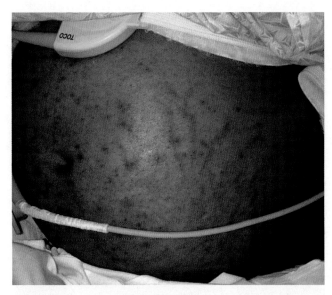

Figure 21.8. Pruritic folliculitis of pregnancy: Follicular erythematous or tan papules on the abdomen. (Courtesy of Dr. Eve Lowenstein.)

Pathology

The histopathology is that of acute folliculitis, with special stains for microorganisms being negative (Fig. 21.13A). The inflammatory infiltrate contains lymphocytes, neutrophils, as well as rare eosinophils, plasma cells, and occasional giant cells (Fig. 21.13B).[19] Intrafollicular pustule formation and destruction of the follicular wall with abscess formation in the dermis have been reported.[18] Nonspecific changes can be seen, such as ulcerations, spongiosis, exocytosis of inflammatory cells, mild dermal edema, and a perivascular infiltrate similar to that observed within the hair follicles (see Fig. 21.13A).[18] DIF is negative.

Laboratory Tests

Serologic tests are negative and levels of sex hormones are normal for gestational age. Increased serum androgen levels[23] have not been confirmed.[24]

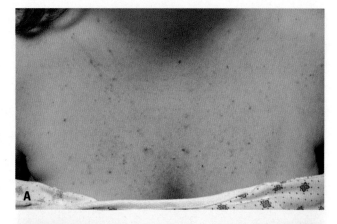

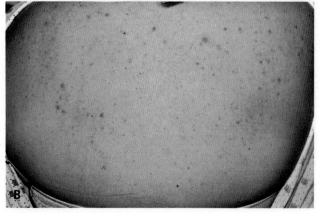

Figure 21.10. Pruritic folliculitis at 13 weeks' gestation (patient's second pregnancy): Acneiform papulopustules (**A**) on the chest and (**B**) the upper back. The patient had developed similar lesions in her first pregnancy and had no history of atopy.

Diagnosis

The characteristic follicular distribution of mildly symptomatic papulopustules and the histopathology of sterile folliculitis are sufficient for the diagnosis.

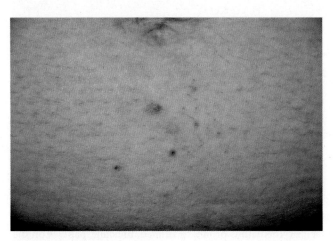

Figure 21.9. Pruritic folliculitis of pregnancy: Close-up of follicular papules on the abdomen.

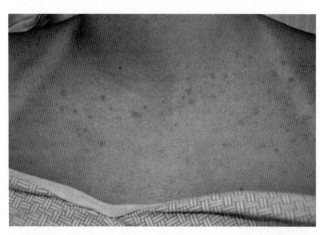

Figure 21.11. *Pityrosporum* folliculitis at 25 weeks' gestation presenting with monomorphous papulopustules on the upper chest. The lesions are clinically indistinguishable from the acneiform presentation of pruritic folliculitis of pregnancy.

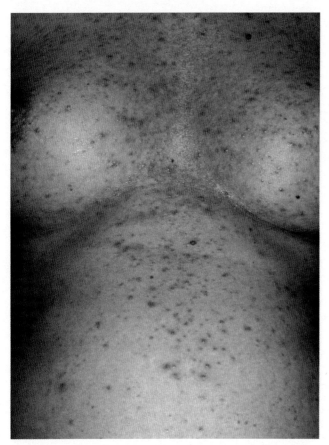

Figure 21.12. A florid presentation of pruritic folliculitis of pregnancy as extensive acneiform papulopustules covering the chest and abdomen. Lesions are shown at 30 weeks' gestation in a 26-year-old primigravida. There was no history of atopy, and the lesions resolved spontaneously postpartum. (Courtesy of Dr. Magdalena Roth.)

Differential Diagnosis

PFP should be differentiated from infectious folliculitis, specific dermatoses, and insect bites (see Table 21.1). Infectious folliculitis can be ruled out by cultures and special stains, such as a Gram stain for bacteria and a periodic acid-Schiff (PAS) stain for fungi. Polymorphic eruption usually starts later in gestation, shows a typical distribution along abdominal striae, and only exceptionally contains follicular lesions. PP primarily shows lesions on the extensor extremities, and its histopathology is not follicular. Obstetric cholestasis demonstrates no primary skin lesions, and elevated serum bile acid levels confirm the diagnosis. The differentiation from AEP may be challenging when PFP presents with papular lesions (Fig. 21.14) but is easy if the presentation of PFP includes acneiform lesions. Insect bites can be suggested by history and the presence of very pruritic lesions.

Pathogenesis

The etiology of PFP remains elusive. PFP may be a heterogeneous group, with the acneiform presentations possibly related to hormonal changes of gestation. It has been

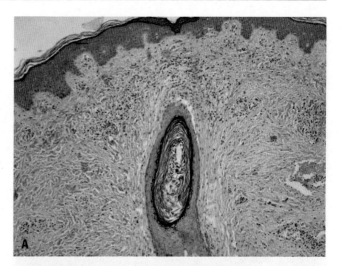
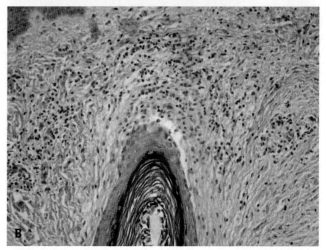

Figure 21.13. Histopathology of pruritic folliculitis of pregnancy. (**A**) Conspicuous follicular-centered lymphohistiocytic infiltrate, mild dermal edema, and superficial perivascular infiltrate (hematoxylin and eosin stain, ×10). (**B**) A higher magnification of the follicular infiltrate shows occasional plasma cells (hematoxylin and eosin stain, ×20). Special stains for bacteria and fungi were negative.

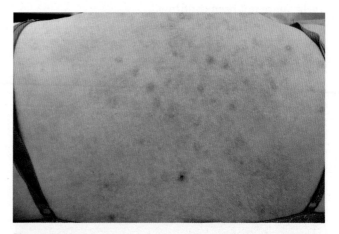

Figure 21.14. Pruritic folliculitis of pregnancy (second trimester): Erythematous or tan, excoriated, follicular papules on the upper back. The patient had an atopic background, and the differentiation from atopic eruption was challenging.

suggested[23] that PFP may be a form of hormonally induced acne, similar to steroid acne, based on clinical similarities with steroid acne, an association with increased serum androgen levels,[23] and a case of PFP in a patient that had a similar eruption while on danazol.[18] Nevertheless, PFP lacks a comedonal component that is typically seen in steroid acne,[25] and a report of 12 PFP patients showed no increase in serum androgen levels when compared to healthy pregnant controls.[24] It has been postulated that PFP may result from end-organ hypersensitivity to increased levels of sex hormones during gestation,[23] but there has been scarce evidence in support of this hypothesis. An association with obstetric cholestasis[26] has not been confirmed. Other authors have postulated that PFP is a variant of PEP[3] because follicular lesions have been reported in PEP,[27] but the clinicopathologic features of PFP differ from those of PEP.

A study classified PFP under AEP based on a history of childhood eczema and a family history of atopy in one patient with PFP.[2] The authors claimed clinical similarities between the papular presentation of PFP and follicular eczema.[9] However, although the papular presentation of PFP may resemble follicular eczema (see Fig. 21.13), common features of follicular eczema, such as significant xerosis, pruritus, confluence of lesions, and keratosis pilaris, have not been reported in PFP. Similarly, follicular spongiosis is not seen on a biopsy in PFP but is a feature in follicular eczema. Because of the rarity of the disease, clinical associations, such as that with atopy, have not been confirmed. However, only 1 of almost 30 reported PFP cases has been associated with a history of atopy. The case reported by these authors[19] as well as other cases (see Figs. 21.9 and 21.11) were not associated with atopy. A suggestion that PFP can be caused by *pityrosporum*[28] was debated.[25] Ambros-Rudolph, Black, and Vaughan Jones suggested classifying only those cases showing a papular presentation and overlap with atopy as PFP and referring to the acneiform presentations as "acneiform eruption" in pregnancy.[9] However, data supporting an overlap with atopy are insufficient.

Maternal and Fetal Risks

There have been no fetal risks, with preterm delivery[21] and threatened preterm labor[3] probably being coincidental in individual cases. An association with decreased birth weight in the largest series[11] needs to be validated.

Management

Treatment is symptomatic because the eruption is self-limited. Low-to-moderate potency topical steroids, oral antihistamines, and other topical antipruritic medications have been only mildly effective, with an incomplete relief of pruritus.[18] Oral and topical antibiotics have been ineffective.[19] Creams containing 10% benzoyl peroxide and 1% hydrocortisone have been helpful.[29] A case was treated successfully with narrowband UVB.[21] The pregnant patient should be counseled that PFP resolves spontaneously by delivery or postpartum and has not been associated with any maternal or fetal risks.

ATOPIC ERUPTION OF PREGNANCY

AEP is a conceptual umbrella that comprises AD, including *new AD* (AD developing for the first time in pregnancy), PP, and PFP.[2] The concept gives emphasis on atopic diathesis being the common denominator of these entities and a possible clinical overlap among them. The AEP concept may facilitate the differentiation among specific dermatoses because AEP starts earlier in gestation than polymorphic eruption and pemphigoid gestationis. However, as discussed previously, it has been challenged whether PP and PFP are always associated with atopy and should be included under AEP.[14,16,30]

Epidemiology

The studies that introduced the concept of AEP showed that AD is the most common pregnancy dermatosis, accounting for 36% to 49.7% of all pregnancy dermatoses. These studies indicated an unexpectedly high incidence of AD, including new AD (up to 79% of AD cases), in pregnancy; only 20% to 30% of patients with AEP have a history of AD prior to gestation.[2] Exacerbation of AD in pregnancy ranged between 52%[31] and 61%[32] in other studies. Still, an older large prospective study had not shown an increased incidence of AD in pregnancy.[3] A history of similar eruptions in previous pregnancies was reported in 34% of patients,[2] a personal history of atopy (asthma, hay fever, or AD), and/or infantile AD in 27% of pregnant females with AD, and a family history of atopy in 50% of cases.[11] Infantile AD was reported in 19% of the offspring.[11]

Clinical Features

Approximately 75% of patients with AEP develop symptoms within the first two trimesters, and the earlier onset of lesions in gestation can help differentiate AEP from specific dermatoses.[2] The study showed that 79% of AEP patients never had AD but were characterized as atopic based on a personal and/or family history of atopy and/or elevated serum IgE levels.[2] AEP comprises patients with both patchy eczematous features (E-type AEP; 67% of AEP) (Fig. 21.15) and papular/prurigo lesions (P-type AEP; 33% of AEP) (Fig. 21.16).[2] Eczematous lesions can be seen, often as an exacerbation of preexisting AD (20% of AEP cases). The P-type shows small pruritic erythematous disseminated papules, at times grouped, exanthematous, or follicular-looking, and/or prurigo lesions on the trunk and extremities that can be clinically indistinguishable from PP (see Figs. 21.16 and 21.17).[2] In these authors' experience, the coexistence of E- and P-types is common (Fig. 21.17). A generalization of lesions is often noticed (see Figs. 21.15 and 21.16), especially with inadequate control of the disease, and an erythrodermic state can be exceptionally seen.[33]

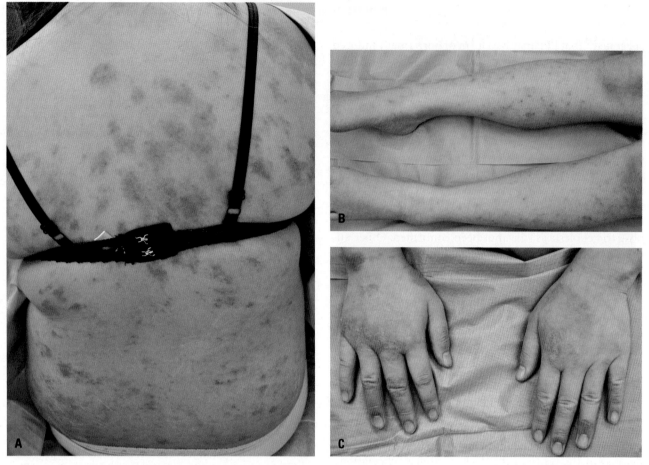

Figure 21.15. E-type of atopic eruption of pregnancy: Generalized eczematous papules and plaques (**A**) on the back, (**B**) the extensor surface of lower extremities, and (**C**) the dorsa of the hands. Excoriations are invariably seen.

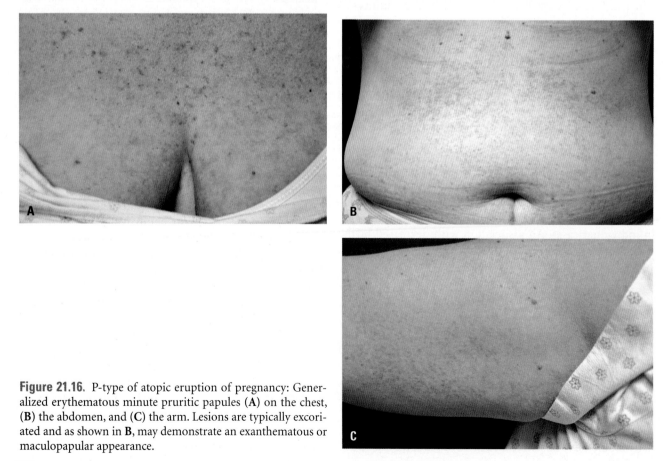

Figure 21.16. P-type of atopic eruption of pregnancy: Generalized erythematous minute pruritic papules (**A**) on the chest, (**B**) the abdomen, and (**C**) the arm. Lesions are typically excoriated and as shown in **B**, may demonstrate an exanthematous or maculopapular appearance.

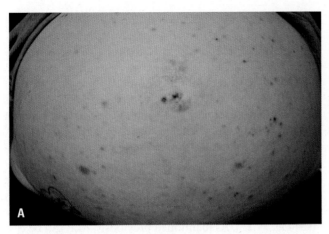 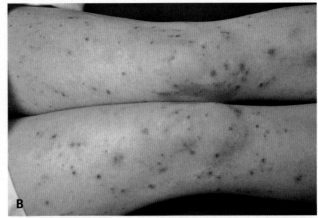

Figure 21.17. A severe, generalized atopic eruption that started at 20 weeks' gestation (lesions shown at 32 weeks) in a primigravida: Numerous excoriated lesions are noticed (**A**) on the abdomen and (**B**) lower extremities. Although P-type lesions predominate, eczematous (E-type) papules and plaques can be also seen. This presentation is clinically indistinguishable from prurigo of pregnancy.

Atopic sites such as the flexural aspects of the extremities (Fig. 21.18), face, neck, and V of the neck/chest are frequently involved.[11] Truncal involvement is also very common (Fig. 21.19), with 68% of cases involving the abdomen.[2] Hand/foot eczema is not uncommon (see Fig. 21.15C), with palms and soles often involved. Less common presentations include follicular eczema, eczema of the nipple and/or areola, and dyshidrosis (for a discussion of these manifestations and superinfected AD, see Ch. 9). The frequency of xerosis, keratosis pilaris, and other minor criteria of atopy[15] has not been reported. Significant postinflammatory hyperpigmentation can be seen, especially in patients of color (Fig. 21.20). Although a history of AEP in previous pregnancies was reported in up to 34% of cases,[2] the postpartum course of AEP, including how often patients with new AD in pregnancy subsequently develop flares in the nonpregnant state, has yet to be established.

Pathology

Skin histopathology shows nonspecific findings, including a perivascular lymphohistiocytic infiltrate and epidermal changes, such as spongiosis, hyperkeratosis, and parakeratosis. Findings vary depending on the stage of the disease and the manipulation of lesions by the patient; changes of lichen simplex chronicus may be seen over time. Such histopathologic features do not allow differentiation from other entities such as polymorphic eruption or PP. Immunofluorescence studies are negative.

Laboratory Tests

Elevated serum IgE levels (uncontrolled) were reported in 18% of patients with AD in pregnancy (PP and PFP cases not included)[11] and subsequently in 71% of AEP patients.[2] There have been no other serologic abnormalities.

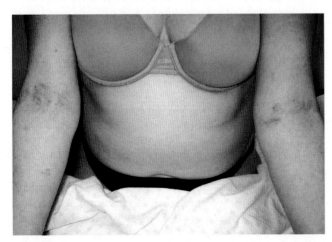

Figure 21.18. An atopic eruption at 12 weeks' gestation: Typical atopic sites, such as the antecubital fossae and chest, are involved. The patient had a history of atopic dermatitis with a similar distribution before pregnancy.

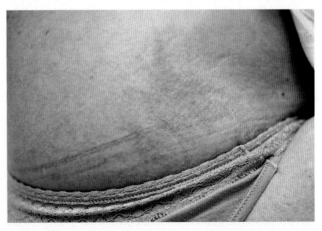

Figure 21.19. An atopic eruption at 18 weeks' gestation: Eczematous (E-type) confluent lesions on the lateral abdomen; the abdomen is involved in 68% of cases of atopic eruption.

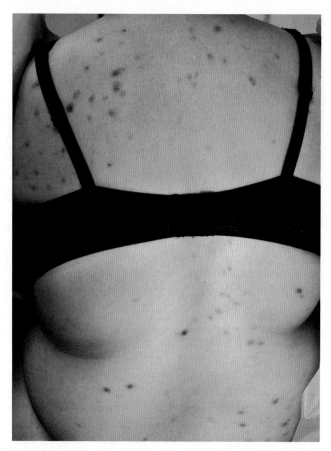

Figure 21.20. Extensive postinflammatory hyperpigmentation on the back secondary to atopic eruption; dyspigmentation is more common in darker skin.

Diagnosis

The diagnosis is clinical, based on the onset of an eczematous eruption early in pregnancy in patients that may have an atopic background (personal or family history of atopy). Two studies on AD in pregnancy[31,32] used Hanifin's and Rajka's criteria[15] and another two[2,11] used the U.K. Working Party criteria.[34] However, these criteria may not reliably differentiate between AEP and other dermatoses, such as polymorphic eruption, when AEP presents in an atypical (nonflexural) distribution because the diagnosis in these cases relies solely on historic information such as personal and/or family history of atopy, history of dry skin, and history of flexural involvement (see Ch. 9).[30]

Differential Diagnosis

AEP should be differentiated from specific dermatoses, obstetric cholestasis, contact dermatitis, drug eruptions, and infestations such as scabies (see Table 21.1). Sparing of the striae distensae, absence of urticarial lesions, and an earlier presentation help differentiate AEP from polymorphic eruption. However, the differentiation between the two entities can be challenging in those AEP cases presenting with nonflexural distribution, because the diagnosis of AEP in

this case depends exclusively on historic data (history of atopy and/or eruption in a flexural distribution).

Regarding PP and PFP, the advocates of the AEP concept suggest including them under the umbrella of AEP. However, as aforementioned, some PP patients satisfied only minor criteria of atopy[2,11] or never had AD[3] (see cases shown in Figs. 21.1 and 21.3), and the association between PP and atopy was not validated in a large prospective study.[3] Ingber indicated that the presentation of pruritic papulonodules on the extensor aspects of the extremities in PP is not the distribution of widespread and papular types of AD[16]; however, the distinction between these entities may not be easily made based solely on clinical grounds (see Fig. 21.17). As mentioned previously, AEP can be easily differentiated from the acneiform presentation of PFP. Nevertheless, because the papular presentation of PFP may resemble follicular eczema, the differentiation can be challenging (see Fig. 21.14). Obstetric cholestasis shows no primary skin lesions, and an elevated serum bile acid level is a clue to the diagnosis. Contact dermatitis can be ruled out by history and response to removal of the offending allergen. Infestations such as scabies can be ruled out by history and the presence of specific signs (i.e., burrows in scabies).

Pathogenesis

The pathogenesis of AEP is thought to be related to the T-helper 2 (Th2)-skewed immunity that characterizes pregnancy (see Ch. 9). Production of interleukin-4, a Th2 cytokine, by the placenta may be critical to the induction of IgE and the exacerbation of AD in pregnancy. Nevertheless, IgE levels did not correlate with the deterioration of AD during pregnancy in a small recent study,[32] and further studies are required in order to determine whether it is the intrinsic (*nonallergic* or *atopiform dermatitis*) and/or the extrinsic (IgE-associated) AD that is affected by pregnancy.[30] Whether patients with AEP will show manifestations of atopy in the nonpregnant state has to be established. It is possible that pregnancy induces a transient *atopiform dermatitis* in a significant number of patients, and these patients may not show signs of atopy, such as IgE-associated reactions to allergens, postpartum.

Maternal and Fetal Risks

The maternal and fetal prognosis is unaffected. Pharmacologic risks related to the use of topical steroids can be minimized with judicious use. Oral steroids should be avoided in the first trimester (see Ch. 23). Maternal risks associated with other immunosuppressants, such as cyclosporine and azathioprine, are also discussed in Chapter 23. Fetal risks are related to a systemic infection, such as a disseminated herpetic infection, when there is superinfection of maternal lesions.

Management

This is discussed in Chapter 9 (Atopic Dermatitis; see Table 9.2) and outlined in Table 21.2.

TABLE 21.2	Summary of Management Options
Disease	**Management**
Prurigo of pregnancy	■ Cooling baths and topical antipruritic medications, such as aqueous cream with 1%–2% menthol[11] ■ Moderately or highly potent topical steroids; intralesional or under occlusion may also be helpful[8,17] ■ Oral H$_1$ antihistamines[17] ■ A short taper of oral steroid in cases of recalcitrant pruritus[10] ■ Narrowband UVB Rx[8]
Pruritic folliculitis of pregnancy	■ Topical antipruritic medications are mildly effective ■ Low-to-moderate potency topical steroids and oral antihistamines are mildly effective[18] ■ Creams containing 10% benzoyl peroxide and 1% hydrocortisone[29] ■ Narrowband UVB Rx[21]
Atopic eruption of pregnancy	■ Emollients, topical antipruritic medications, topical steroids, oral H$_1$ antihistamines[30,35] ■ Short taper of oral steroid for severe cases[30] ■ UVB phototherapy[35] ■ Topical calcineurin inhibitors on small areas (face, neck, intertriginous areas)[35] ■ Cyclosporine is the safest systemic Rx in severe cases not responding to oral steroids[30]

Rx, therapy/treatment; UVB, ultraviolet light B.

MATERNAL RISKS

Prurigo: None
Pruritic folliculitis: None
Atopic eruption: Risks from superinfection of lesions; risks from pharmacologic treatment

FETAL RISKS

Prurigo: None
Pruritic folliculitis: Preterm delivery (one case); decreased birth weight (case series)
Atopic eruption: Risks from superinfection of lesions; risks from pharmacologic treatment

KEY POINTS

■ Prurigo of pregnancy has an incidence between 1 in 300 and 1 in 450 pregnancies and presents as pruritic papules and nodules predominantly on the extensor aspects of the extremities.

■ The treatment of prurigo includes topical corticosteroids, oral antihistamines, and narrowband UVB phototherapy; a short course of oral corticosteroid may be required in recalcitrant cases.

■ Pruritic folliculitis of pregnancy is a rare entity that presents with pruritic follicular papules or acneiform papulopustules on the upper trunk and extremities; treatment includes topical medications, such as creams containing 10% benzoyl peroxide and 1% hydrocortisone, and narrowband UVB.

■ The concept of atopic eruption of pregnancy emphasizes that atopic dermatitis is the most common pregnancy dermatosis and often develops for the first time during gestation, and that specific dermatoses, such as prurigo and pruritic folliculitis, are possibly associated with atopy.

■ Atopic eruption starts earlier in pregnancy, with 75% of cases manifesting in the first two trimesters, which helps differentiate it from a polymorphic eruption and pemphigoid gestationis.

■ The treatment of atopic eruption includes emollients, topical corticosteroids, and oral antihistamines; UVB phototherapy is a safe second-line treatment option; if systemic agents other than oral steroids are needed for severe disease, cyclosporine is the safest option.

REFERENCES

1. Kroumpouzos G, Cohen LM. Specific dermatoses of pregnancy: an evidence-based systematic review. *Am J Obstet Gynecol.* 2003;188:1083–1092.
2. Ambros-Rudolph CM, Müllegger RR, Vaughan-Jones SA, et al. The specific dermatoses of pregnancy revisited and reclassified: results of a retrospective two-center study on 505 pregnant patients. *J Am Acad Dermatol.* 2006;54:395–404.
3. Roger D, Vaillant L, Fignon A, et al. Specific pruritic dermatoses of pregnancy. A prospective study of 3192 women. *Arch Dermatol.* 1994;130:734–739.
4. Besnier E, Brocq L, Jacquet L. *La Pratique Dermatologique.* Vol. 1. Paris, France: Masson; 1904:75.
5. Nurse D. Prurigo of pregnancy. *Australas J Dermatol.* 1968;9: 258–267.
6. Spangler AS, Reddy W, Bardawill WA, et al. Papular dermatitis of pregnancy. *JAMA.* 1962;181:577–581.
7. Holmes RC, Black M. The specific dermatoses of pregnancy. *J Am Acad Dermatol.* 1983;8:405–412.
8. Ingber A. Prurigo of pregnancy. In: Ingber A, ed. *Obstetric Dermatology.* Berlin, Germany: Springer-Verlag; 2009:151–156.
9. Ambros-Rudolph CM, Black MM, Vaughan Jones S. The papular and pruritic dermatoses of pregnancy. In: Black MM,

Ambros-Rudolph C, Edwards L, et al., eds. *Obstetric and Gynecologic Dermatology*. 3rd ed. London, England: Mosby Elsevier; 2008:73–77.

10. Wen-ge F, Yun Q. Prurigo gestationis. *Chin Med J*. 2010;123: 638–640.

11. Vaughan Jones SA, Hern S, Nelson-Piercy C, et al. A prospective study of 200 women with dermatoses of pregnancy correlating the clinical findings with hormonal and immunopathological profiles. *Br J Dermatol*. 1999;141:71–81.

12. Cicek D, Kandi B, Demir B, et al. Intrahepatic cholestasis occurring with prurigo of pregnancy. *Skinmed*. 2007;6:298–301.

13. Bos JD. Reappraisal of dermatoses of pregnancy. *Lancet*. 1999; 354:1140–1142.

14. Cohen LM, Kroumpouzos G. Pruritic dermatoses of pregnancy: to lump or to split? *J Am Acad Dermatol*. 2007;56:708–709.

15. Hanifin JM, Rajka G. Diagnostic features of atopic eczema. *Acta Derm Venereol (Stockh)*. 1980;92:S44–S47.

16. Ingber A. Atopic eruption of pregnancy. *J Eur Acad Dermatol Venereol*. 2010;24:974.

17. Kroumpouzos G, Cohen LM. Dermatoses of pregnancy. *J Am Acad Dermatol*. 2001;45:1–19.

18. Zoberman E, Farmer ER. Prutitic folliculitis of pregnancy. *Arch Dermatol*. 1981;117:20–22.

19. Kroumpouzos G, Cohen LM Pruritic folliculitis of pregnancy. *J Am Acad Dermatol*. 2000;43:132–134.

20. Fox GN. Prutitic folliculitis of pregnancy. *Am Fam Physician*. 1989;39:189–193.

21. Reed J, George S. Pruritic folliculitis of pregnancy treated with narrowband (TL-01) ultraviolet B phototherapy. *Br J Dermatol*. 1999;141:177–179.

22. Walters J, Clark DC. Pruritic rash during pregnancy. *Am Fam Physician*. 2005;71:1380–1382.

23. Wilkinson SM, Buckler H, Wilkinson N, et al. Androgen levels in pruritic folliculitis of pregnancy. *Clin Exp Dermatol*. 1995; 20:234–236.

24. Vaughan Jones SA, Hern S, Black MM. Neutrophil folliculitis and serum androgen levels. *Clin Exp Dermatol*. 1999;24: 392–395.

25. Kroumpouzos G. Pityrosporum folliculitis during pregnancy is not pruritic folliculitis of pregnancy. *J Am Acad Dermatol*. 2005;53:1098–1099.

26. Esteve E, Vaillant L, Bacq Y, et al. [Pruritic folliculitis of pregnancy: role of associated intrahepatic cholestasis?] *Ann Dermatol Venereol*. 1992;119:37–40.

27. Borrego L. Follicular lesions in polymorphic eruption of pregnancy. Follicular lesions in polymorphic eruption of pregnancy. *J Am Acad Dermatol*. 2000;42:146.

28. Parlak AH, Boran C, Topçuoglu MA. Pityrosporum folliculitis during pregnancy: a possible cause of pruritic folliculitis of pregnancy. *J Am Acad Dermatol*. 2005;52:528–529.

29. Black MM. Progress and new directions in the investigation of the specific dermatoses of pregnancy. *Keio J Med*. 1997;46: 40–41.

30. Koutroulis I, Papoutsis J, Kroumpouzos G. Atopic dermatitis in pregnancy: current status and challenges. *Obstet Gynecol Surv*. 2011;66:654–663.

31. Kemmett D, Tidman MJ. The influence of menstrual cycle and pregnancy on atopic dermatitis. *Br J Dermatol*. 1991;125: 59–61.

32. Cho S, Kim HJ, Oh SH, et al. The influence of pregnancy and menstruation on the deterioration of atopic dermatitis symptoms. *Ann Dermatol*. 2010;22:180–185.

33. Roth MM. Atopic eruption of pregnancy: a new disease concept. *J Eur Acad Dermatol Venereol*. 2009;23:1466–1467.

34. Williams HC, Burney PGJ, Hay RJ, et al. The U.K. Working Party's diagnostic criteria for atopic dermatitis. I: derivation of a minimum set of discriminators for atopic dermatitis. *Br J Dermatol*. 1994;131:383–396.

35. Weatherhead S, Robson SC, Reynolds NJ. Eczema in pregnancy. *BMJ*. 2007;335:152–154.

CHAPTER **22** # Drug Safety

Kudakwashe Mutyambizi ■ Bonnie T. Mackool

INTRODUCTION

Certain drugs have deleterious effects on the fetus and/or the mother. The strength of evidence varies for each drug but is nonetheless crucial in a physician's treatment decisions and the provision of informed consent for the pregnant patient. Of equal importance is knowledge of those systemic medications in the dermatologic repertoire for which safety has been well documented.[1] In this chapter, we will review medication interactions precipitating contraceptive failure; key differences in the drug metabolism in the pregnant patient; and maternal, fetal, and neonatal risks associated with commonly used systemic medications in dermatology. In addition to emerging medications, we will also review established medications, some of which have significant toxicity profiles.

CONTRACEPTIVE FAILURE

Contraceptive failure has been conclusively determined with the concomitant use of oral contraceptive pills and rifampin[2] or griseofulvin,[3] as well as concomitant use of nonsteroidal anti-inflammatory drugs (NSAIDs) and intrauterine devices[4] (Table 22.1). However, the data are equivocal with other potentially implicated medications.[2–4]

DRUG METABOLISM IN PREGNANCY

Pregnancy alters the rate and extent of drug metabolism, although the underlying molecular mechanisms are incompletely understood. Estradiol has been shown to upregulate the P450 CYP2B6 and CYP2A6 enzymes in human hepatocytes.[5,6] This induction of the P450 system can result in a more rapid metabolism of CYP2B6 substrates, such as lidocaine, some coumarins, cyclophosphamide, and amitriptyline.[7]

DETERMINING MATERNAL AND FETAL RISKS

The period of organogenesis (14 to 60 days gestational age) is maximally sensitive to teratogens. Animal testing and human epidemiologic studies are the mainstay in categorizing teratogenicity and maternal–fetal morbidity[8]; however, animal studies are imperfect in their extrapolation to humans. Furthermore, well-powered, controlled, human epidemiologic studies are generally lacking because of ethical constraints. Typically, the more definitive data that exist arise from unintended human exposure as in the case of inadvertent pregnancy while on or newly exposed to a medication. With the dual goal of protecting pregnant women from inadvertent harm and centralizing information, pregnancy registries are being developed for emerging medications, such as the biologics. The interpretation of data can pose challenges. For example, fetal toxicity from the medication versus the disease cannot always be distinguished, particularly in cases of high morbidity. Another factor that can make interpretation of data challenging is background rates of major congenital malformations. Estimates of congenital malformations are approximately 2% in all pregnancies; an additional 3% of children within the first few years of life will have evidence of congenital malformations.[9] Maternal risk factors such as age and family history also contribute to the risk of malformation confounded with medication risk. As study methodology and assay sensitivity improve, data from older studies are increasingly questioned. Yet, nearly 50% of pregnancies in the United States are unplanned with subsequent significant risk for exposure of the fetus to potentially teratogenic medications.[10]

The U.S. Food and Drug Administration (FDA) designated a five-letter pregnancy labeling system (outlined in Table 22.2), which provides physicians with information to guide medication choices for a pregnant patient. Drug companies are required to produce this data on their products. Criticisms of this system are that it does not impart the different magnitudes of risk for developmental toxicity and that it focuses too much on animal data. Additionally, the revision process of a medication's rating is inconsistent as new safety data become available. The differential risk at various time points in the gestational period is not addressed. Finally, the teratogenic risks with topical versus systemic formulations of the same medication are incompletely differentiated. In response to these shortcomings, a revision of the FDA labeling system, including explanatory statements, has been proposed and is under consideration. Schaefer has proposed an evidence-based system to guide medication risk counseling in pregnancy that takes into consideration the duration of a medication on the market

TABLE 22.1	Systemic Dermatologic Medications Implicated in Contraceptive Failure	
Medication	**Contraception**	**Mechanism**
Rifampin[2]	OCPs	Hepatic microsomal enzyme induction resulting in ↑ estrogen metabolism
Griseofulvin[3]	OCPs, Mirena IUD	Hepatic microsomal enzyme induction resulting in ↑ estrogen metabolism
Tetracycline[1]	OCPs	Controversial; ↓ enterohepatic circulation of estrogens
Sulfonamides[1]	OCPs	Controversial; ↓ enterohepatic circulation of estrogens
NSAIDs[4]	IUD	Unknown
Azathioprine[4]	IUD	Unknown

↑, increased; ↓, reduced; IUD, intrauterine device; NSAID, nonsteroidal anti-inflammatory drug; OCP, oral contraceptive pill.

(Adapted from Leachman SM, Reed B. The use of dermatologic drugs in pregnancy and lactation. *Dermatol Clin.* 2006;24:167–197.)

TABLE 22.2	U.S. Food and Drug Administration Use-in-Pregnancy Ratings	
Category	**Description**	**Comments**
A	Well-controlled human studies show no fetal risk	Safe medications; <1% of drugs are category A
B	Animal studies show fetal risk not confirmed by human studies *or* animal studies do not show fetal risk and well-controlled human studies are lacking	No evidence of risk in humans; the chance of fetal harm is remote but remains a possibility
C	Well-controlled human studies are lacking and animal studies are lacking or show fetal risk	Risk cannot be ruled out; the potential benefits from the drug may outweigh the potential fetal risk; two-thirds of all drugs in the United States are category C
D	Human studies or investigational or postmarketing data show fetal risk	Positive evidence of risk; potential benefits may outweigh risk (i.e., in a life-threatening situation or serious disease for which safer drugs cannot be used or are ineffective)
X	Animal/human studies or investigational or postmarketing data show fetal risk that clearly outweighs any possible benefit	Contraindicated in pregnancy

TABLE 22.3	Lactation Risk Categories by Hale[12] and Codes by Weiner and Buhimischi[13]
Hale Categories	
L1	Safest
L2	Safer
L3	Probably safe
L4	Possibly hazardous
L5	Contraindicated
Weiner & Buhimschi Codes	
S	Safe
U	Unknown
NS	Not safe

and the period of fetal exposure.[11] Schaefer's system is a promising approach but has not included a classification of all existing medications. Useful databases are the Teratogen Information System (TERIS), the Reprotox database, and the *U.S. Pharmacopeia Dispensing Information,* Volume 1.

LACTATION CONSIDERATIONS

Currently, drug companies are not required to study the use of medications during lactation, and most lactation data are accrued from case reports or retrospective studies. Thus, a large proportion of safety recommendations are not evidence-based but rather founded on expert opinion. A contemporary and comprehensive resource for drug safety in lactation is the *LactMed* database, published by the National Library of Medicine. Additionally, the *UpToDate* database includes lactation information on all drugs included in its database. The American Academy for Pediatrics (AAP) provides a compatibility rating with breastfeeding for many medications, with further guidelines published by the World Health Organization (WHO) and the Centers for Disease Control and Prevention (CDC). These resources have been referenced in Tables 22.4 to 22.18, under Lactation, Comments and Recommendations. Two lactation safety assessment systems are increasingly referenced (Table 22.3). For ease of comparison, the Hale and Weiner lactation safety categorizations are also represented here (see Table 22.3).[12,13]

In general, low molecular weight, lipid soluble, nonionized, weakly basic medications are more likely to pass into breast milk.[1] Multiple pharmacodynamic considerations influence the likelihood of toxicity. In the first 72 hours' postpartum, immature tight junctions are more permissive to the entry of high–molecular-weight compounds into the milk compartment. Premature infants and neonates with an immature renal and hepatic system are more likely to accrue metabolites to toxic levels due to higher drug bioavailability and slower drug clearance. Maternal adverse effects are an important clue to the fact that the mother may have higher than normal serum drug concentrations, with increased toxic risk to the infant even in cases involving medications that are classified as safe in lactation.

DERMATOLOGIC DRUGS AND FERTILITY

The teratogenic effects of paternal exposure to a drug on a subsequently conceived fetus are poorly defined. Drugs associated with particular controversy in this area include acitretin and methotrexate. The theoretical mechanisms by which teratogenicity and spontaneous abortion could be induced are through direct effects on the fertilizing sperm, or through the absorption of the drug vaginally from the male ejaculate.[14] Nevertheless, the acitretin ejaculate concentration is very small when compared to therapeutic blood levels. Unlike acitretin, methotrexate has been shown to decrease the sperm count in exposed males. The data remain inconclusive regarding the teratogenic potential of preconceptual paternal methotrexate exposure in humans, although generally, physicians advise a 3-month methotrexate-free interval in the male before attempting conception. Thalidomide has been identified in seminal fluid and on the spermatozoa of male rabbits, with congenital malformations observed in rabbit neonates fathered by male rabbits exposed to thalidomide for prolonged courses. In humans, thalidomide has been detected in semen 4 weeks after receiving 100-mg daily doses.[15] A theoretical risk of congenital malformation following paternal exposure to thalidomide thus exists. The manufacturer recommends contraceptive barrier protection for men even after a vasectomy; it further advises against sperm donation.

The FDA rating and lactation safety assessment with explanatory recommendations for commonly used dermatologic medications are listed in Tables 22.4 to 22.18. The safest medications in each medication category are summarized in Table 22.19.

TABLE	22.4	**Category X Medications**

Dermatologic Medication	Pregnancy			Lactation	
	Animal & Human Studies	FDA Category	Comments & Recommendations	Category	Comments & Recommendations
Acitretin	*Animals*: Embryotoxic, teratogenic at subtherapeutic doses *Humans*: NTDs, craniofacial anomalies, CV defects[14]	X	Black box warning regarding birth defects; avoid pregnancy for 3 years after completion of Rx (P.A.R.T.); avoid alcohol during and 2 months after Rx because alcohol intake results in formation of etretinate that has longer half-life than acitretin, and therefore, prolongs period of teratogenicity	U	Small amounts in breast milk; compatible with breastfeeding as per AAP; not rec by manufacturer prior to or during breastfeeding
Estrogen	*Animals*: DES assoc with NTDs, embryolethal *Humans*: Synthetic DES teratogenic; no clear evidence of teratogenicity in retrospective studies of estrogen-containing OCPs; no well-controlled studies	X	No clear evidence of fetal harm with currently available estrogen-containing OCPs when inadvertently taken early in pregnancy[13]; contraindicated during pregnancy	S (OCPs), L3	Small amounts in breast milk, effects on infant appear minimal[12]; ↓ quantity/quality of breast milk; some authors suggest estrogen-containing OCPs not be started until after the sixth week of lactation,[13] and others wait at least 1 week postpartum prior to instituting progesterone Rx[12]; estradiol compatible with breastfeeding as per AAP; manufacturer rec caution
Finasteride	*Animals*: Hypospadias, ↓ fertility in male offspring[1] *Humans*: No studies	X	Exposure to medication is also possible through contact with broken or crushed tablets or semen from male partner; however, systemic levels after these exposures do not seem clinically relevant		Unknown if it enters breast milk; contraindicated per manufacturer
5-Fluorouracil	*Animals*: Systemic form teratogenic; no studies with topical *Humans*: No well-controlled studies, reports of oral cleft, VSDs, and miscarriages with systemic and topical formulations[1]	X (topical) D (systemic)	Absorption of topical is low (<6%)	U, L5	Unknown if it enters breast milk; not rec by manufacturer; no AEs reported in exposed infant[2]; if used, monitor neonatal CBC; topical should pose negligible risk to breastfeeding infant; avoid application to breast

| TABLE | 22.4 | **Category X Medications** *(continued)* |

| Dermatologic Medication | Pregnancy | | | Lactation | |
	Animal & Human Studies	FDA Category	Comments & Recommendations	Category	Comments & Recommendations
Isotretinoin	*Animals*: Teratogen, primates more sensitive to teratogenic effects than rodents *Humans*: Among others, craniofacial, ear, skeletal, CV, thymic, NTDs, and CNS defects, spont abortion, premature birth, and mental retardation[1]	X	Black box warning regarding severe birth defects; wide range of maternal AEs; restricted distribution through iPLEDGE program; two forms of effective contraception required 1 month before, during, and 1 month following Rx; no recommendations regarding paternal exposure	NS, L5	Unknown if it enters breast milk but because it is lipid soluble, concentration in milk may be significant[12]; not rec by manufacturer
Methotrexate	*Animals*: Embryotoxicity and teratogenicity *Humans*: Embryotoxicity and teratogenicity (craniofacial, musculoskeletal, CV, GI, and skin anomalies)[16]	X	Black box warning; critical period is 6–8 weeks gestational age at doses >10 mg/week; after Rx, females should avoid pregnancy for 1 ovulatory cycle, and males should avoid causing pregnancy for 3 months	NS, L3 (acute), L5 (chronic)	Low levels in breast milk; contraindicated given risk of neonatal immunosuppression
Thalidomide	*Animals*: Amelia, micromelia, CNS malformations *Humans*: Phocomelia, multiple organ abnormalities, fetal demise[15,17]	X	Black box warning regarding severe birth defects and fetal death; wide range of maternal AEs; restricted distribution through S.T.E.P.S.; abstinence or two forms of contraception in females 1 month before, during, and 1 month after Rx; manufacturer rec barrier protection in males even after a vasectomy, no sperm donation (fetal risk from exposure to semen of male patient taking thalidomide is unknown)	U	No human data; unknown whether it enters breast milk, but excretion is possible because of drug's low molecular weight; rec discontinuation of breastfeeding or medication

Note: Category X medications are known and often potent teratogens with any potential benefit eclipsed by the teratogenic risk in desired pregnancies. Several of these medications are available to women of childbearing age only through restricted distribution programs requiring compliance with effective contraception. If pregnancy occurs during treatment, the medication should be immediately discontinued and the patient should be referred to an obstetrician/gynecologist experienced in reproductive toxicity for further evaluation and counseling.

↓, reduced; AAP, American Academy of Pediatrics; AE, adverse effect; assoc, associated; CBC, complete blood cell count; CNS, central nervous system; CV, cardiovascular; DES, diethylstilbestrol; FDA, U.S. Food and Drug Administration; GI, gastrointestinal; NTD, neural tube defect; OCP, oral contraceptive pill; P.A.R.T., pregnancy prevention actively required during and after treatment; rec, recommended/recommends; Rx, treatment; spont, spontaneous; S.T.E.P.S., system for thalidomide education and prescribing safety; VSD, ventricular septal defect.

TABLE 22.5	**Analgesics**					

		Pregnancy			Lactation	
Dermatologic Medication	**Animal & Human Studies**	**FDA Category**	**Comments & Recommendations**	**Category**	**Comments & Recommendations**
Acetaminophen	*Animals*: No teratogenicity, constricts *ductus arteriosus* *Humans*: Long experience, no well-controlled studies; nephro- and hepato-toxic to infant and mother at high doses; third trimester *ductus arteriosus* constriction (case reports)[18]	B	Preferred analgesic in pregnancy; absorption and bioavailability retarded due to delayed gastric emptying	S, L1	Breast milk levels much lower than infant dosing; assoc between frequent exposure to drug and childhood asthma not validated[19]
Acetaminophen with codeine	*Animals*: No reproduction studies *Humans*: Inconsistent assoc with congenital malformations[1]	C	Neonatal withdrawal symptoms may be observed when used late in pregnancy	S, L3	Risk of fetal over-dose; death in infant breastfed by mother who was an ultra-rapid metabolizer of codeine to high levels of morphine[20]
Aspirin	*Animals*: Known teratogen *Humans*: Fetal demise, IUGR, neonatal acidosis, fetal/neonatal hemorrhage, premature closure of *ductus arteriosus* perinatally[1]	D	Assoc with maternal anemia, hemorrhage, prolonged gestation, and labor	S, L3	Metabolite salicylic acid excreted in breast milk to dis-proportionately high levels; metabolic acidosis, thrombocytopenia in breastfed infants, hemolysis in G6PD-deficient infants, risk of Reye syndrome; occasional doses safe per WHO, avoid long-term Rx
Gabapentin	*Animals*: Teratogenicity[21] *Humans*: No well-controlled studies	C	Crosses human placenta; no evidence of teratogenicity in a small postmarketing study[13]	S, L3	Low levels in breast milk; monitor for drowsiness, weight gain

TABLE 22.5	Analgesics *(continued)*

| Dermatologic Medication | Pregnancy | | | Lactation | |
	Animal & Human Studies	FDA Category	Comments & Recommendations	Category	Comments & Recommendations
NSAIDs	*Animals*: Ibuprofen blocks blastocyte implantation *Humans*: No teratogenicity; assoc with oral clefts, CV anomalies (premature closure of *ductus arteriosus*), ↑ risk spont abortion in first trimester	C	NSAIDs close to conception assoc with miscarriage; assoc with IUD failure	S, L1 (ibuprofen), S, L3 (L4 with chronic use) (naproxen)	Low levels in breast milk, no AEs with ibuprofen; a case of prolonged bleeding, hemorrhage and acute anemia in an infant with naproxen; not rec by manufacturer
Opioid narcotics	*Animals*: No teratogenicity with isolated use except morphine (CNS abnormalities with maternotoxic doses) *Humans*: No teratogenicity, neonatal neurobehavioral defects[1]	C	Neonatal respiratory depression from high dose near time of delivery; neonatal withdrawal symptoms with prolonged gestational exposure	S, L3	Withdrawal on breastfeeding cessation; not rec by manufacturer
Tramadol	*Animals*: No teratogenicity, no well-controlled studies *Humans*: No well-controlled studies	C	Withdrawal with gestational exposure[20]	S, L3	Levels achieved in breast milk much lower than infant dosing; not rec by manufacturer

Note: Of the analgesics, acetaminophen appears the safest in both pregnancy and lactation, with limited reports of adverse events. When hepatic derangements limit acetaminophen use during lactation, NSAIDs such as ibuprofen are considered second-line agents.

↑, increased; AE, adverse effect; assoc, associated; CNS, central nervous system; CV, cardiovascular; FDA, U.S. Food and Drug Administration; G6PD, glucose-6-phosphate dehydrogenase; IUD, intrauterine device; IUGR, intrauterine growth restriction; NSAID, nonsteroidal anti-inflammatory drug; rec, recommended/recommends; Rx, treatment; spont, spontaneous; WHO, World Health Organization.

TABLE	22.6	**Antibiotics**

| Dermatologic Medication | Pregnancy | | | Lactation | |
	Animal & Human Studies	FDA Category	Comments & Recommendations	Category	Comments & Recommendations
Azithromycin	*Animals*: No teratogenicity *Humans*: No teratogenicity; less history with newer macrolides than erythromycin[22,23]	B	First-line antibiotic in pregnancy; use in penicillin-allergic patient	U, L2	Low levels in breast milk, unlikely clinically relevant; GI AEs; manufacturer rec caution
Cephalosporins	*Animals*: No teratogenicity *Humans*: No teratogenicity[22]	B	First-line antibiotic in pregnancy; maternal AEs include drug eruptions, anaphylaxis, pseudomembranous colitis, diarrhea, transaminitis	S, L1–L2	Low levels in breast milk, may disrupt GI flora, observe for diarrhea
Clindamycin	*Animals*: No teratogenicity *Humans*: No teratogenicity or IUGR; no well-controlled studies	B	Second-line antibiotic in pregnancy due to maternal AEs including diarrhea and pseudomembranous colitis; however, the latter has been only exceptionally reported in gestation (not clinically relevant)	S, L3	Low levels in breast milk, more GI AEs than others; topical application safe, may cause infant diarrhea if applied to maternal nipple, cream/gel rec for nipple application given risk of licking/paraffin exposure with ointment; not rec by manufacturer
Clofazimine	*Animals*: Teratogenic at supratherapeutic doses *Humans*: Reports of hyperpigmentation in infants following prolonged intrauterine exposure[22]	C	WHO rec continuation in pregnancy when treating Hansen disease where benefits outweigh risks	U, L3	Relatively large amounts in breast milk with pink discoloration, discolors infant skin, no permanent toxicity
Dapsone	*Animals*: None *Humans*: Uncontrolled data	C	Stopping Rx for Hansen disease in last month of gestation may minimize theoretical kernicterus risk[24]	S, L4	Low levels in breast milk; monitor for signs of hemolysis in G6PD-deficient newborn and premature infants; not rec by manufacturer

TABLE 22.6	Antibiotics *(continued)*				

Dermatologic Medication	Pregnancy			Lactation	
	Animal & Human Studies	FDA Category	Comments & Recommendations	Category	Comments & Recommendations
Doxycycline	*Animals*: As for tetracycline (see the following) *Humans*: ↑ cleft palate, esophageal atresia only with oxytetracycline (precursor of drug)	D	Crosses placenta; similar effects on teeth and maternal risks as with tetracycline (see the following)	NS, L3 (L4 with chronic use)	Less bound to calcium in breast milk thus slightly ↑ absorption than other tetracyclines, yet relative amount of tooth staining lower than with other tetracyclines; avoid prolonged or repeated courses during nursing; not rec by manufacturer
Erythromycin ethylsuccinate and base	*Animals*: No teratogenicity *Humans*: Considered safe (no well-controlled studies); reports of cardiac malformations, negated by more recent multicenter trials[23]	B	Erythromycin estolate is category C (should be avoided) because second trimester use assoc with reversible maternal hepatotoxicity (10%)	S, L1 (L3 for early postnatally)	Low levels in breast milk, mild GI AEs; early postnatal intake assoc with pyloric stenosis[25] (not confirmed); topical application safe, may cause infant diarrhea if applied to maternal nipple, cream/gel rec for nipple application given risk of licking/paraffin exposure with ointment; manufacturer rec caution
Fluoroquinolones	*Animals*: No teratogenicity, cartilage and tendon damage in immature animals, ↑ spont abortion *Humans*: Suboptimal, small, short studies show no evidence of teratogenesis or adverse events[22]	C	Avoid because of animal evidence of risk to developing tendons and joints	S (possibly), L3 (ciprofloxacin), S (likely), L3 (levofloxacin)	Low levels in breast milk with ofloxacin but variable with ciprofloxacin (the former preferred); arthropathy considered unlikely[12]; dose-related alteration in bowel flora; a case of pseudomembranous colitis; not rec by manufacturer; if used, avoid breastfeeding 4–6 hours after dose

(continued)

| TABLE | 22.6 | **Antibiotics** *(continued)* |

Dermatologic Medication	Pregnancy			Lactation	
	Animal & Human Studies	FDA Category	Comments & Recommendations	Category	Comments & Recommendations
Metronidazole	*Animals*: No teratogenicity *Humans*: No teratogenicity (no well-controlled studies), effects on organogenesis unknown[22]	B	Avoid in first trimester; second-line antibiotic	S, L2	Measurable levels in breast milk, but lower than therapeutic doses used to treat infants; may cause GI AEs, ↑ *Candida* load; not rec by manufacturer
Minocycline	*Animals*: As for tetracycline (see the following) *Humans*: No teratogenicity (no well-controlled data)[22]	D	Crosses placenta; similar effects on teeth and maternal risks as with tetracycline (see the following)	U, L2 (acute)/ L4 (chronic)	Black breast milk reported, theoretical risk of dental staining; not rec by manufacturer
Penicillins	*Animals*: No teratogenicity *Humans*: Studies performed, long clinical experience; traverse placenta but no teratogenicity or IUGR[22]	B	First-line antibiotic; physiologic changes in second/third trimester may alter pharmacokinetics and require higher dosing[26]	S, L1	Single maternal dose of 4 million units penicillin G produces low levels in breast milk; AEs in the infant include changes in GI flora and allergic reactions
Rifampin	*Animals*: Teratogenicity *Humans*: No well-controlled studies; almost never used as monotherapy, unclear if reported malformations secondary to rifampin or other components of multidrug regimens[27]	C	Assoc with contraceptive failure; first-line Rx for active tuberculosis; peripartum vitamin K prophylaxis b/o assoc with hemorrhagic disease of the newborn	S, L2	Low levels in breast milk, therefore, no AEs expected; not rec by manufacturer

TABLE 22.6	**Antibiotics** *(continued)*

Dermatologic Medication	Pregnancy			Lactation	
	Animal & Human Studies	FDA Category	Comments & Recommendations	Category	Comments & Recommendations
Tetracycline	*Animals*: Fetal dental staining, no teratogenicity; evidence of fetal toxicity (such as retardation of skeletal development) *Humans*: Fetal dental staining, no teratogenesis; no well-controlled data[1]	D	Crosses placenta; assoc with maternal hepatotoxicity, pseudotumor cerebri; reliable contraception encouraged for women on extended Rx for acne; contraindicated ≥15 wks' gestation due to bone inhibition, teeth discoloration, maternal hepatitis; second-line antibiotic up to 14 wks	S, L2	Rash, mild GI AEs; theoretical risk of dental enamel or bone deposition but absorption inhibited by calcium in breast milk (low serum levels in infant); avoid prolonged or repeated courses during nursing; not rec by manufacturer
Trimethoprim–sulfamethoxazole	*Animals*: ↑ oral clefts *Humans*: Possible assoc with CV, UT, NTDs, oral clefts; data inconclusive[28]	C	Second-line antibiotic during pregnancy; trimethoprim is a folate antagonist: avoid in first trimester; peripartum sulfonamide use assoc with ↑ risk of hyperbilirubinemia	U, L3	Avoid in G6PD-deficient, premature infants, and ill neonates due to ↑ risk of hyperbilirubinemia; per manufacturer, all sulfonamides contraindicated given kernicterus risk
Vancomycin	*Animals*: No teratogenicity or IUGR *Humans*: No teratogenicity (no well-controlled data)	C	Crosses placenta; risk of ototoxicity not substantiated[13]	S, L1	Low levels in breast milk and poor absorption from infant's GI tract

Note: Of the antibiotics, penicillins and cephalosporins appear the safest to use during pregnancy and lactation. For the penicillin-allergic mother, azithromycin is preferred.

↑, increased; AE, adverse effect; assoc, associated; b/o, because of; CV, cardiovascular; FDA, U.S. Food and Drug Administration; G6PD, glucose-6-phosphate dehydrogenase; GI, gastrointestinal; IUGR, intrauterine growth restriction; NTD, neural tube defect; rec, recommended/recommends; Rx, treatment; spont, spontaneous; UT, urinary tract; WHO, World Health Organization.

TABLE 22.7	Antifungal Agents, Systemic

Dermatologic Medication	Pregnancy			Lactation	
	Animal & Human Studies	FDA Category	Comments & Recommendations	Category	Comments & Recommendations
Amphotericin B	*Animals*: No teratogenicity *Humans*: No large studies but long experience, no teratogenicity[29]	B	Wide spectrum of severe maternal AEs (fever, tachycardia, hypertension, GI upset); risk of transient neonatal renal dysfunction	U, L3	Unknown if it enters breast milk but given that it is virtually non-absorbable orally, it is unlikely that the amount in milk would be clinically relevant to a breastfeeding infant[12]
Fluconazole	*Animals*: Weak teratogen (dose-dependent ossification defects) *Humans*: Skeletal malformations at higher, prolonged doses[1]	C	Wide spectrum of maternal AEs (GI upset, headache, dizziness, dysgeusia) and drug interactions; high dose prolonged fluconazole Rx in pregnancy should be used only in a life-threatening situation when there are no alternative Rxs[29]	NS, L2	Enters breast milk; AEs include facial flushing, GI upset, mucous stools; not rec by manufacturer; compatible with lactation as per AAP
Griseofulvin	*Animals*: ↓ spermatogenesis, fetal demise, growth retardation, skeletal abnormalities *Humans*: No well-controlled data, unsubstantiated reports of conjoined twins[1]	C	Crosses placenta; males to wait 6 months before attempting conception, females should wait 1 month; ↑ hepatic metabolism of OCPs; wide spectrum of maternal AEs; manufacturer rec avoidance	U, L2	Unknown whether excreted in breast milk; manufacturer rec caution
Itraconazole	*Animals*: Dose-related embryotoxicity and teratogenicity secondary to adrenal effects,[30] oral cleft, and skeletal defects *Humans*: No well-controlled studies; no teratogenicity in a cohort	C	Thought to have the lowest risk of teratogenicity of systemic azole antifungal agents given minimal effect on steroid hormones[1]; wide spectrum of maternal AEs and drug interactions	U, L2	Enters human milk, limited data; highest M:P = 1.77; absorption in an infant via breastfeeding is somewhat unlikely because drug requires an acidic milieu for absorption (unlikely in a diet high in milk)[12]

TABLE 22.7	Antifungal Agents, Systemic *(continued)*					
	Pregnancy			**Lactation**		
Dermatologic Medication	**Animal & Human Studies**	**FDA Category**	**Comments & Recommendations**	**Category**	**Comments & Recommendations**	
Ketoconazole	*Animals*: Syndactyly and oligodactyly at supratherapeutic doses[30] *Humans*: No well-controlled studies; limb defects, may interfere with implantation and maintenance of early pregnancy[1]	C	Wide spectrum of drug interactions[12]; to be avoided, especially in first trimester	S, L2	Enters breast milk; limited published data; not rec by manufacturer	
Nystatin	*Animals*: No studies *Humans*: No studies	C	Well-tolerated, may cause oral irritation and sensitization	S, L1	Unknown if it enters breast milk; however, absorption into infant circulation is unlikely especially because maternal absorption is poor	
Terbinafine	*Animals*: No teratogenicity[1] *Humans*: No studies	B	Elective use not rec by manufacturer	NS, L2	Manufacturer reports M:P = 7:1 after oral administration and rec against systemic or topical use, although no data suggesting problems with topical form; systemic form potentially toxic; AEs unlikely in older infants, monitor neonates for jaundice and signs of liver toxicity	
Voriconazole	*Animals*: Embryotoxicity, teratogenicity *Humans*: No well-controlled studies	D	Known animal teratogen, avoid in pregnancy	U	Unknown if it enters breast milk; not rec by manufacturer	

Note: Despite a wide spectrum of AEs, amphotericin B appears to be the safest systemic antifungal during pregnancy from a teratogenesis standpoint. Data are quite limited regarding safety in lactation, and although it is anticipated that amphotericin B would probably be safe in lactation, only ketoconazole is known to be safe in lactation, bearing the designation of lactation category S. Of note, the AAP considers fluconazole compatible with breastfeeding, yet its lactation safety rating remains NS.

↑, increased; ↓, reduced; AAP, American Academy of Pediatrics; AE, adverse effect; FDA, U.S. Food and Drug Administration; GI, gastrointestinal; M:P, milk-to-maternal plasma ratio; OCP, oral contraceptive pill; rec, recommended/recommends; Rx, treatment.

TABLE 22.8   Antifungal Agents, Topical

| Dermatologic Medication | Pregnancy | | | Lactation | |
	Animal & Human Studies	FDA Category	Comments & Recommendations	Category	Comments & Recommendations
Ciclopirox	*Animals*: No teratogenicity *Humans*: No studies[1]	B	Manufacturer rec use if benefit to mother justifies fetal risk	S, L3	Limited data, unlikely that infant would be affected; manufacturer rec caution
Clotrimazole	*Animals*: No fetal harm with intravaginal application *Humans*: Use for vaginitis in first trimester assoc with slightly ↑ risk of spont abortions[31] but finding debated[29]	B	Poor systemic absorption following topical and vaginal administration	S, L1	Unknown if it enters breast milk; unlikely that infant would be affected; manufacturer rec caution
Econazole	*Animals*: No teratogenicity *Humans*: No well-controlled data[1]; unknown if it crosses placenta	C	Inhibits placental aromatase; assoc with spont abortions (one study); manufacturer rec first-trimester use only if essential to welfare of mother; use during the second and third trimesters only if clearly needed[32]	S	Unknown if it enters breast milk; manufacturer rec caution
Ketoconazole	*Animals*: No studies *Humans*: No well-controlled studies	C	Not detectable in plasma following chronic use of 2% shampoo	S, L2	Systemic absorption likely low; avoid topical application to breast
Miconazole	*Animals*: No fetal harm with intravaginal application; dystocia in rats at supratherapeutic doses *Humans*: No teratogenicity[33]; use for vaginitis in first trimester assoc with slightly ↑ risk of spont abortions,[31] but finding is debated[29]	C	Small amounts absorbed following vaginal application; safe but caution rec for first trimester[31,33]	S, L2	Unknown if it enters breast milk; manufacturer rec caution

TABLE 22.8	Antifungal Agents, Topical *(continued)*

Dermatologic Medication	Animal & Human Studies	Pregnancy FDA Category	Pregnancy Comments & Recommendations	Lactation Category	Lactation Comments & Recommendations
Naftifine	*Animals*: No teratogenicity *Humans*: No well-controlled studies	B	4% absorbed following topical administration; manufacturer rec use only if clearly needed	S, L3	Unknown if it enters breast milk; manufacturer rec caution
Nystatin	*Animals*: No studies *Humans*: No studies	C	Not absorbed following topical application to intact skin	S, L1	Unknown if it enters breast milk; however, absorption into infant circulation is unlikely especially because maternal absorption is poor
Selenium sulfide	*Animals*: Embryotoxicity, teratogenicity at supratherapeutic doses *Humans*: No studies	C	Minimal systemic absorption, unlikely to reach clinically relevant serum level; not rec by manufacturer given lack of studies	S	Unknown if it enters breast milk; manufacturer rec caution
Terbinafine	*Animals*: No teratogenicity[1] *Humans*: No studies	B	Manufacturer rec use only when need clearly established	L2	Manufacturer rec against breastfeeding, although no data suggest risk; AEs unlikely in older infants, monitor neonates for jaundice and signs of liver toxicity

Note: Ciclopirox, clotrimazole, naftifine, and nystatin are all considered safe in pregnancy and lactation. Of the topical antifungals, the longest experience has been with clotrimazole and clinical studies have been performed, whereas data are limited for ciclopirox and naftifine. Thus, clotrimazole appears to be the safest topical antifungal in pregnancy.

↑, increased; AE, adverse effect; assoc, associated; FDA, U.S. Food and Drug Administration; rec, recommends/recommended; spont, spontaneous.

| TABLE 22.9 | **Antihistamines** |

| Dermatologic Medication | Pregnancy | | | Lactation | |
	Animal & Human Studies	FDA Category	Comments & Recommendations	Category	Comments & Recommendations
Cetirizine[a]	*Animals*: No teratogenicity *Humans*: Relative safety in first trimester[34]	B	Safe in pregnancy	U, L2	Enters breast milk (3% of dose)[12]; use lowest dose; drowsiness with higher doses and prolonged use
Chlorpheniramine	*Animals*: No teratogenicity *Humans*: Has not been associated with teratogenesis[35]	B	Preferred by some authors above second-generation H_1 antihistamines in first trimester[35]	NS (possibly), L3	Unknown if it enters breast milk; no AEs with small occasional doses, larger doses may ↓ milk supply; observe for sedation and irritability
Cyproheptadine	*Animals*: No teratogenicity or IUGR[36] *Humans*: Rate of malformations equal to that of control groups	B	Limited data in humans, longer experience with diphenhydramine (preferred)	U, L3	Unknown if it enters breast milk; may interfere with lactation, cause sedation and irritability; not rec by manufacturer
Diphenhydramine	*Animals*: No teratogenicity or IUGR *Humans*: Assoc with oral cleft has not been confirmed	B	Long h/o uneventful use in pregnancy; reports of infantile depression when administered during labor[37]	S, L2	May enter breast milk at very low levels; no AEs with small occasional doses, larger doses may ↓ milk supply, cause sedation, and irritability; not rec by manufacturer
Doxepin[b]	*Animals*: Low fetal weight and structural abnormalities at supratherapeutic doses *Humans*: No well-controlled studies	C	Second-generation antihistamines preferred	NS, L5	Small amounts enter breast milk; metabolite of medication has a long half-life; fetal LBW and apnea reported in breastfed infants; not rec by manufacturer

| TABLE 22.9 | **Antihistamines** *(continued)* |

| Dermatologic Medication | Pregnancy | | | Lactation | |
	Animal & Human Studies	FDA Category	Comments & Recommendations	Category	Comments & Recommendations
Fexofenadine[a]	*Animals*: No teratogenicity, ↓ pup weight gain and survival with supratherapeutic doses *Humans*: No well-controlled studies	C	Loratadine preferred	S (likely) L2	A metabolite of terfenadine, was found at very low levels in breast milk in a terfenadine study; no AEs with small occasional doses, larger doses may ↓ milk supply, cause sedation, and irritability; manufacturer rec caution
Hydroxyzine	*Animals*: Teratogenic in supratherapeutic doses *Humans*: No teratogenicity in small studies	C	Monitor for infant withdrawal symptoms	U, L1	Unknown if it enters breast milk; case report of neonatal seizures with withdrawal from chronic intrauterine exposure[38]; no AEs with small occasional doses, larger doses may ↓ milk supply, cause sedation, and irritability
Loratadine[a]	*Animals*: Teratogenic in supratherapeutic doses *Humans*: ↑ risk of hypospadias not confirmed[39]	B	Most extensively studied second-generation antihistamine	S, L1	Very low levels in breast milk; safest antihistamine in lactation, nonsedating

Note: Of the antihistamines, loratadine and diphenhydramine at their lowest doses are the safest to use in pregnancy and lactation. Although both loratadine and diphenhydramine are pregnancy category B (safe), loratadine is preferred given that it is nonsedating. An association between exposure during the last 2 weeks of pregnancy to antihistamines and retrolental fibroplasia in premature infants has been reported.

[a] A second-generation H_1 antihistamine.

[b] Topical doxepin is pregnancy category B.

↑, increased; ↓, reduced; AE, adverse effect; assoc, associated; h/o, history of; FDA, U.S. Food and Drug Administration; IUGR, intrauterine growth restriction; LBW, low birth weight; rec, recommended/recommends.

| TABLE | 22.10 | **Antiparasitic Agents** | | | |

		Pregnancy		Lactation	
Dermatologic Medication	**Animal & Human Studies**	**FDA Category**	**Comments & Recommendations**	**Category**	**Comments & Recommendations**
Crotamiton	*Animals*: No studies *Humans*: No studies	C	Little data; not as effective as permethrin		Unknown if it enters breast milk; no AEs reported
Ivermectin	*Animals*: Teratogenic at high doses (oral cleft, clubbed forepaws) *Humans*: No well-controlled studies; mass Rx programs for onchocerciasis have not identified teratogenicity[40]	C	No adverse pregnancy outcomes in community-based Rx programs for onchocerciasis; medication blocks P-glycoprotein–mediated efflux[13]; manufacturer rec against use	S, L3	Enters breast milk in low concentrations (highest M:P = 0.57); no problems identified in infants in large third-world populations; CDC and manufacturer do not rec use in lactation
Lindane	*Animals*: No teratogenicity, no IUGR at doses equivalent to human exposure; incoordination of uterine contractions[13] *Humans*: AEs including neurotoxicity with use on traumatized skin, case report of stillborn infant; no well-controlled studies[41]	C	Black box warning regarding neurotoxicity; questionable assoc with hypospadias, risks of maternal neurotoxicity, and aplastic anemia; most AEs involve misuse; not to be used on traumatized/ scratched or inflamed skin because systemic absorption can be high	S (likely), L4	Enters breast milk at low concentrations; manufacturer rec interruption of breastfeeding with expression and discard of milk for 24 hours and other sources rec bottle-feeding for 2 days following use[13]
Malathion	*Animals*: No teratogenicity *Humans*: No teratogenicity, possible assoc with shortened gestational duration[42]	B	Percutaneous absorption in acetone vehicle is 8% but that of lotion formulation has not been studied; use only if clearly needed		Unknown if it enters breast milk; risk of neonatal respiratory depression; manufacturer rec caution

TABLE 22.10	**Antiparasitic Agents** *(continued)*

| Dermatologic Medication | Pregnancy | | | Lactation | |
	Animal & Human Studies	FDA Category	Comments & Recommendations	Category	Comments & Recommendations
Permethrin	*Animals*: No teratogenicity or IUGR *Humans*: No well-controlled studies	B	Drug of choice for lice infestation and scabies during pregnancy; <2% absorbed after single application with rapid metabolism to inactive metabolites; long history of use with minimal AEs[43]; some authors rec shorter application (2 hours) in pregnancy; manufacturer rec use only if clearly needed	S (likely), L2	Enters breast milk but kinetics unclear; unlikely that systemic concentration in neonate would be clinically relevant; as per manufacturer, consider discontinuing nursing temporarily or withhold medication while nursing
Precipitated sulfur	*Animals*: No studies *Humans*: Old literature indicating animal and human fatalities when applied to abraded skin, not borne out by subsequent clinical experience[44]		Unregulated; <1% is absorbed; thought to be safe but less effective than permethrin		No data on lactation; most authors consider it safe
Thiabendazole	*Animals*: No teratogenicity or IUGR at doses equivalent to human exposure *Humans*: No well-controlled studies	C	Wide spectrum of maternal AEs; manufacturer rec use only if benefit to mother outweighs fetal risk	U, L3	Unknown if it enters breast milk; not rec by manufacturer
Spinosad	*Animals*: No teratogenicity *Humans*: No studies	B	FDA-approved for head lice; topical spinosad not absorbed systemically; manufacturer rec use only if clearly needed		Not present in human milk, however, suspension formula includes benzoyl alcohol, which is absorbed and may enter breast milk; manufacturer rec caution, consider avoiding breastfeeding and discard milk for 8 hours following application

Note: Permethrin appears to be the safest antiparasitic agent in both pregnancy and lactation. Some providers use precipitated sulfur as first-line agent with the caveat that data are very limited, and medication remains unrated in both the pregnancy and lactation classification systems.

AE, adverse effect; assoc, associated; CDC, Centers for Disease Control and Prevention; FDA, U.S. Food and Drug Administration; IUGR, intrauterine growth restriction; M:P, milk-to-maternal plasma ratio; rec, recommends/recommended; Rx, treatment.

TABLE 22.11   Antiviral Agents

Dermatologic Medication	Animal & Human Studies	Pregnancy FDA Category	Comments & Recommendations	Lactation Category	Comments & Recommendations
Acyclovir	*Animals*: No teratogenicity, IUGR, and malformations at maternotoxic doses *Humans*: Long experience without AEs; data from small pregnancy registry shows no teratogenicity[45]	B	Prompt IV acyclovir Rx when strong suspicion for *eczema herpeticum* or disseminated herpes infection; prophylaxis to prevent recurrences initiated at 36 weeks[1]; manufacturer rec caution	S, L2	Enters breast milk, no AEs; neonatal AEs unlikely with topical application away from breast; if applying to breast, avoid ointment given risk of mineral paraffin exposure with licking; manufacturer rec caution
Cidofovir	*Animals*: Embryotoxicity, teratogenicity, and assoc with hypospermia *Humans*: No well-controlled studies	C	Males: Barrier contraception during and 3 months after Rx; females: effective contraception during and 1 month after Rx	U	Unknown if it enters breast milk; not rec by manufacturer
Foscarnet sodium	*Animals*: Skeletal anomalies *Humans*: No well-controlled studies	C	Monitoring amniotic fluid volumes by ultrasound weekly after 20 weeks rec to detect oligohydramnios	U, L4	Unknown if it enters breast milk; not rec by manufacturer
Ganciclovir	*Animals*: Teratogenicity, inhibits spermatogenesis *Humans*: No well-controlled studies	C	Males: Barrier contraception during and 3 months following Rx; females: effective contraception during Rx	S (likely)	Unknown if it enters breast milk; not rec by manufacturer
Famciclovir	*Animals*: No teratogenicity, causes benign tumors *Humans*: Pregnancy registry exists, no well-controlled studies[46]	B	Prodrug of penciclovir; manufacturer rec use only when maternal benefit clearly outweighs fetal risk	U, L2	Unknown if it enters breast milk; neonatal AEs unlikely with topical application away from breast; not rec by manufacturer
Valacyclovir	*Animals*: No teratogenicity *Humans*: Data from small pregnancy registry shows no teratogenicity[45,46]	B	Prodrug of acyclovir, first-line Rx for genital HSV and herpes zoster in pregnancy and lactation; HSV prophylaxis at 36 weeks ↓ risk of recurrence and need for cesarean section[1]	S, L1	Levels of acyclovir achieved in breast milk higher than with administration acyclovir directly but remains <1% infant Rx dose, no AEs expected; report of elevated transaminases in infant whose mother also on HAART[47]; manufacturer rec caution

Note: Of the antiviral agents, acyclovir and its prodrug valacyclovir appear to be the safest in both pregnancy and lactation. Although famciclovir also appears safe, there is a limited experience with this medication. Given its long history of safe use, acyclovir is typically preferred.

↓, reduced; AE, adverse effect; assoc, associated; FDA, U.S. Food and Drug Administration; HAART, highly active antiretroviral therapy; HSV, herpes simplex virus; IUGR, intrauterine growth restriction; IV, intravenous; rec, recommends/recommended; Rx, treatment.

TABLE	22.12	**Biologic Agents**

| Dermatologic Medication | Animal & Human Studies | Pregnancy | | Lactation | |
		FDA Category	Comments & Recommendations	Category	Comments & Recommendations
Adalimumab	*Animals*: No teratogenicity *Humans*: No well-controlled studies; case reports of uneventful pregnancies[48,49]; pregnancy registry established	B	Manufacturer rec use in pregnancy only when clearly needed	L3	Low levels in breast milk; no AEs; not rec by manufacturer
Alefacept	*Animals*: No teratogenicity *Humans*: No studies; pregnancy registry for women becoming pregnant on Rx or within 8 weeks of Rx	B	Manufacturer rec use in pregnancy only if benefit to mother justifies fetal risk		Unknown if it enters breast milk; not rec by manufacturer
Etanercept	*Animals*: No evidence of harm *Humans*: Pregnancy registry established, no well-controlled studies; reports of VACTERL assoc with tumor necrosis factor antagonists[50] but assoc debated	B	Manufacturer rec use only when clearly needed	L3	Low levels in breast milk; AEs unlikely; not rec by manufacturer
Infliximab	*Animals*: No studies *Humans*: Short-term data from two registries show no teratogenesis[51,52]	B	Does not actively cross placenta in first trimester, maximum transplacental transport in third trimester (levels up to 3× maternal serum levels); some authors rec stopping at week 30 and resuming after delivery; detectable in infant's serum for up to 6 months	S (likely), L2	Unknown if it enters breast milk (high molecular weight, not orally absorbed); unlikely to affect breastfed infant, not rec by manufacturer

(continued)

TABLE 22.12	Biologic Agents *(continued)*					
	Pregnancy				**Lactation**	
Dermatologic Medication	**Animal & Human Studies**	**FDA Category**	**Comments & Recommendations**	**Category**	**Comments & Recommendations**	
Rituximab	*Animals*: Immuno-suppression *Humans*: Premature birth, neonatal hematologic abnormalities, infections[53]	C	Manufacturer rec effective contraception during and for 12 months following Rx		Unknown if it enters breast milk; manufacturer rec stop breastfeeding until drug levels are no longer detectable	
Ustekinumab	*Animals*: No teratogenicity *Humans*: No well-controlled studies[54]	B	Manufacturer rec use only if benefit justifies fetal risk		Unknown if it enters breast milk; manufacturer rec caution and that unknown risks to the infant from GI or systemic exposure should be weighed against the benefits of breastfeeding	

Note: Infliximab and etanercept may be considered the safest of the biologic agents in pregnancy because they have been on the market the longest with the best characterization to date. The biologic agents are relatively new medications, which makes some providers cautious in prescribing them to the pregnant patient despite their overall favorable FDA rating. Patients who start or decide to continue etanercept or adalimumab treatment during gestation should be encouraged to enroll in existing pregnancy registries. As new medications, alefacept, rituximab, and ustekinumab have not been rated in lactation. Adverse events can be life threatening when they occur, in particular, severe infections and malignancies. The most recent data regarding teratogenesis suggest that the biologic drugs are, in fact, the safest systemic medication for the diseases for which they are FDA approved, with particular reference to psoriasis for the dermatologist. The FDA rating does not currently evaluate for novel risks, such as potential effects on the fetal or neonatal immune system, and may become clearer with a longer history of use.

AE, adverse effect; assoc, associated; GI, gastrointestinal; rec, recommends/recommended; Rx, treatment; VACTERL, vertebral abnormalities, anal atresia, cardiac defect, tracheoesophageal, renal, and limb anomalies.

TABLE 22.13	Corticosteroids

		Pregnancy		Lactation	
Dermatologic Medication	Animal & Human Studies	FDA Category	Comments & Recommendations	Category	Comments & Recommendations
Corticosteroids, general topical	*Animals*: More potent steroids teratogenic, assoc with oral cleft *Humans*: Case-control study showed ↑ odds ratio of oral cleft with first-trimester use[55] but four other case-control studies[56] and a recent cohort[57] did not confirm the association; use of very potent steroids over large body surface areas assoc with LBW[1,58] but an analysis stratified by potency did not confirm the finding[59]	C	Use may be considered safe if applied on small body surface areas and/or for a short period of time[1]; minimize use of moderate and high-potency steroids in first trimester	S (likely) or U	Insufficient data; however, unlikely that systemic levels would be clinically relevant; should not be applied to breast until cessation of breastfeeding (case of infantile hypertension with use on the areola)
Corticosteroids, general systemic	*Animals*: Oral cleft, placental insufficiency, spont abortion, IUGR *Humans*: Placental insufficiency, adrenal suppression, oral cleft in several studies[57,60] supported by meta-analysis[61] but not a recent cohort,[57] spont abortion,[62] LBW,[61,62] and prematurity[61,62]	C (see the following)	Risks related to daily dose, but most importantly, duration of Rx; avoid in first trimester; fetal risks also include HPA suppression (especially important if used near time of delivery), immunosuppression, and congenital cataract; maternal risks include gestational diabetes and pregnancy-induced hypertension	See the following; U, L3 (dexamethasone) U (cortisone)	Prednisone and prednisolone found at low levels in breast milk, peaking 2 hours after maternal dose; delay nursing to 3–4 hours after intake of >20 mg/d prednisone to minimize exposure; AAP rates them compatible with breastfeeding
Betamethasone (systemic)	*Animals*: See *Corticosteroids, general systemic* (previous) *Humans*: See *Corticosteroids, general systemic* (previous)	C	As previous; peripartum betamethasone injection can delay milk production; betamethasone is often used in premature labor to stimulate fetal lung maturation	U, L3	May enter breast milk because of low molecular weight; manufacturer rec caution

(continued)

TABLE 22.13	**Corticosteroids** *(continued)*

| Dermatologic Medication | Animal & Human Studies | Pregnancy | | Lactation | |
		FDA Category	Comments & Recommendations	Category	Comments & Recommendations
Hydrocortisone (systemic)	*Animals*: Oral cleft, IUGR, and cataract *Humans*: See *Corticosteroids, general systemic* (previous)	C	See *Corticosteroids, general systemic* (previous)	S (likely)	Enters breast milk; manufacturer rec caution
Methylpred-nisolone, prednisolone	*Animals*: See *Corticosteroids, general systemic* (previous) *Humans*: Oral cleft and LBW	C	Converted by placental enzymes to inactive prednisone or less active cortisone, thus only 10% of maternal dose reaches fetus	S (likely), L2	Enters breast milk (see previous); manufacturer rec caution; AAP rates compatible, also suggested by long clinical experience
Prednisone	*Animals*: See *Corticosteroids, general systemic* (previous) *Humans*: Oral cleft, LBW, prematurity, abortion,[61] and congenital cataract[63]	C	No ↑ risk of congenital anomalies with doses 40–80 mg/d for short periods of time as per several authors[1] but no controlled data; short courses can be considered in second and third trimesters	S, L2	Enters breast milk (see previous); compatible; substitute prednisolone if long-term Rx or required dose >20 mg/d
Triamcinolone (topical)	*Animals*: Oral cleft *Humans*: IUGR in mother using equivalent of 40 mg/d through topical application[64]	C	Limited use in daily practice is considered safe; manufacturer rec use only if potential benefit outweighs fetal risk	U, L3	Unknown if it enters breast milk but levels would likely be low; manufacturer rec caution; observe growth rate; infantile hypertension following application to nipples

Note: All topical corticosteroids are labeled as category C regardless of strength. Given the other variables related to absorption, such as location, skin integrity, and size of area treated, the risk of topical steroid absorption is difficult to quantify. The risk of oral cleft with first-trimester exposure to topical steroids has been debated. In clinical practice, the lowest potency efficacious topical steroid is used for limited duration. Prednisolone appears to be the safest systemic steroid in pregnancy and lactation. As per some sources, first-trimester use of systemic steroids is pregnancy category D. The evidence for major congenital malformations, other than oral cleft, associated with first-trimester exposure to systemic corticosteroids in various studies, is weak. No consistent pattern of major congenital malformations was noted in the studies that reported an increased overall risk of major anomalies.[60]

↑, increased; AAP, American Academy of Pediatrics; assoc, associated; FDA, U.S. Food and Drug Administration; HPA, hypothalamus–pituitary axis; IUGR, intrauterine growth restriction; LBW, low birth weight; rec, recommends; Rx, treatment; spont, spontaneous.

TABLE 22.14	Immunomodulators, Systemic Nonsteroidal				
		Pregnancy		**Lactation**	
Dermatologic Medication	**Animal & Human Studies**	**FDA Category**	**Comments & Recommendations**	**Category**	**Comments & Recommendations**
Auranofin	*Animals*: Orofacial, limb, skeletal malformations, and hydrocephalus *Humans*: No teratogenicity in small studies, no long-term follow-up	C	AEs include cytopenias, eosinophilia, GI side effects, nephrotic syndrome, and mucocutaneous reactions	U	Enters breast milk; not rec by manufacturer
Chloroquine, hydroxy-chloroquine	*Animals*: Studies on chloroquine show teratogenicity at supratherapeutic doses and accumulation in fetal ocular melanin structures *Humans*: Pregnancy registry available; no teratogenicity in small studies; large clinical series in malaria and SLE are reassuring[65]	C	Risk of SLE flare greater than risk of AEs, continue medication during pregnancy	S, L3 (chloroquine) S, L2 (hydroxy-chloroquine)	Low levels in breast milk; AAP considers them compatible with breastfeeding
IVIG	*Animals*: No studies *Humans*: No studies, no reported AEs	C	Used in treatment of pregnancy-related autoimmune conditions, rubella postexposure prophylaxis		Unknown if it enters breast milk; manufacturer rec caution
Phenytoin	*Animals*: Reproduced fetal hydantoin syndrome (constellation of malformations) *Humans*: Fetal hydantoin syndrome, isolated reports of neuroblastoma, and coagulation defects	D	Monitor maternal serum levels if used; folic acid and vitamin K coadministration in last month of pregnancy	S, L2	Low levels in breast milk; not rec by manufacturer

Note: Thalidomide is presented in Table 22.4. IVIG has proven to be safe in several case series. There have been no reports of adverse outcomes; however, it is rated as category C due to a lack of animal and human studies. The high cost of IVIGs limits its use. Antimalarials, similarly, have a long history of reassuring clinical experience with the benefits outweighing the risks in pregnancy and lactation in indicated conditions.

AAP, American Academy of Pediatrics; AE, adverse effect; FDA, U.S. Food and Drug Administration; GI, gastrointestinal; IVIG, intravenous immunoglobulin; rec, recommended/recommends; SLE, systemic lupus erythematosus.

TABLE 22.15	Immunomodulators, Topical				

Dermatologic Medication	Animal & Human Studies	FDA Category	Comments & Recommendations	Category	Comments & Recommendations
		Pregnancy		**Lactation**	
Imiquimod	*Animals*: No teratogenicity, reduced pup weight, and delayed ossification at maternotoxic levels *Humans*: Unclear if it crosses placenta, no studies on systemic absorption[1]	C	Manufacturer rec use in pregnancy only if benefit outweighs fetal risk	U	Unknown if it enters breast milk, unlikely significant; manufacturer rec caution
Pimecrolimus	*Animals*: No toxicity, no teratogenicity, and no IUGR with supratherapeutic doses *Humans*: Inadequate data, unclear if it crosses placenta, and unlikely that maternal systemic concentration reaches clinically relevant level	C	Debated risk of lymphoma	U, L2/L4 (nipple)	Unknown if it enters breast milk; use contraindicated by manufacturer
Tacrolimus	*Animals*: No studies; systemic tacrolimus assoc with malformations and maternal toxicity *Humans*: Inadequate data; systemic tacrolimus assoc with neonatal hyperkalemia and renal dysfunction, placental levels may be higher than maternal serum[66]	C	Debated risk of lymphoma; systemic tacrolimus continued in transplanted women during pregnancy	NS, L3	Systemic tacrolimus achieves low levels in breast milk; topical tacrolimus presents low risk, is poorly absorbed, but avoid application to breast; reports that its use may be compatible with breastfeeding; contraindicated by manufacturer

Note: There are no well-controlled human studies for medications in this class, which are subsequently category C. Thus, topical immunomodulators are best avoided in pregnancy and other medication classes are considered unless the benefit to the mother of a specific agent in this class outweighs the potential fetal risk. With the exception of imiquimod, use in lactation is discouraged by the manufacturer. With all agents, application to the breast is to be avoided if breastfeeding.

assoc, associated; FDA, U.S. Food and Drug Administration; IUGR, intrauterine growth restriction; rec, recommends.

TABLE 22.16	Immunosuppressive Agents

Dermatologic Medication	Pregnancy			Lactation	
	Animal & Human Studies	FDA Category	Comments & Recommendations	Category	Comments & Recommendations
Azathioprine	*Animals*: Teratogenic, causes azoospermia, and IUGR *Humans*: No well-controlled studies; no teratogenicity, sporadic congenital anomalies[67]; report of congenital anomalies in child of father on long-term Rx[68]; IUGR reported, but unclear if it reflects drug or disease[67]; neonatal leukopenia or pancytopenia[69]	D	Medication seems safer than previously thought and should not be withheld if medically indicated[67,70]; unclear whether paternal periconception use carries risk; IUD failure reported; neonatal leukopenia/thrombocytopenia can be prevented with reduction of dose in the third trimester	U, L3	Enters breast milk; older literature cited concern for immunosuppression, more recent evidence shows that risk is low and drug can continue with breastfeeding; no long-term follow-up studies; not rec by manufacturer
Bleomycin	*Animals*: Teratogenicity and abortifacient effects *Humans*: No well-controlled studies	D	Should be used only if the benefit justifies potential fetal risk; not rec by manufacturer	U	Unknown if it enters breast milk; not rec by manufacturer
Colchicine	*Animals*: No AEs *Humans*: Limited data; use in FMF has not shown teratogenicity	C	Should be used only if the benefit outweighs fetal risk	S, L4	Enters breast milk, manufacturer rec caution; highest levels achieved 6–8 hours after dose, can avoid breastfeeding in this range; AAP rates if compatible
Cyclophosphamide	*Animals*: Embryotoxicity, teratogenicity *Humans*: No well-controlled studies; fetal malformations and neonatal secondary malignancies reported; male and female sterility may be irreversible[71]	D	Should be used only if the benefit outweighs fetal risk; not rec by manufacturer	NS, L5	Enters breast milk in high concentration, neonatal neutropenia reported; not rec by manufacturer

(continued)

TABLE 22.16	Immunosuppressive Agents *(continued)*					

Dermatologic Medication	Animal & Human Studies	Pregnancy			Lactation	
		FDA Category	Comments & Recommendations	Category	Comments & Recommendations
Cyclosporine	*Animals*: Nephrotoxicity, VSDs with supratherapeutic dose *Humans*: IUGR and prematurity but unclear whether these AEs reflect effects of medication or underlying disease; isolated reports of malformation with inconsistent pattern[72]	C	Medication is relatively safe if used judiciously and for the shortest duration possible; wide spectrum of drug interactions; rec by manufacturer only if benefit outweighs fetal risk	S (likely), L3	Low levels in breast milk; AAP rec breast-feeding can be considered; not rec by manufacturer
Hydroxyurea	*Animals*: IUGR and embryotoxic and teratogenic at subtherapeutic doses *Humans*: No well-controlled studies	D	Should be used only if the benefit outweighs fetal risk; not rec by manufacturer	NS (possibly), L2	Enters breast milk; not rec by manufacturer
Mycophenolate mofetil	*Animals*: Wide range of malformations *Humans*: ↑ first-trimester pregnancy loss, oral clefts, skeletal, external ear, and visceral anomalies	D	Negative pregnancy test prior to starting Rx, counseling, and effective contraception; registry established	L4	Not rec by manufacturer
Sulfasalazine	*Animals*: No teratogenicity *Humans*: Agranulocytosis, oligospermia, and male infertility[73]; potential for kernicterus	B	Rec for male patients considering conception to avoid sulfasalazine; folate supplementation required	S, L3	Enters breast milk; risk of kernicterus, folate supplementation required

Note: Methotrexate is presented in Table 22.4. Cyclosporine appears to be the safest immunosuppressant in both pregnancy and lactation. Azathioprine is possibly safer than previously thought and currently used extensively in pregnancy. Although sulfasalazine carries the same pregnancy and lactation ratings as cyclosporine, the indications for these two medications are likely to differ. Moreover, sulfasalazine's association with male infertility and antifolate properties render it less desirable.

↑, increased; AAP, American Academy of Pediatrics; AE, adverse effect; FDA, U.S. Food and Drug Administration; FMF, familial Mediterranean fever; IUD, intrauterine device; IUGR, intrauterine growth restriction; rec, recommended/recommends; Rx, treatment; VSD, ventricular septal defect.

TABLE 22.17	**Miscellaneous Medications, Systemic**

| Dermatologic Medication | Pregnancy | | | Lactation | |
	Animal & Human Studies	FDA Category	Comments & Recommendations	Category	Comments & Recommendations
Bisphosphonates (alendronate sodium/ pamidronate)	*Animals*: Bone density, skeletal and tooth abnormalities, prolonged labor, and fetal death due to hypocalcemia *Humans*: No well-controlled studies; case reports of reversible hypocalcemia in newborn following maternal exposure to pamidronate[74]	C	Manufacturer rec against use unless benefit outweighs maternal and fetal risks	U, L3 (alendronate) S, L2 (pamidronate)	Unknown if they enter breast milk; no published experience; manufacturer rec caution
Methoxsalen	*Animals*: No teratogenicity studies *Humans*: No well-controlled studies; in one limited study, no defects, and LBW infants	C	Wide range of AEs; unknown if it crosses placenta; several studies have shown no evidence of increased fetal risks with PUVA Rx in pregnancy[75]; manufacturer rec use only if clearly indicated	U	Unknown if it enters breast milk; no published experience; manufacturer rec caution
Penicillamine	*Animals*: Teratogenic at supratherapeutic doses *Humans*: No well-controlled studies; assoc with congenital cutis laxa and assoc defects, rare severe penicillamine embryopathy[76]; no teratogenicity with low-dose penicillamine[13]	D	Contraindicated in pregnancy except in Wilson disease and some cases of cystinuria[13]	U, L4	Unknown if it enters breast milk; not rec by manufacturer
Spironolactone	*Animals*: Antiandrogen and feminizes male rat fetuses *Humans*: No well-controlled studies, unknown if it crosses placenta; case report of high dose Rx yielded normal male infant[77]	D	Maternal AEs include hyperkalemia, agranulocytosis, and hepatotoxicity; manufacturer rec use only if benefit outweighs fetal risks	S, L2	Low levels in breast milk; not rec by manufacturer

Note: Bisphosphonates incorporate into bone matrix, with gradual release over years. Alendronate, for example, has a half-life of approximately 10 years, although it is not pharmacologically active. Clinical experience has overall been reassuring, although there is a theoretical risk of fetal harm, particularly skeletal, when a woman becomes pregnant after a course of bisphosphonate therapy. Systemic PUVA Rx takes the C pregnancy category of methoxsalen. Topical PUVA Rx may provide a safer option during pregnancy because systemic methoxsalen levels are undetectable with topical use for localized disease (i.e., affecting palms and soles [see Table 22.18]).

AE, adverse effect; assoc, associated; FDA, U.S. Food and Drug Administration; LBW, low birth weight; PUVA, psoralen plus ultraviolet light A (UVA); rec, recommends/recommended; Rx, treatment.

TABLE 22.18	**Miscellaneous Medications, Topical**				
	Pregnancy			Lactation	
Dermatologic Medication	**Animal & Human Studies**	**FDA Category**	**Comments & Recommendations**	**Category**	**Comments & Recommendations**
Anthralin	*Animals*: No studies *Humans*: No studies	C	Manufacturer rec use only if clearly needed	U	Unknown if it enters breast milk but unlikely that the neonate would ingest a clinically relevant amount; manufacturer rec caution
Coal tars	*Animals*: Carcinogenic and mutagenic *Humans*: Systemic absorption with shampoo reported and no teratogenicity[48,78]	C[a]	Unregulated products; rec avoidance in first trimester, restricted use in second and third trimesters		Neonatal absorption with skin-to-skin contact but not present in breast milk; avoid application to breast during breastfeeding
Mechlorethamine HCl (topical nitrogen mustard)	*Animals*: Teratogenic *Humans*: No controlled data	D	Unknown if it crosses placenta; although most reports have not shown fetal AEs, drug should not be used in first trimester		Unknown if it enters breast milk; systemic form is category U; breastfeeding should be discontinued while mother is receiving Rx
Methoxsalen (topical)	*Animals*: No teratogenicity studies *Humans*: No controlled data	C	Undetectable blood levels with topical PUVA Rx for localized disease (i.e., palms and soles)[75]; washing off the skin after topical PUVA Rx can minimize blood levels[75]		No data; however, it is unlikely that drug enters breast milk at clinically relevant levels after topical PUVA Rx for localized disease; manufacturer rec caution
Minoxidil	*Animals*: No teratogenicity or IUGR, systemic embryotoxicity at high oral doses, and fetal hypertrichosis *Humans*: No well-controlled studies	C	Fetal hypertrichosis reported with maternal topical use	S, L2	Excreted into breast milk after oral administration; topical minoxidil unlikely to achieve clinically relevant levels in breast milk[79]
Podofilox	*Animals*: No teratogenicity or IUGR *Humans*: No well-controlled data with podofilox; podophyllum resin assoc with placental infarction, fetal death, and stillbirth following extensive maternal Rx of vulvar wart[80]	C X (podophyllum resin)	Applications of 0.1–1.5 mL produce peak serum levels <17 ng/mL, therefore, it is unlikely the maternal systemic concentration will reach a clinically relevant level after Rx of small warts[13]	S (likely)	Unknown if podofilox enters breast milk but unlikely that neonatal levels would be clinically relevant

TABLE 22.18	Miscellaneous Medications, Topical *(continued)*

| Dermatologic Medication | Pregnancy | | | Lactation | |
	Animal & Human Studies	FDA Category	Comments & Recommendations	Category	Comments & Recommendations
Potassium iodide (SSKI)	*Animals*: No teratogenicity (limited data) *Humans*: No well-controlled data	D	Crosses placenta; potential risk of fetal hypothyroidism (second/third trimesters)	S, L4	Limited data; excreted in breast milk; AAD classifies it compatible with lactation
Sulfa/sodium sulfacetamide	*Animals*: No teratogenicity *Humans*: No teratogenicity	C	Systemic absorption after topical administration unknown; kernicterus not reported; manufacturer rec use only if clearly needed	U	Unknown if they enter breast milk; manufacturer rec caution
Vitamin D analogues (calcipotriene, calcitriol)	*Animals*: Incomplete ossification and other skeletal abnormalities at high oral doses *Humans*: No well-controlled studies; no AEs reported	C	Should be used only if benefit outweighs fetal risk	U, L3 (calcipotriene)	Unknown if they enter breast milk; manufacturer rec caution

Note: 5-Fluorouracil is presented in Table 22.4. In recent years, FDA categorization for topical formulations of medications has been incorporated. However, this process is incomplete and the same designation is given in some instances in both topical and systemic formulations without supporting data. Additionally, it is difficult to extrapolate the systemic absorption of a topical medication in the general population to the pregnant population given the increase in circulating blood volume, generalized vasodilation, and increased metabolism in the pregnant state, which may all contribute to an increase in systemic absorption. The risk of significant systemic absorption increases with application over large body surface areas, for extended periods of time, and with occlusion and to mucosal surfaces, and pregnant women should be counseled accordingly. For example, podophyllum resin has been implicated in fetal demise with extensive vulvar application for the treatment of warts.[80] For most topical medications, application to the breast during breastfeeding should be avoided given the risk of direct fetal ingestion, although the risk of systemic uptake by this route is likely low. Furthermore, ointments confer the additional risk of paraffin toxicity to nursing infants when applied to the breast.

[a] Categorization applies only to coal tar bath products; other coal tar products are not categorized.[75]

AAD, American Academy of Pediatrics; AE, adverse effect; assoc, associated; FDA, U.S. Food and Drug Administration; IUGR, intrauterine growth restriction; PUVA, psoralen plus ultraviolet light A (UVA); rec, recommends; Rx, treatment; SSKI, saturated solution of potassium iodide.

TABLE 22.19	Safest Medications in Pregnancy and Lactation	
Medication Category	**Safest in Pregnancy**	**Safest in Lactation**
Analgesics	Acetaminophen	Acetaminophen
Antibiotics	Penicillins, cephalosporins, azithromycin, erythromycin base or ethylsuccinate	Penicillins, cephalosporins, azithromycin
Antifungal agents, systemic	Amphotericin B, nystatin	Amphotericin B (likely), ketoconazole, nystatin
Antifungal agents, topical	Clotrimazole, nystatin	Clotrimazole, nystatin
Antihistamines	Loratadine > diphenhydramine	Loratadine > diphenhydramine
Antiparasitic agents	Permethrin > precipitated sulfur	Permethrin > precipitated sulfur
Antiviral agents	Acyclovir > valacyclovir	Acyclovir > valacyclovir
Biologic agents	Infliximab, etanercept	Infliximab, etanercept
Corticosteroids, systemic	Prednisolone > prednisone	Prednisolone > prednisone
Corticosteroids, topical	Low-potency steroids	Low-potency steroids
Immunomodulators, systemic nonsteroidal	IVIG > hydroxychloroquine	Hydroxychloroquine
Immunomodulators, topical	None	Tacrolimus
Immunosuppressive agents	Cyclosporine > azathioprine	Colchicine, azathioprine, cyclosporine

Note: With few exceptions, the medications found to be the safest in pregnancy are also the safest in lactation. In some instances, such as with azathioprine, lactation is not recommended by the manufacturer, yet in clinical practice, the medication is considered safe to use, with safety endorsement by guideline setting entities such as the American Academy of Pediatrics. In such cases, these guidelines bear greater weight than the manufacturer's recommendations. Safety data for several of the topical medications in lactation are incomplete and are often extrapolated from the systemic forms, but need to take into consideration not only concentration of the agent in breast milk, but ingestion exposure from suckling. Providers are advised to reference the continually updated resources described in this text, because revisions of pregnancy and lactation ratings occur with the generation of contemporary data.

>, safer than; IVIG, intravenous immunoglobulin.

KEY POINTS

- Physicians should be aware of drugs that can have deleterious effects to the fetus as well as medication interactions that can affect male and female fertility and/or that may precipitate contraceptive failure.
- Knowledge of those medications for which safety in pregnancy and/or lactation has been well documented (summarized in Table 22.19) is crucial.
- If a patient is pregnant and needs a medication that places her or her fetus at risk, the physician should use the available databases in order to delineate this risk and go through a risk/benefit discussion.
- Inadequate data or controversy among sources over drug safety in pregnancy and lactation may make the physician's decision on treatment challenging; informed patient consent requires that the physician review conflicting data with the patient.
- When inadvertent pregnancy occurs in women receiving medications for dermatologic conditions, the opportunity to enroll in existing drug registries should be offered in addition to supportive counseling and facilitating access to resources.
- In using topical medications with unknown risk profiles, the extent of the body surface area application should be considered and direct application to the nipple in the breastfeeding mother should be avoided.
- Adverse maternal effects may indicate higher than normal serum drug concentrations with an increased toxic risk to the infant, even in cases involving medications classified as safe in lactation.

REFERENCES

1. Leachman SM, Reed B. The use of dermatologic drugs in pregnancy and lactation. *Dermatol Clin.* 2006;24:167–197.
2. Reimers D, Jezek A. Simultaneous use of rifampin and other antituberculous agents with oral contraceptives. *Prax Clin Pneumol.* 1971;25:255–262.
3. Van Dijke CPH, Weber JCP. Interaction between oral contraceptives and griseofulvin. *Br Med J (Clin Res Ed).* 1984;288:1125–1126.

4. Papiernik E, Rozenbaum H, Amblard P, et al. Intra-uterine device failure: relation with drug use. *Eur J Obstet Gynecol Reprod Biol*. 1989;32:205–212.

5. Koh K, Jurkovic S, Yang K, et al. Estradiol induces cytochrome P450 2B6 expression at high concentrations: implications in estrogen-mediated gene regulation in pregnancy. *Biochem Pharmacol*. 2012;84:93–103.

6. Higashi E, Fukami T, Itoh M, et al. Human CYP2A6 induced by estrogen via estrogen receptor. *Drug Metab Dispos*. 2007;35:1935–1941.

7. Ekins S, Kharasch E. Molecular characterization of CYP2B6 substrates. *Curr Drug Metab*. 2008;9:363–373.

8. Stockton D, Paller A. Drug administration to the pregnant or lactating woman: a reference guide for dermatologists. *J Am Acad Dermatol*. 1990;23:87–103.

9. Richmond S, Atkins J. A population-based study of the prenatal diagnosis of congenital malformation over 16 years. *BJOG*. 2005;112:1349–1357.

10. Han JY, Nava-Ocampo AA, Koren G. Unintended pregnancies and exposure to potential human teratogens. *Birth Defects Res A Clin Mol Teratol*. 2005;73:245–248.

11. Schaefer C, Peters P, Miller RK, eds. *Drugs during Pregnancy and Lactation: Treatment Options and Risk Assessment*. 2nd ed. London, England: Elsevier Academic Press; 2007.

12. Hale TW, ed. *Medications and Mother's Milk*. 11th ed. Amarillo, TX: Pharmasoft Publishing; 2004.

13. Weiner CP, Buhimschi CS, eds. *Drugs for Pregnant and Lactating Women*. 2nd ed. Philadelphia, PA: Saunders Elsevier; 2009.

14. Cordier S. Evidence for a role of paternal exposures in developmental toxicity. *Basic Clin Pharmacol Toxicol*. 2008;102:176–181.

15. Teo SK, Harden JL, Burke AB, et al. Thalidomide is distributed into human semen after oral dosing. *Drug Metab Dispos*. 2001;29:1355–1357.

16. Nguyen C, Duhl A, Escallon CS, et al. Multiple anomalies in a fetus exposed to low-dose methotrexate in the first trimester. *Obstet Gynecol*. 2002;99:599–602.

17. Hallene K, Oby E, Lee BJ, et al. Prenatal exposure to thalidomide, altered vasculogenesis, and CNS malformations. *Neuroscience*. 2006;142:267–283.

18. McElhatton P, Sullivan F, Volans G. Paracetamol overdose in pregnancy analysis of the outcomes of 300 cases referred to the Teratology Information Service. *Reprod Toxicol*. 1997;11:85–94.

19. Bakkenheim E, Mowinkel P, Carlsen C. Paracetamol in early infancy: the risk of childhood allergy and asthma. *Acta Paediatr*. 2011;100:90–96.

20. Handal M, Engeland A, Furu K. Use of prescribed opioid analgesics and co-medication with benzodiazepines in women before, during, and after pregnancy: a population based cohort study. *Eur J Clin Pharmacol*. 2011;67:953–960.

21. Prakash P, Rai R, Pai M, et al. Teratogenic effects of the anticonvulsant gabapentin in mice. *Singapore Med J*. 2008;49:47–53.

22. Mylonas I. Antibiotic chemotherapy during pregnancy and lactation period: aspects for consideration. *Arch Gynecol Obstet*. 2011;283:7–18.

23. Bar-Oz B, Weber-Schoendorfer C, Berlin M, et al. The outcomes in pregnancy of women exposed to the new macrolides in the first trimester: a prospective, multicenter, observational study. *Drug Saf*. 2012;35:689–698.

24. Thornton YS, Bowe ET. Neonatal hyperbilirubinemia after treatment of maternal leprosy. *S Med J*. 1989;82:668.

25. Cooper W, Ray W, Griffin M. Prenatal prescription of macrolide antibiotics and infantile hypertrophic pyloric stenosis. *Obstet Gynecol*. 2002;100:101.

26. Andrew A, Easterling T, Carr DB, et al. Amoxicillin pharmacokinetics in pregnant women: modeling and simulations of dosage strategies. *Clin Pharmacol Ther*. 2007;81:547–556.

27. Holdiness M. Teratology of the antituberculosis drugs. *Early Hum Dev*. 1987;15:61–74.

28. Wen S, Zhou J, Walker M. Maternal exposure to folic acid antagonists and placenta-medicated adverse pregnancy outcomes. *CMAJ*. 2008;179:1263–1268.

29. Sobel JD. Use of antifungal drugs in pregnancy: a focus on safety. *Drug Saf*. 2000;23:77–85.

30. Van Cauteren H, Lampo A, Vandenberghe J, et al. Safety aspects of oral antifungal agents. *Br J Clin Pract Suppl*. 1990;71:47–49.

31. Rosa FW, Baum C, Shaw M. Pregnancy outcomes after first-trimester vaginitis drug therapy. *Obstet Gynecol*. 1987;69:751–755.

32. Econazole nitrate cream [E. Fougera & Co. A division of Fougera Pharmaceuticals Inc.]. DailyMed Web site. http://dailymed.nlm.nih.gov/dailymed/lookup.cfm?setid=b0bb5206-3698-4a6b-9100-40bb86f1a0ca. Revised June 2012. Accessed September 3, 2012.

33. Czeizel AE, Kazy Z, Puhó E. Population-based case-control teratologic study of topical miconazole. *Congenit Anom (Kyoto)*. 2004;44:41–45.

34. Weber-Schoendorfer C, Schaefer C. The safety of cetirizine during pregnancy. A prospective observational cohort study. *Reprod Toxicol*. 2008;26:19–23.

35. Briggs GC, Freeman RK, Yaffe SY, eds. *Drugs in Pregnancy and Lactation*. 9th ed. Philadelphia, PA: Wolters Kluwer; 2011.

36. Weinstein D, Ornoy A, Ben-Zur Z, et al. Teratogenicity of cyproheptadine in pregnant rats. *Arch Int Pharmacodyn Ther*. 1975;215:345–349.

37. Miller A. Diphenhydramine toxicity in a newborn: a case report. *J Perinatol*. 2000;20:390–391.

38. Serreau R. Neonatal seizures associated with maternal hydroxyzine hydrochloride in late pregnancy. *Reprod Toxicol*. 2005;20:573–574.

39. Schwarz EB, Moretti ME, Nayak S, et al. Risk of hypospadias in offspring of women using loratadine during pregnancy: a systematic review and meta-analysis. *Drug Saf*. 2008;31:775–788.

40. Pacqué M, Munoz B, Poetschke G, et al. Pregnancy outcome after inadvertent ivermectin treatment during community-based distribution. *Lancet*. 1990;336:1486–1489.

41. Friedman SJ. Lindane neurotoxic reaction in nonbullous congenital ichthyosiform erythroderma. *Arch Dermatol*. 1987;123:1056–1058.

42. Eskenazi B, Harley K, Holland N. Association of in utero organophosphate pesticide exposure and fetal growth and length of gestation in an agricultural population. *Environ Health Perspect*. 2004;112:1116–1124.

43. Meinking TL, Taplin D. Safety of permethrin vs. lindane for the treatment of scabies. *Arch Dermatol*. 1996;132:959–962.

44. Rasmussen JE. The problem of lindane. *J Am Acad Dermatol*. 1981;5:507–516.

45. Stone KM, Reiff-Eldridge R, White AD, et al. Pregnancy outcomes following systemic prenatal acyclovir exposure: conclusions from the International Acyclovir Pregnancy Registry, 1984–99. *Birth Defects Res*. 2004;70:201–207.

46. Pasternak B, Hviid A. Use of acyclovir, valacyclovir and famciclovir in the first trimester of pregnancy and the risk of birth defects. *JAMA*. 2010;304:859–866.

47. Drake A, Roxby A, Kiarie J, et al. Infant safety during and after maternal valacyclovir therapy in conjunction with antiretroviral HIV-1 prophylaxis in a randomized clinical trial. *PLoS One*. 2012;7:e34635.

48. Bae YS, Voorhees AS, Hsu S, et al. Review of treatment options for psoriasis in pregnant or lactating women: from the Medical

Board of the National Psoriasis Foundation. *J Am Acad Dermatol.* 2012;67:459–477.

49. Berthelot J, De Bandt M, Goupille P, et al. Exposition to anti-TNF drugs during pregnancy: outcome of 15 cases and review of literature. *Joint Bone Spine.* 2009;76:28–34.

50. Carter JD, Valeriano J, Vasey B. Tumor necrosis factor alpha inhibition and VATER association: a causal relationship? *J Rheumatol.* 2006;33:1014–1017.

51. Singh JA, Wells GA, Christensen R, et al. Adverse effects of biologics: a network meta-analysis and Cochrane overview. *Cochrane Database Syst Rev.* 2011;(2):CD008794.

52. Katz JA, Antoni C, Keenan GF, et al. Outcome of pregnancy in women receiving infliximab for the treatment of Crohn's disease and rheumatoid arthritis. *Am J Gastroenterol.* 2004;99:2385–2392.

53. Pham T, Fautrel B, Gottenberg JE, et al. Rituximab (MabThera) therapy and safety management. Clinical tool guide. *Joint Bone Spine.* 2008;75:S1–S99.

54. Stelara (ustekinumab) injection, solution [Janssen Biotec, Inc.]. DailyMed Web site. http://dailymed.nlm.nih.gov/dailymed/lookup.cfm?setid=c77a9664-e3bb-4023-b400-127aa53bca2b. Revised June 2012. Accessed September 3, 2012.

55. Edwards M, Agho K, Attia J, et al. Case-control study of cleft lip or palate after maternal use of topical corticosteroids during pregnancy. *Am J Med Genet A.* 2003;120A:459–463.

56. Pradat P, Robert-Gnansia E, Di Tanna GL, et al. First trimester exposure to corticosteroids and oral clefts. *Birth Defects Research A Clin Mol Teratol.* 2003;67:968–970.

57. Hviid A, Mølgaard-Nielsen D. Corticosteroid use during pregnancy and risk of orofacial clefts. *CMAJ.* 2011;183:796–804.

58. Mahe A, Perret J, Dumont A, et al. The cosmetic use of skin-lightening products during pregnancy in Dakar, Senegal: a common and potentially hazardous practice. *Trans R Soc Trop Med Hyg.* 2007;101:183–187.

59. Mygind H, Thulstrup AM, Pedersen L, et al. Risk of intrauterine growth retardation, malformations and other birth outcomes in children after topical use of corticosteroid in pregnancy. *Acta Obstet Gynecol Scand.* 2002;81:234–239.

60. Rodríguez-Pinilla E, Martínez-Frías ML. Corticosteroids during pregnancy and oral clefts: a case-control study. *Teratology.* 1998;58:2–5.

61. Park-Wyllie L, Mazzotta P, Pastuszak A, et al. Birth defects after maternal exposure to corticosteroids: prospective cohort study and meta-analysis of epidemiological studies. *Teratology.* 2000;62:385–392.

62. Gur C, Diav-Citrin O, Ornoy A. Pregnancy outcome after first trimester exposure to corticosteroids: a prospective controlled study. *Reprod Toxicol.* 2004;18:93–101.

63. Kraus AM. Congenital cataract and maternal steroid ingestion. *J Pediatr Ophthalmol.* 1975;12:107–108.

64. Katz FH, Thorp JM Jr, Bowes WA Jr. Severe symmetric intrauterine growth retardation associated with the topical use of triamcinolone. *Am J Obstet Gynecol.* 1990;162:396–397.

65. Hydroxychloroquine sulphate tablet, film coated [Mylan Pharmaceuticals Inc.]. DailyMed Web site. http://dailymed.nlm.nih.gov/dailymed/lookup.cfm?setid=b5869e45-27fc-4f33-80db-4a509b8256c1. Revised August 2012. Accessed September 3, 2012.

66. Expert Group on Renal Transplantation. European Best practice guidelines for renal transplantation. Section IV; Long-term management of the transplant recipient. IV.10. Pregnancy in renal transplant patients. *Nephrol Dial Transplant.* 2002;17(suppl 4):50–55.

67. Ostensen M, Khamashta M, Lockshin M, et al. Anti-inflammatory and immunosuppressive drugs and reproduction. *Arthritis Res Ther.* 2006;8:209.

68. Tallent M, Simmons R, Najarian J. Birth defects in child of male recipient of kidney transplant. *JAMA.* 1970;211:1854–1855.

69. Davison JM, Dellagrammatikas H, Parkin JM. Maternal azathioprine therapy and depressed haemopoiesis in the babies of renal allograft patients. *Br J Obstet Gynaecol.* 1985;92:233–239.

70. Viktil KK, Engeland A, Furu K. Outcomes after anti-rheumatic drug use before and during pregnancy: a cohort study among 150,000 pregnant women and expectant fathers. *Scand J Rheumatol.* 2012;41:196–201.

71. Amato D. Neutropenia from cyclophosphamide in breast milk. *Med J Aust.* 1977;1:383–384.

72. Lamarque V, Leleu M, Krupp P, et al. Analysis of 629 pregnancy outcomes in renal transplant recipients with Sandimmune. *Transplant Proc.* 1997;29:2480.

73. Levi A, Fisher A, Hendry W. Male infertility due to sulphasalazine. *Lancet.* 1979;2:276–278.

74. Stathopoulos IP, Liakou CG, Katsarila A, et al. The use of bisphosphonates in women prior to or during pregnancy and lactation. *Hormones (Athens).* 2011;10:280–291.

75. Tauscher AE, Fleischer AB Jr, Phelps KC, et al. Psoriasis and pregnancy. *J Cutan Med Surg.* 2002;6:561–570.

76. Pinter R, Hogge WA, McPherson E. Infant with severe penicillamine embryopathy born to a woman with Wilson disease. *Am J Med Genet A.* 2004;128A:294–298.

77. de Arriba G, Sanchez-Heras M, Basterrechea MA. Gitelman syndrome during pregnancy: a therapeutic challenge. *Arch Gynecol Obstet.* 2009;280:807–809.

78. Franssen ME, van der Wilt GJ, de Jong PC, et al. A retrospective study of the teratogenicity of dermatological coal tar products. *Acta Derm Venereol.* 1999;79:390–391.

79. Valdivieso A, Valdes G, Spiro TE, et al. Minoxidil in breast milk. *Ann Intern Med.* 1985;102:135.

80. Chamberlain MJ, Reynolds AL, Yeoman WB. Medical memoranda. Toxic effect of podophyllum application in pregnancy. *Br Med J.* 1972;3:391–392.

CHAPTER 23

Skin Care Products, Cosmetics, and Cosmeceuticals

George Kroumpouzos ■ Zoe Draelos

INTRODUCTION

This chapter reviews the use of skin care products, cosmetics, and cosmeceuticals in pregnancy, with an emphasis on safety data. The systemic absorption of these products is discussed as well as limitations of animal studies and biases in pregnancy warnings. The U.S. Food and Drug Administration (FDA) pregnancy categories are discussed in Chapter 22 (see Table 22.2).

QUALITY OF DATA

Safety data regarding the use of skin care products in human pregnancy are scarce, in part because of ethical constraints in performing randomized controlled studies in gestation. Also, safety data on cosmetics and cosmeceuticals are limited because these products are not regulated. Some data exist for topical retinoids, products used in the treatment of acne, and skin-lightening agents. There are insufficient data for most common "offenders" in media, such as phthalates, parabens, fragrance, formaldehyde, sodium lauryl sulphate, toluene, mineral oil, synthetic colors, dihydroxyacetone, and chemicals used in hair care.

BIASES IN PREGNANCY WARNINGS

Since data are scarce, biases often arise in the literature and media regarding the safety of skin care and cosmetic products in pregnancy. Biases may include, among others, sample size, recall, retrospective ascertainment, and citation bias (systematic ignoring of papers that contain content conflicting with a claim) as well as bias against the null hypothesis (media publicize more "positive" than "negative" studies).[1] Translating animal studies to human topical application is also a source of bias. Many authorities and cosmetic companies have adopted a zero tolerance policy mandating that a cosmetic ingredient should not be used in pregnancy if there is evidence of risk from animal studies. However, exclusion of an ingredient by teratology screening does not mean that it has been proven harmful to humans through normal topical use.

ANIMAL STUDIES

There is a lack of experimental animal studies designed to simulate topical application of skin care products in humans. Conclusions regarding teratogenicity and genotoxicity generated from studies with bottle-fed animals, especially at maternally toxic dose levels, are not applicable to humans. Furthermore, the subcutaneous injection of a cosmetic in animal studies may not accurately reflect in vivo epidermal absorption in humans. Only a few animal studies involving the topical application of a cosmetic ingredient (e.g., mineral oils, dibutyl adipate, hair dyes, formaldehyde) have been performed, and in them there has been no evidence of significant systemic absorption.

TOPICAL RETINOIDS

Tretinoin (all-*trans* retinoic acid; pregnancy category C) is a naturally occurring form of vitamin A that represents an oxidized form of all-*trans* retinol. The natural conversion of all-*trans* retinol to tretinoin in the skin is tightly regulated and thus only a small portion of all-*trans* retinol is metabolized to tretinoin by human keratinocytes. Tretinoin is also synthesized from endogenous all-*trans* retinol that is delivered via the bloodstream to basal keratinocytes. The percutaneous absorption of a single dose is <1% with tretinoin 0.1% in microsphere gel and 2% with emollient 0.05% cream; the absorption does not alter the systemic endogenous retinoid levels.[2] The topical application of vitamin A preparation in females also does not affect plasma concentrations of retinol, retinyl esters, or retinoic acids.[3] Tretinoin can cross the human placenta, but there are no well-controlled studies. Topical tretinoin has demonstrated a lack of teratogenic potential in animal models.[4]

There have been four case reports of malformations (ear, limb reduction, central nervous system abnormalities) associated with first-trimester tretinoin use.[5–8] In three of the four, the ear involvement was suggestive of *retinoid acid embryopathy*, although the role of tretinoin in these cases remains unclear. Furthermore, a retrospective[9] and two small prospective studies[10,11] showed no difference in minor malformations, including those associated with *retinoid embryopathy*, between patients exposed in the first trimester and in controls. Nevertheless, extensive publicity of case reports of malformations may have caused a bias against the null hypothesis. Controlled studies with a larger sample size are needed, but for the time being, the topical application of tretinoin should be avoided during the first trimester.[12] Because the previous studies of tretinoin did not reveal risks and because only a small proportion of *all*-trans *retinol* is metabolized to tretinoin in the human skin, nonregulated products containing retinol may be considered safe. In an animal study, *retinyl palmitate*, a common ingredient in cosmetic products, showed no genotoxic effects.[13] Retinyl palmitate is readily hydrolyzed to retinol in the skin, and its in vitro percutaneous absorption is 18% within 30 hours. However, it is unlikely that percutaneous absorption changes systemic endogenous retinoid levels.

Adapalene (pregnancy category C) is a synthetic retinoid that is used in the treatment of acne vulgaris. It has not been clarified whether adapalene crosses the placenta. Animal studies have not revealed teratogenic effects with oral doses representing up to six times the maximum recommended human dose, and there is a lack of well-controlled studies in pregnant women. The percutaneous absorption of adapalene is negligible (0.01%), and its penetration into the deep epidermis and dermis is very limited. A case report associated cutaneous exposure to adapalene in early pregnancy with fetal anophthalmia and agenesis of optic chiasma.[14] For the time being, the use of adapalene in pregnancy is not recommended.

Tazarotene (pregnancy category X) is a synthetic retinoid that is used in the treatment of acne and psoriasis but has also shown some efficacy in the treatment of photoaging. Following topical application, tazarotene is rapidly converted to its active metabolite, tazarotenic acid, in human keratinocytes. Systemic absorption of the active metabolite and parent drug is low (≤6%) following cutaneous application of 0.05% and 0.1% gel, and there is no significant systemic accumulation following multiple topical applications.[15] The drug and its metabolites are rapidly eliminated from the plasma via the urine and feces. The use of tazarotene in pregnancy is prohibited by the FDA based on associations with teratogenicity and postimplantation fetal loss in studies in rats and rabbits at oral doses producing 0.7 and 13 times, respectively, the systemic exposure in psoriasis patients when extrapolated for topical treatment of 20% of body surface area.[16] However, no teratogenicity has been observed in animal studies from topical tazarotene. Also, tazarotene-related fetal abnormalities have not been reported in humans, and there may be less systemic exposure in the treatment of facial acne. Furthermore, plasma levels of tazarotene and tazarotenic acid after topical application are comparable to those reported after tretinoin and adapalene treatment and similar to those of endogenous retinoids.[16] Well-controlled human studies are required before drawing conclusions about its safety in pregnancy.

Safety data on regulated topical retinoids are summarized in Table 23.1.

NONRETINOID TOPICAL MEDICATIONS

Topical Antibacterials

Clindamycin and **erythromycin** (pregnancy category B) have been used as topical treatments for acne, and their use in pregnancy has been determined to be safe. Erythromycin shows minimal percutaneous absorption, and in studies of topical 2% erythromycin, there were no detectable serum levels.[17] The percutaneous absorption of topical clindamycin is ≤5%.[18] Urine levels have been detected following the topical application of clindamycin hydrochloride, but not clindamycin phosphate,[19] and the latter should be preferred in order to minimize systemic exposure. An association with pseudomembranous colitis has been exceptionally reported in nonpregnant women. However, in several studies, an effect of clindamycin on intestinal microflora has not been demonstrated.[20]

Benzoyl Peroxide and Salicylic Acid

There have been no reported adverse effects in human pregnancy associated with benzoyl peroxide or salicylic acid use (pregnancy category C). Although the percutaneous absorption of benzoyl peroxide is concentration dependent, only 3% of a benzoyl peroxide 10% preparation shows percutaneous penetration.[21] After conversion to benzoic acid in the skin, it enters systemic absorption and is rapidly excreted as benzoate in the urine. Cautious use of benzoyl peroxide can be considered safe in pregnancy. Absorption of salicylic acid 5% to 10% can be as high as 25%[22] and varies with vehicle and duration of contact as well as mode of application. When applied under occlusion, the time of peak concentration is 5 hours. The maximum strength of salicylic acid in nonregulated acne products in the United States is 2%, and minimal absorption should be expected with application on small areas, such as the face. Salicylate toxicity, associated with serum levels of 200 to 400 μg per milliliter, is unlikely with topical application but possible if the drug is applied over a large surface area for prolonged periods of time.[15]

Topical Dapsone

Dapsone 5% gel (pregnancy category C) has been approved for the treatment of acne vulgaris. Use of the medication near term is not recommended because a risk of hyperbilirubinemia and kernicterus, especially in premature babies, has been reported with systemic administration (see Ch. 22, Table 22.6). Although small quantities of topical application to the mother are likely harmless to the fetus, the medication should be used in pregnancy only if the potential benefit justifies the potential fetal risk.

Skin-Lightening Agents

Hydroquinone (pregnancy category C) shows dermal absorption in human skin in both aqueous and alcoholic formulations and is excreted mainly as glucuronide or sulfate conjugates. The in vivo bioavailability for a 24-hour

TABLE 23.1	**Topical Retinoids**					
	Pregnancy			**Lactation**		
Dermatologic Medication	**Animal & Human Studies**	**FDA Category[a]**	**Comments & Recommendations**	**Category[a]**	**Comments & Recommendations**	
Tretinoin	*Animals*: No teratogenicity; dose-related IUGR in some studies *Humans*: Three studies showed no difference in malformations between patients exposed in first trimester and controls[9–11]	C	Low percutaneous absorption does not change endogenous levels[2]; four cases of malformations with first-trimester use[5–8]; application should be avoided in first trimester	U, L3	Minimal amounts in breast milk are not thought to be harmful to infants; animal studies show no AEs during lactation[15]	
Adapalene	*Animals*: No teratogenicity with oral doses up to 6× MRHD *Humans*: Lack of well-controlled studies	C	Negligible percutaneous absorption[15]; case report of fetal anophthalmia and agenesis of optic chiasma[14]; use in pregnancy not rec	U, L3	Unknown whether it enters human breast milk, but levels would be extremely low to represent any risk to the infant	
Tazarotene	*Animals*: Teratogenicity and postimplantation fetal loss with oral administration *Humans*: No AEs reported[16]; lack of well-controlled studies	X	Low percutaneous absorption[15]; use in pregnancy is prohibited	U, L3	Excreted in rodent milk but unknown whether it enters human milk; however, unlikely that neonate could ingest any clinically relevant amounts	

[a] U.S. FDA pregnancy and lactation categories are outlined in Chapter 22, Tables 22.2 and 22.3.

AEs, adverse effects; IUGR, intrauterine growth restriction; MRHD, maximum recommended human dose; rec, recommended.

application of a 2% cream is 45%.[23] Animal studies involving parenteral administration at maternally toxic doses showed fetal growth restriction, but no animal studies with topical application have been conducted. A study on hydroquinone use in human pregnancy showed no increase in adverse effects[24]; however, the small sample size decreases its reliability. Leave-on bleaching creams containing hydroquinone should not be used in pregnancy, and melasma should be treated postpartum. It remains to be clarified whether hydroquinone included in hair dyes and nail additives at low concentrations (<1%) poses any fetal risks at all. **Kojic acid** is not toxic in reproductive and genotoxicity studies, and its slow absorption into human skin makes fetal risks unlikely, at least at the low concentrations (1% to 4%) in leave-on cosmetics.[25] **Azelaic acid** (pregnancy category B), a topical medication primarily used in acne vulgaris and rosacea, has a mild skin-lightening effect and is safe during pregnancy. Percutaneous absorption is

approximately 4% for the cream and up to 8% for gel formulation.[15] Safety data for the previous nonretinoid topical medications are summarized in Table 23.2.

Topical Corticosteroids

Noncosmetic use of steroids (pregnancy category C) on large body surface areas may be associated with risks similar to those of systemic steroids (i.e., intrauterine growth restriction).[26] A small cohort study showed an association between potent topical steroid use and small babies,[24] a finding that was not confirmed (see Ch. 22, Table 22.13).[27] A small case-control study[28] showed an increased odds ratio for cleft lip/palate with first-trimester noncosmetic use, which was not confirmed by several other studies.[29] It is implausible that steroids found in cosmetics can be associated with fetal risks, especially because they are applied to small surface areas.

| TABLE 23.2 | **Nonretinoid Topical Medications** | | | | |

		Pregnancy		Lactation	
Dermatologic Medication	**Animal & Human Studies**	**FDA Category**[a]	**Comments & Recommendations**	**Category**[a]	**Comments & Recommendations**
Erythromycin	*Animals*: No teratogenicity or IUGR *Humans*: No well-controlled studies; no AEs reported	B	Safe in pregnancy		Oral form enters human breast milk, and is S, L1 Category (L3 for early postnatal); no AEs reported in infants with topical
Clindamycin	*Animals*: No teratogenicity or IUGR *Humans*: No well-controlled studies; no AEs reported	B	Urine levels detected with clindamycin hydrochloride but not phosphate,[19] and the latter should be preferred		Systemic form enters human breast milk, and is S (likely), L3 Category; no AEs reported in infants with topical; manufacturer rec discontinuation
Benzoyl peroxide	*Animals*: No studies *Humans*: No studies; no AEs reported	C	Low percutaneous absorption[21]; cautious use can be considered safe; to be used only if clearly needed		Unknown whether it enters human breast milk; no AEs reported in infants
Salicylic acid	*Animals*: No reproduction studies with topical *Humans*: No well-controlled studies; no AEs reported	C	Salicylate toxicity unlikely[15]; not to be applied over large area[22]; to be used only if clearly needed		Unknown whether it enters human breast milk; no AEs reported in infants
Dapsone	*Animals*: Embryocidal with oral doses resulting in a systemic exposure 500 or 800× that observed with topical MRHD *Humans*: No well-controlled studies; no AEs reported	C	Risk of hyperbilirubinemia and kernicterus, especially in premature infants, reported with systemic administration; to be used only if clearly needed		Oral form enters human breast milk, and is S (likely), L4 Category; no AEs reported in infants with topical
Hydroquinone	*Animals*: No reproduction studies with topical formulation *Humans*: No studies; no AEs reported[24]	C	Substantial dermal absorption[23]; use in pregnancy not rec	S (likely)	Unknown whether it enters human breast milk; no AEs reported in infants
Azelaic acid	*Animals*: No teratogenicity or IUGR *Humans*: No well-controlled studies; no AEs reported	B	Endogenous levels not altered by amount absorbed[15]	L3	No AEs reported; unlikely to enter human breast milk or produce AEs in the infant

[a] U.S. FDA pregnancy and lactation categories are outlined in Chapter 22, Tables 22.2 and 22.3.

AEs, adverse effects; IUGR, intrauterine growth restriction; MRHD, maximum recommended human dose; rec, recommends/recommended.

NONREGULATED SKIN CARE PRODUCTS

α-Hydroxy Acid Products

Glycolic acid is present in products used to treat acne, photodamage, hyperpigmentation, and other cosmetic problems. Risks have been reported in animal studies with doses much higher than those used in cosmetic products. No studies have been performed in human pregnancy; however, its systemic absorption is minimal.[30] Therefore, topical glycolic acid use in pregnancy can be considered safe. Other α-hydroxy acids, such as *lactic acid*, *malic acid*, and *citric acid*, have negligible systemic absorption and are also deemed safe at their current concentrations.

Sunscreens

Studies in humans show minimal dermal absorption of sunscreen ingredients. Also, recent data show that insoluble nanoparticles used in titanium dioxide- or zinc oxide-containing sunscreens do not show dermal absorption, and, therefore, pose no fetal risks.[31] Finally, the use of sunscreen for the prevention or treatment of gestational melasma has not been associated with fetal adverse effects. Reported risks with oxybenzone, titanium oxide, zinc oxide, and octyl methoxycinnamate in animal studies may not be extrapolated to humans. Oxybenzone has been linked to reduced numbers of live births in animal studies[32] and may have harmful estrogenic effects[33]; although this data may not translate to human topical application.

Self-Tanning Agents

Self-tanning products contain dihydroxyacetone 1% to 15% (a color additive). Dihydroxyacetone binds to amino acids in the stratum corneum, but systemic levels with topical application are extremely low (0.5%).[34] Therefore, occasional use in pregnancy can be considered safe.

Hair Care Products

In a controlled study, maternal hair dye use during pregnancy was associated with a mildly increased risk of neuroblastoma. The study, however, was not adjusted for confounders.[35] Animal studies did not reveal any risk of teratogenicity with aminophenols, phenylenediamine, and ethanolamine when used in high oral or subcutaneous doses. There were no risks from percutaneous absorption of hair dyes.[36] There is currently no evidence of fetal risks to exposed hairdressers, such as demise, preterm delivery, small-for-gestational age infants, and malformations. It can be concluded that the risks about hair product use have been exaggerated. There is negligible systemic absorption from occasional use unless there are burns or abscesses on the scalp. Still, studies in humans are needed. It is believed that there are no fetal adverse effects from receiving hair treatments three to four times during pregnancy.[37]

Depilatory and Bleaching Agents

Thioglycolic acid <5% is often used in depilatory products.[38] There has been no evidence of mutagenicity or carcinogenicity with high oral doses in rat studies. Sodium, calcium, and potassium hydroxide in depilatory creams disassociate into the respective ions, and therefore are safe in pregnancy. Hydrogen peroxide is found in low concentrations in hair-bleaching creams. Once absorbed, it is rapidly metabolized, and, therefore, it is unlikely that substantial amounts are absorbed after topical application.

Phthalates

A number of cosmetic products contain diethyl phthalate and/or dibutyl phthalate. Personal care product use predicts urinary levels of some phthalate monoesters.[39] Significant exposure to phthalates during pregnancy has been demonstrated.[40] An association between urine phthalate levels and pregnancy loss was shown in a small study,[41] but the source of phthalates was not specified. Concerns about phthalate levels associated with the use of personal care products in pregnancy have been raised but not well substantiated. The contribution of personal care products to phthalate levels has not been established because phthalates are also used in food packaging and processing materials. The contribution of cosmetic versus noncosmetic sources to phthalate levels needs to be determined, and further studies in pregnancy are needed.

Preservatives

Concerns have been raised about the estrogenicity of *parabens*. However, it has been revealed to be not as potent as previously thought. The estrogen-sensitive period of implantation in animal studies is not vulnerable to paraben exposure.[42] Comparisons with human data (17beta-estradiol or diethylstilbestrol) indicate that it is implausible that parabens could increase the risk of any estrogen-mediated effects. Although exposure to *formaldehyde* has been associated with adverse pregnancy outcomes in population studies and toxicity in animal studies, a contribution of cosmetic use to these outcomes has not been reported. Exposure to formaldehyde is via multiple routes (oral, inhalation, topical), which makes it impossible to draw conclusions about risks of cosmetic use. However, percutaneous application was not associated with any embryotoxic effects in an animal study that involved topical application.[43]

Botanical Products

There have been no documented adverse effects in human pregnancy from the topical application of herbal products. Risks from aloe vera (embryonic death and skeletal anomalies)[44] and rosemary (fetal death)[45] in animals that received oral doses of these ingredients are not appropriately extrapolated to topical application in humans.

Risks similar to those reported with the oral intake of some herbal medicines have not been reported with topical application.

PATIENT COUNSELING

Providing good information and ensuring that communication with the patient is successful is the most important aspect of counseling. Extrapolating experimental animal data to humans should not be included in counseling, because these data are often not representative of topical cosmetic application in humans. The healthcare provider should focus on advising as to whether an exposure places the patient at higher risk, but the final decision about using the cosmetic or skin care product rests with the patient. However, physicians may stress that, with specific exceptions, use of cosmetics is safe during pregnancy.

KEY POINTS

- Due to insufficient data on the use of skin care products and cosmetics in human pregnancy, more studies are needed to help to minimize biases in pregnancy warnings.

- Animal studies involving bottle-fed animals or animals fed through a tube do not translate to topical application in humans.

- Judicious use of cosmetics and cosmeceuticals is not associated with significant systemic absorption.

- Prescription strength topical retinoids should not currently be used in pregnancy, especially in the first trimester; more studies are required.

- Over-the-counter skin care products used for acne are safe in pregnancy; although salicylic acid should not be applied over a large surface area.

- Skin-lightening creams containing hydroquinone should be avoided in pregnancy.

- With the exception of skin-lightening creams and first-trimester use of prescription strength topical retinoids, all skin care products and cosmetics are considered safe in gestation.

- Pregnant women may continue using their cosmetics in pregnancy and look their best without risking the health of the fetus.

REFERENCES

1. Koren G, Nickel S. Sources of bias in signals of pharmaceutical safety in pregnancy. *Clin Invest Med.* 2010;33:E349–E355.
2. Kochhar DM, Christian MS. Tretinoin: a review of the nonclinical developmental toxicology experience. *J Am Acad Dermatol.* 1997;36:S47–S59.
3. Latriano L, Tzimas G, Wong F, et al. The percutaneous absorption of topically applied tretinoin and its effect on endogenous concentrations of tretinoin and its metabolites after single doses or long-term use. *J Am Acad Dermatol.* 1997;36:S37–S46.
4. Nohynek GJ, Meuling WJ, Vaes WH, et al. Repeated topical treatment, in contrast to single oral doses, with Vitamin A-containing preparations does not affect plasma concentrations of retinol, retinyl esters or retinoic acids in female subjects of child-bearing age. *Toxicol Lett.* 2006;163:65–76.
5. Lipson AH, Collins F, Webster WS. Multiple congenital defects associated with maternal use of topical tretinoin. *Lancet.* 1993;341:1352–1353.
6. Camera G, Pregliasco P. Ear malformation in baby born to mother using tretinoin cream. *Lancet.* 1992;339:687.
7. Navarre-Belhassen C, Blanchet P, Hillaire-Buys D, et al. Multiple congenital malformations associated with topical tretinoin. *Ann Pharmacother.* 1998;32:505–506.
8. Selcen D, Seidman S, Nigro MA. Otocerebral anomalies associated with topical tretinoin use. *Brain Dev.* 2000;22:218–220.
9. Jick SS, Terris BZ, Jick H. First trimester topical tretinoin and congenital disorders. *Lancet.* 1993;341:1181–1182.
10. Loureiro KD, Kao KK, Jones KL, et al. Minor malformations characteristic of the retinoic acid embryopathy and other birth outcomes in children of women exposed to topical tretinoin during early pregnancy. *Am J Med Genet A.* 2005;136:117–121.
11. Shapiro L, Pastuszak A, Curto G, et al. Safety of first-trimester exposure to topical tretinoin. *Lancet.* 1997;350:1143–1144.
12. Krautheim A, Gollnick H. Transdermal penetration of topical drugs used in the treatment of acne. *Clin Pharmacokinet.* 2003;42:1287–1304.
13. Dufour EK, Whitwell J, Nohynek GJ, et al. Retinyl palmitate is non-genotoxic in Chinese hamster ovary cells in the dark or after pre-irradiation or simultaneous irradiation with UV light. *Mutat Res.* 2009;672:21–26.
14. Autret E, Berjot M, Jonville-Bera AP, et al. Anophthalmia and agenesis of optic chiasma associated with adapalene gel in early pregnancy. *Lancet.* 1977;350:339.
15. Akhavan A, Bershad S. Topical acne drugs: review of clinical properties, systemic exposure, and safety. *Am J Clin Dermatol.* 2003;4:473–492.
16. Menter A. Pharmacokinetics and safety of tazarotene. *J Am Acad Dermatol.* 2000;43:S31–S35.
17. Schmidt JB, Knobler R, Neumann R, et al. [External erythromycin therapy of acne]. *Z Hautkr.* 1983;58:1754–1760.
18. Barza M, Goldstein JA, Kane A, et al. Systemic absorption of clindamycin hydrochloride after topical application. *J Am Acad Dermatol.* 1982;7:208–214.
19. Stoughton RB, Cornell RC, Gange RW, et al. Double-blind comparison of topical 1 percent clindamycin phosphate (Cleocin T) and oral tetracycline 500 mg/day in the treatment of acne vulgaris. *Cutis.* 1980;26:424–425, 429.
20. Van Hoogdalem EJ. Transdermal absorption of topical anti-acne agents in man; review of clinical pharmacokinetic data. *J Eur Acad Dermatol Venereol.* 1998;11:S13–S19.
21. Yeung D, Nacht S, Dan Bucks BS, et al. Benzoyl peroxide: percutaneous penetration and metabolic disposition. II: effect of concentration. *J Am Acad Dermatol.* 1983;9:920–924.
22. Schwarb FP, Gabard B, Rufli T, et al. Percutaneous absorption of salicylic acid in man after topical administration of three different formulations. *Dermatology.* 1999;198:44–51.
23. Wester RC, Melendres J, Hui X, et al. Human in vivo and in vitro hydroquinone topical bioavailability, metabolism and disposition. *J Toxicol Environ Health A.* 1998;54:301–317.

24. Mahe A, Perret JL, Ly F, et al. The cosmetic use of skin-lightening products during pregnancy in Dakar, Senegal: a common and potentially hazardous practice. *Trans R Soc Trop Med Hyg*. 2007; 101:183–187.

25. Burnett CL, Bergfeld WF, Belsito DV, et al. Final report of the safety assessment of Kojic acid as used in cosmetics. *Int J Toxicol*. 2010;29:244S–273S.

26. Katz VL, Thorp JM Jr, Bowes WA Jr. Severe symmetric intra-uterine growth retardation associated with the topical use of triamcinolone. *Am J Obstet Gynecol*. 1990;162:396–397.

27. Mygind H, Thulstrup AM, Pedersen L, et al. Risk of intrauterine growth retardation, malformations and other birth outcomes in children after topical use of corticosteroid in pregnancy. *Acta Obstet Gynecol Scand*. 2002;81:234–239.

28. Edwards MJ, Agho K, Attia J, et al. Case-control study of cleft lip or palate after maternal use of topical corticosteroids during pregnancy. *Am J Med Genet A*. 2003;120A:459–463.

29. Czeizel AE, Rockenbauer M. Population-based case-control study of teratogenic potential of corticosteroids. *Teratology*. 1997; 56:335–340.

30. Andersen FA. Final report on the safety assessment of glycolic acid, ammonium, calcium, potassium, and sodium glycolates, methyl, ethyl, propyl, and butyl glycolates, and lactic acid, ammonium, calcium, potassium, sodium and TEA-lactates, methyl, ethyl, isopropyl, and butyl lactates, and lauryl, myristyl, and cetyl lactates. *Int J Toxicol*. 1998;17:S1–S241.

31. Nohynek GJ, Dufour EK. Nano-sized cosmetic formulations or solid nanoparticles in sunscreens: a risk to human health? *Arch Toxicol*. 2012;86:1063–1075.

32. Gulati DK, Mounce R, Chapin RE, et al. *Final Report on the Reproductive Toxicity of 2-Hydroxy-4-Methoxybenzophenone (CAS no. 131-57-7) in CD-1-Swiss Mice*. National Technical Information Service Report/PB91-158477. Research Triangle Park, NC: National Institute of Environmental Health Sciences; 1990.

33. Schlumpf M, Cotton B, Conscience M, et al. In vitro and in vivo estrogenicity of UV screens. *Environ Health Perspect*. 2001; 109:239–244.

34. Yourick JJ, Koenig ML, Yourick DL, et al. Fate of chemicals in skin after dermal application: does the in vitro skin reservoir affect the estimate of systemic absorption? *Toxicol Appl Pharmacol*. 2004;195:309–320.

35. McCall EE, Olshan AF, Daniels JL. Maternal hair dye use and risk of neuroblastoma in offspring. *Cancer Causes Control*. 2005; 16:743–748.

36. Burnett C, Goldenthal EI, Harris SB, et al. Teratology and per-cutaneous toxicity studies on hair dyes. *J Toxicol Environ Health*. 1976;1:1027–1040.

37. Chua-Gocheco A, Bozzo P, Einarson A. Safety of hair products during pregnancy: personal use and occupational exposure. *Can Fam Physician*. 2008;54:1386–1388.

38. Bozzo P, Chua-Gocheco A, Einarson A. Safety of skin care products during pregnancy. *Can Fam Physician*. 2011;57:665–667.

39. Duty SM, Ackerman RM, Calafat AM, et al. Personal care product use predicts urinary concentrations of some phthalate monoesters. *Environ Health Perspect*. 2005;113:1530–1535.

40. Just AC, Adibi JJ, Rundle AG, et al. Urinary and air phthalate concentrations and self-reported use of personal care products among minority pregnant women in New York city. *J Expo Sci Environ Epidemiol*. 2010;20:625–633.

41. Toft G, Jönsson BA, Lindh CH, et al. Association between pregnancy loss and urinary phthalate levels around the time of conception. *Environ Health Perspect*. 2012;120:458–463.

42. Shaw J, deCatanzaro D. Estrogenicity of parabens revisited: impact of parabens on early pregnancy and an uterotrophic assay in mice. *Reprod Toxicol*. 2009;28:26–31.

43. Overman DO. Absence of embryotoxic effects of formaldehyde after percutaneous exposure in hamsters. *Toxicol Lett*. 1985; 24:107–110.

44. Nath D, Sethi N, Skingh RK, et al. Commonly used abortifacient plants with special reference to their teratologic effect in rats. *J Ethnopharmacol*. 1992;36:147–154.

45. Nusier MK, Bataineh HN, Daradkah HM. Adverse effects of rosemary (Rosmarinus officinalis L.) on reproductive function in adult male rats. *Exp Biol Med (Maywood)*. 2007;232:809–813.

Kachiu C. Lee ■ Raymond Dufresne

INTRODUCTION

Performing dermatologic surgery on pregnant patients requires careful consideration. Maternal and fetal health can influence surgical timing, use of antibiotics and anesthetic agents, and the type of procedure. Maternal medications and comorbidities also need extensive review because these factors can affect dermatologic surgery. The surgeon must weigh the risks and benefits to both the patient and fetus prior to proceeding. This chapter addresses pertinent issues when considering surgery in the pregnant patient.

RELEVANT PHYSIOLOGIC CHANGES

Respiratory, cardiovascular, renal, and gastrointestinal physiologic changes can all influence aspects of the surgical procedure. In order to meet fetal oxygen demands, maternal minute respiration increases, which causes a state of compensated respiratory alkalosis.[1] Cardiovascular changes, including increased cardiac output and stroke volume with decreased peripheral vascular resistance, help meet the oxygenation needs of the fetus. Because of decreased peripheral vascular resistance and increased production of coagulation factors, such as those produced by the liver (factors VII, VIII, IX, and X), patients are at higher risk of thromboembolic events. Patients reclining for long procedures may consider using compression stockings to decrease this risk. Over time, the gravid uterus enlarges to compress the inferior vena cava and the lower aorta in the supine position. Also, a supine position during surgery may worsen the already increased acid reflux that is secondary to a progesterone-induced decrease of the gastroesophageal sphincter tone. Any episodes of maternal hypotension can compromise uterine blood flow, and blood pressure should be monitored closely during any procedure.[1]

Patients need to take breaks during long procedures because of frequent urination secondary to increased renal flow, glomerular filtration rate, and increased bladder pressure as a result of the enlargement of gravid uterus. Frequent snacking will help with the hypoglycemia of pregnancy that is typically secondary to continuous glucose demands of the fetus and will prevent ketosis. Ligamentous laxity may cause muscle cramps and pelvic or lower back discomfort, and repositioning breaks during surgical procedures will offer relief to the patient.

INITIAL EVALUATION

Prior to the surgical procedure, a detailed personal and family history needs to be taken, with a focus on comorbidities and current medications, and a physical examination should be performed.

History

A history should focus on factors that may influence the metabolism of lidocaine, the most commonly used anesthetic in dermatologic surgery. Lidocaine is metabolized by the liver enzyme P450 CYP1A2; therefore, liver dysfunction increases the risk of toxicity.[2] This medication is also protein bound, and low-protein states may increase risk. Medications that can affect lidocaine levels include inhibitors of P450 CYP1A2, such as cimetidine, ciprofloxacin, fluoroquinolones, and inducers of P450, such as clonidine, phenytoin, tobacco, theophylline, warfarin, acetaminophen, naproxen, and beta-blockers. Patients with a personal or family history of thrombosis or clotting factor deficiencies may need thromboprophylaxis, such as subcutaneous heparin and pneumatic leg compression, if undergoing lengthy or complex procedures.[1]

A review of systems should focus on infectious and hepatic symptoms, such as fever, chills, malaise, jaundice, nausea, vomiting, and light-colored stools. Diseases affecting liver function, such as obstetric cholestasis, biliary disease, hepatitis, and acute fatty liver of pregnancy, need to be ruled out. Acute fatty liver of pregnancy is a rare condition of the third trimester or immediate postpartum period that presents with nausea, vomiting, and malaise. Due to high mortality, patients suspected of having the disorder should seek immediate care through their obstetrician, and skin surgery should be delayed. Eclampsia presents with hypertension, seizures, headaches, and lethargy. HELLP (hemolysis, elevated liver enzymes, and low platelets) syndrome, which presents with right upper quadrant or epigastric pain, nausea, vomiting, and malaise, also needs to be ruled out. Hypertension and proteinuria are clues that liver function may be compromised, and caution is recommended when treating patients with possible preeclampsia.

Physical Examination

Baseline vital sign measurements can uncover poor tolerability for surgery or underlying infections if there is significant elevation of the white blood with bands. It should be noted that the white blood cell count is naturally slightly elevated during pregnancy, and this should not be mistaken for symptoms of inflammation.[1] Normal blood pressure rules out preeclampsia. Excessive edema or signs of liver disease, such as jaundice or right upper quadrant pain, warrants an additional workup.

INDICATIONS AND SPECIAL CONSIDERATIONS

Minimally invasive procedures, such as a skin biopsy or shave removal of a bleeding *granuloma gravidarum*, should not be deferred, especially if the procedure is performed to rule out malignancy.[3] The American College of Obstetrics and Gynecology (ACOG) recommends surgical clearance from the patient's obstetrician prior to any procedure.[4] Regarding the timing of nonemergent surgery, most authors concur that this should not be performed during the first or third trimester and recommend scheduling it during the second trimester or postpartum in order to minimize maternal and fetal risks.[1] Maternal and fetal risks of skin surgery in pregnancy are shown in the box.

Dysplastic Nevi and Melanoma

A biopsy of any suspicious lesion is warranted regardless of pregnancy trimester. Concerning lesions must be treated with the same urgency compared to lesions in nonpregnant patients. Biopsy-proven melanoma should be excised with appropriate margins. Regarding staging of melanoma, a sentinel lymph node biopsy with lymphoscintigraphy is considered safe during pregnancy because fetal exposure to radiation from the dye tracer (technetium-99) is <5 mGy, which is considered harmless.[5] The risk of an allergic reaction to blue dye is minimal (≤2%), and a life-threatening anaphylactic reaction occurs in 0.7% to 1.1% (see Ch. 15); anaphylaxis has been reported in patients with negative skin-prick testing.[6] Because of these risks, some authors suggest using radiocolloid alone in the first trimester. An effort should be made to avoid general anesthesia when performing sentinel lymph node biopsy in pregnancy; however, performing the procedure under local anesthesia may be difficult in certain anatomic locations, such as the axilla (deep nodes in proximity to the thoracodorsal nerve) or the inguinal/pelvic region with deep lymph nodes.[7]

Using X-ray and computed tomography (CT) scans should be deferred in the first trimester, and if possible, avoided all together due to fetal radiation exposure. Non-contrast magnetic resonance imaging is preferred because it does not use radiation.[2] Ultrasound is safe but has low sensitivity and specificity in detecting melanoma metastasis. A chest X-ray delivers approximately 1.4 mGy, whereas an abdominal CT scan delivers 25 mGy. Table 24.1 lists common radiologic procedures and their associated fetal radiation exposures.[8] Table 24.2 reviews noncancer radiation-related fetal risks.[9] Fetal exposures to diagnostic radiation in doses <100 mGy are not considered a reason for a termination of pregnancy.[10] Fetal risk is minimal with doses <10 mGy, whereas fetuses exposed to a cumulative dose >50 mGy may be at risk.[11] The childhood estimates of cancer risk related to radiation exposure at dose of 0 to 50 mGy, 50 to 500 mGy, or >500 mGy are 0.3% to 1%, 1% to 6%, and >6%, respectively, when compared with a background exposure risk of 0.3%.[9]

TABLE 24.1	Fetal Exposure to Common Radiologic Diagnostic Procedures	
Procedure	**Range of Fetal Dose (mGy)**	**Risk of Childhood Cancer per Examination**[a]
X-ray chest or skull; CT head and/or neck	0.001–0.01	<1 in 1,000,000
CT pulmonary angiogram	0.01–0.1	1 in 100,000 to 1 in 1,000,0000
X-ray abdomen or pelvis/hip; CT chest/liver	0.1–1.0	1 in 10,000 to 1 in 100,000
X-ray lumbar spine; CT abdomen; 18F-FDG PET tumor scan	1.0–10	1 in 1,000 to 1 in 10,000
CT pelvis or abdomen/pelvis or chest/abdomen/pelvis; 18F-FDG PET/CT whole body	10–50	1 in 200 to 1 in 1,000

[a] Background exposure risk is 0.3%.[9]

CT, computed tomography; 18F-FDG PET, 18F-fluorodeoxyglucose positron emission tomography.

(Modified from Wall BF, Meara JR, Muirhead CR, et al. *Protection of Pregnant Patients During Diagnostic Medical Exposures to Ionizing Radiation.* United Kingdom: Health Protection Agency, The Royal College of Radiologists, and College of Radiographers; 2009.)

TABLE 24.2	Noncancer Radiation-Related Health Risks to the Fetus	
	Acute Radiation Dose to the Embryo/Fetus	
Time Postconception	**50–500 mGy**[a]	**>500 mGy**
<2 weeks	↑ Failure to implant	↑↑ Failure to implant
2–7 wks	GR possible; slightly ↑ major malformations	↑ Miscarriage; GR likely; ↑↑ major malformations (CNS, motor deficiencies)
8–15 wks	GR possible, ↓ in IQ possible; ↑ severe MR (≤20%)	↑ Miscarriage; GR likely; ↓ in IQ possible; ↑ severe MR (>20%); ↑ major malformations
16–25 wks		↑ Miscarriage; GR possible; ↓ in IQ possible; severe MR possible; ↑ major malformations
≥26 wks		Miscarriage and neonatal death, depending on dose

[a] No risks at any stage of gestation with doses <50 mGy. This table provides only approximations of risks because risks are dose dependent within the same gestational period.

↑, increased incidence of; ↑↑, substantially increased incidence of; ↓, reduction; CNS, central nervous system; GR, growth retardation; IQ, intelligence quotient; MR, mental retardation.

(Data from the Centers for Disease Control and Prevention. Radiation and pregnancy: A fact sheet for clinicians. www.bt.cdc.gov/radiation/prenatalphysician.asp. Published November 29, 2011. Accessed May 31, 2012.)

Nonmelanoma Skin Cancer

Although nonmelanoma skin cancer can be safely treated during pregnancy, treatment can arguably be deferred until the postpartum period. In assessing the need for treatment of nonmelanoma skin cancer in pregnant women, the risks of surgery should be weighed against the risks of increased defect size. In a study of 219 nonmelanoma skin cancers that were treated with Mohs surgery, a 1-year delay between initial examination and surgery was associated with a doubling of defect size.[12]

SURGICAL PREPARATION

To decrease the risk of aspiration, all patients should be advised to fast prior to surgery as well as to take an antacid, such as an H_2 antihistamine or proton pump inhibitor. The enlarged uterus may compress the stomach, thus causing gastroesophageal reflux.

Positioning

The left lateral decubitus position, also referred to as the left lateral tilt position, is recommended for increased venous return (Fig. 24.1, see Table 24.3). During the second trimester, the enlarged fetus compresses the mother's inferior vena cava and the lower aorta in the supine position. By the third trimester, cardiac output can decrease by up to 24%. Women compensate by increasing systemic vascular resistance and heart rate or by increasing venous return through paravertebral and azygos systems. However, during anesthesia, these compensatory mechanisms are reduced, resulting in an increased risk of hypotension.

In the left lateral decubitus position, obstruction of the lower aorta and its branches are minimized, thus providing maximum venous return to the cardiac structures.

Antibiotics and Antiseptics

Penicillin and its derivatives are most commonly used, but cephalosporins, and nonestolate erythromycin are also safe (all are pregnancy category B) (see Ch. 22, pregnancy and lactation categories are outlined in Tables 22.2 and 22.3).[13] Levels of ciprofloxacin, clindamycin, levofloxacin, and vancomycin were of the same magnitude or higher in amniotic fluid as in maternal blood.[13] Amoxicillin, gentamicin, and penicillin G and VK showed lower concentrations in pregnant women than in nonpregnant women, suggesting that a shorter dosing interval or increased maternal dose may be required in pregnancy.[13] Pregnancy category C antibiotics

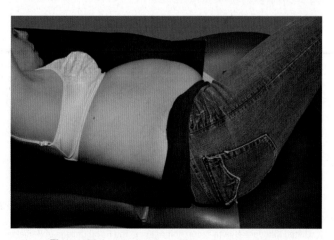

Figure 24.1. The left lateral decubitus position.

TABLE 24.3	**Summary of Management Options**
First trimester	■ Biopsy any suspicious lesions ■ Preferential use of category B medications ■ Avoid, if possible, all diagnostic radiation (especially if ≥50 mGy) ■ Defer nonessential surgical procedures ■ Avoid use of povidone–iodine on or near mucosal surfaces
Second trimester	■ Biopsy any suspicious lesions ■ Preferential use of category B medications ■ Minimize diagnostic radiation ■ Assess for pregnancy-associated comorbidities (i.e., preeclampsia, cholestasis) ■ Position patient in left lateral decubitus position in surgical procedures
Third trimester	■ Biopsy of any suspicious lesions ■ Preferential use of category B medications ■ Minimize diagnostic radiation ■ Assess for pregnancy-associated comorbidities (see previous) ■ Position patient in left lateral decubitus position in surgical procedures ■ Consider deferring nonessential procedures to postpartum period
Postpartum	■ Preferential use of category B medications in breastfeeding mothers ■ Counsel patient on heavy lifting restrictions after surgery if sutures or staples are used ■ Cosmetic procedures may be performed

(chloramphenicol, gentamicin, rifampin, fluoroquinolones) should be used only if the benefit justifies the potential fetal risk, whereas clindamycin and vancomycin (both are pregnancy category B) should be avoided in the first trimester because of a possible small risk (limited data).

Topical alcohol preparations are safe in pregnancy, but because they are flammable, they must dry out before electrocautery or laser procedures. Chlorhexidine gluconate is safe to use topically; however, the risk of corneal damage mandates caution when used around the eyes. Povidone–iodine absorption through mucosal membranes may pose a risk to the fetus. In pregnant women who received povidone–iodine to the vaginal mucosa, a measurable increase in both maternal and neonatal urinary excretion of iodine was noted, although short-term variations in maternal and neonatal thyroid hormones were less consistent.[14,15] The use of povidone–iodine near mucosal surfaces should be avoided and might be considered with caution during the first trimester.[15] Still, questions such as the difference in absorption of povidone–iodine between the vaginal mucosa and the skin and whether a single povidone–iodine application can affect fetal cognitive maturation need to be addressed.[15] The use of hexachlorophene is not recommended because of reports of fetal central nervous system toxicity.[4]

Anesthesia

Although the ACOG does not provide recommendations for use of anesthesia in nonobstetric procedures, it is generally accepted that general anesthesia should be avoided in the first trimester because of possible adverse effects of

anesthetics, such as nitrous oxide, during organogenesis. Nevertheless, most intravenous anesthetics, muscle relaxants, and analgesics are considered safe. Recommendations for local anesthesia during the first trimester have been less specific.[16] Therefore, it is advisable to wait until the second trimester before performing dermatologic surgery. Lidocaine and prilocaine are safe local anesthetics for skin surgery in pregnancy (pregnancy category B) (Fig. 24.2). Lidocaine, with molecular weight <500 Daltons, crosses the placental barrier via simple diffusion that is driven by the concentration gradient between fetal and maternal circulation. Amide anesthetics also cross more readily into

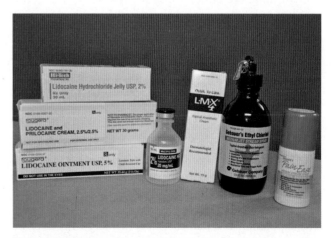

Figure 24.2. Lidocaine and prilocaine are safe in gestation (pregnancy category B). Skin coolants, such as those containing ethyl chloride or pentafluoropropane, can be used in order to minimize discomfort.

fetal circulation given their high lipid solubility. The acid–base status of the mother or fetus can change anesthetic concentrations by altering the ratio of ionized to nonionized forms. Nonionized forms cross the placental barrier more readily than ionized forms. If the fetus is acidotic, then amide anesthetics (the pH of which is near the maternal physiologic pH) are more ionized than nonionized when compared to maternal blood, leading to "ion trapping" within the fetal department. In this condition, there is poor back-diffusion of the ionized form of the amide anesthetic into the maternal circulation. Thus, increased fetal drug concentration can result.[16,17]

Topical Anesthetics

Lidocaine 2.5%/Prilocaine 2.5% Cream (EMLA)

The safety of lidocaine 2.5%/prilocaine 2.5% combination cream (pregnancy category B) is reinforced by the pediatric literature, in which it has been used as early as 26 weeks' gestation.[18,19] Caution is needed with the application near ocular surfaces due to a risk of ocular chemical injury. Although rare, the most important concern relates to the development of methemoglobinemia with high doses of systemically absorbed prilocaine.[20] The milk to plasma ratio of lidocaine is 0.4 but that of prilocaine is unknown. Therefore, the medication should be used with caution in lactation. In a comparison study of liposomal lidocaine, nonliposomal lidocaine, and lidocaine 2.5%/prilocaine 2.5%, liposomal lidocaine showed a longer duration of analgesia.[21]

Tetracaine 1% or 2% Cream, 1% Ointment, 0.5% Ophthalmic Solution

Tetracaine (pregnancy category C) is a long-acting ester anesthetic. Because tetracaine shows limited absorption on intact skin and lidocaine preparations can cause corneal abrasions and ulcerations, tetracaine is preferred on the eyelid or periocular procedures and laceration suturing.[1] It is not known whether tetracaine is excreted in human milk; therefore, it may be used in breastfeeding mothers only when strongly indicated.

Benzocaine

The topical application of benzocaine (pregnancy category C) has been associated with methemoglobinemia in infants and children.[22] There are no reports of methemoglobinemia in pregnancy. However, given the theoretical risk of systemic absorption, it is recommended that this medication be avoided in pregnant females. It is not known whether benzocaine is excreted in human milk; therefore, caution is recommended when using it in nursing patients.

Skin Coolants

The application of a skin coolant containing ethyl chloride or pentafluoropropane is associated with negligible systemic absorption and is considered safe in pregnancy (see Fig. 24.2). Skin coolants can minimize the discomfort of local anesthesia; however, they need to be used with caution in order to minimize their local adverse effects (frostbite, irritation near

mucosal surfaces). Also, because ethyl chloride is flammable, one should ensure that it is not exposed to heat.

Injectable Anesthetics

Lidocaine

The ability of lidocaine to cross tissue barriers through passive diffusion warrants prudent use during pregnancy. Inadvertent arterial injection or large volumes of lidocaine or other anesthetics may put the fetus at risk for cardiac or central nervous system toxicity, and the mother may develop signs of systemic toxicity that mimic aortocaval compression, such as light-headedness, tachycardia, diaphoresis, and headache.[1] Caution is recommended with using injectable anesthetics in end-stage pregnancy when the cardiac output is increased and blood transfusion to the site of anesthetic injection increases, which results in a rapid transfer of the anesthetic into the circulation. The recommended maximum lidocaine dose in the United States is 4.5 mg per kilogram, or 300 mg.[23] Lidocaine binds with low affinity, but high capacity, to breast milk. Because of "ion trapping," given the low pH of breast milk (6.24) and the high pKa of lidocaine (7.9), a dermatologic surgeon should treat breastfeeding patients with the same considerations as pregnant patients. A study found that, following maternal perineal infiltration, lidocaine was detected in neonatal urine for at least 48 hours after delivery.[24] Considering the dose and route of administration, it is unlikely that neonatal levels would be clinically significant. Lidocaine is safe in lactation (lactation category S, L2) when used as directed.

Epinephrine

Epinephrine (pregnancy category C) used in combination with local anesthetics, such as lidocaine, slows their systemic absorption, thus decreasing peak maternal drug levels of these anesthetics. However, a proportional decrease in fetal absorption rate has not been demonstrated. In high levels, epinephrine can cause decreased uterine blood flow or uterine artery spasm, inducing fetal distress. Nevertheless, it is unlikely that such risks could be seen with the dilutions used in dermatologic surgery and the small amounts that are injected. Many authors indicate that the benefit of local vasoconstriction in skin surgery outweighs the potential risk.[1] There have been no teratogenic effects.[25] There have been no pediatric concerns with use in lactation (lactation category S, L1), but one should observe for brief stimulation.

Mepivacaine

Mepivacaine (pregnancy category C) should be used with extreme caution due to the risk of fetal bradycardia. An additional risk includes preterm labor via increased oxytocin-induced contractions.[26] Compared to lidocaine, bupivacaine, and ropivacaine, mepivacaine has the highest fetal–maternal ratio of placental drug transfer.[27] Although there have been no reports of pediatric concerns when the medication was administered in breastfeeding mothers (lactation category S, L3), other medications, such as bupivacaine, enter breast milk in exceedingly low levels and should be preferred.

Tumescent Anesthesia

The effects of tumescent anesthesia on pregnancy have not been evaluated. Concentrations of lidocaine <1% may result in lower total drug used, slower peak onset, and longer duration times.[28,29] There are no reported cases of large volume tumescent anesthesia used during pregnancy.

SURGICAL PROCEDURE

As far as the design of the procedure, determining the skin tension lines may be difficult in certain areas such as the distended abdomen. However, the vector of least tension becomes easier to determine after a circular excision. Although electrocautery is considered safe, concerns have been raised about fetal exposure to potentially harmful or mutagenic particles in electrocautery smoke based on experimental data.[30] Therefore, placing a mask on the patient is recommended. For procedures performed on the extended abdomen, one may need to use a slowly absorbing buried suture with increased strength and knot security.[1] Due to slower wound healing associated with pregnancy, sutures may need to remain longer in the skin. Risk of dehiscence decreases with staged suture removal, especially on the distended abdomen.[1]

POSTOPERATIVE COMPLICATIONS

Possible postoperative complications include infection, wound dehiscence, bleeding, hematoma, and pain. For suspected infection, the physician should swab the wound for a Gram stain and culture. Upon choosing an antibiotic, care should be placed in prescribing a nonteratogenic medication (see Antibiotics and Antiseptics). For wound dehiscence and bleeding, a routine surgical protocol applies. In the case of hematoma, the surgeon needs to carefully evaluate for any signs of hemodynamic compromise. Acetaminophen (pregnancy category B) is the analgesic of choice in pregnancy and can help minimize postoperative pain. It can also be used safely in lactation (lactation category S, L1).

COSMETIC PROCEDURES

Removal of Benign Lesions

The removal of benign lesions, such as seborrheic keratoses, exophytic nevi, and skin tags, for cosmetic or medical reasons can be safely performed in pregnancy. Procedures such as shaving, electrodessication, curettage, radiosurgery (destruction or shaving) (Fig. 24.3), and cryotherapy

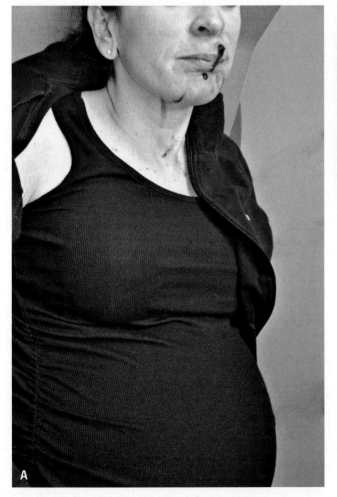

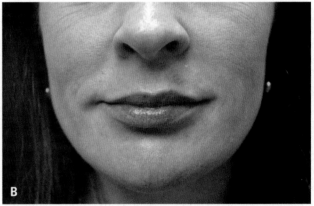

Figure 24.3. (**A**) A large pyogenic granuloma (*granuloma gravidarum*) on the left side of the upper lip bleeding profusely at 26 weeks' gestation. (**B**) Excellent healing shown 4 weeks after shaving the lesion with a radiofrequency device. (Surgitron FFPF EMC, Ellman International Inc.)

pose no significant maternal or fetal risks when performed judiciously. As aforementioned, an effort should be made to minimize patient exposure to smoke during procedures such as electrocautery and radiosurgery, and thus reduce any fetal risks.

Botulinum Toxin Type A

The cosmetic use of botulinum toxin type A (pregnancy category C) has not been studied in pregnancy; however, the drug has been used in pregnancy for medical reasons (i.e., cervical dystonia, blepharospasm). Although it has low systemic toxicity, cases of systemic weakness with doses >600 units have been reported.[31,32] Lower doses may be safe during pregnancy. In one report, a woman with idiopathic cervical dystonia received 300 units every 3 to 6 months preconception and throughout pregnancy without evidence of cognitive or developmental delay in any of her four children.[33] In a survey, 18 women were injected with botulinum toxin once during the first trimester without fetal complications.[34] One case report describes a woman who received 500 units at 4 weeks' gestation with fetal demise of a twin gestation at 10 weeks.[35] However, the association between the drug and miscarriage was unclear because the patient had other risk factors for miscarriage. The avoidance of cosmetic use during pregnancy is recommended.[36]

Sclerotherapy

Varicose veins and telangiectasias may develop or increase in size in pregnancy but often improve postpartum. Therefore, it is recommended that pregnant patients wait until at least 6 to 12 months after pregnancy prior to treating these conditions. Sclerosing solutions can cross the placenta, and their effects on the fetus are unknown. There was no difference in pregnancy outcomes between groups of 45 patients treated with sclerotherapy and 56 patients treated conservatively.[37] Due to the lack of additional studies, definitive conclusions on the safety of sclerotherapy cannot be reached. However, there is an absolute contraindication for sclerotherapy in the first trimester and after the 36th week.[38]

Lasers

The use of 585-nm pulsed dye laser for treatment of symptomatic pyogenic granulomas and warts during pregnancy is considered safe.[39] The laser's microscopic level of penetration minimizes fetal risks unless there is direct exposure, which is very unlikely with appropriate use of the device.[39] Treatment of *condylomata acuminata* with a carbon dioxide laser prior to delivery in order to prevent neonatal recurrent respiratory papillomatosis has not been associated with harmful fetal effects.[40,41] Concerns regarding eye safety are no different than those in the nonpregnant patient. Because there are no studies on

the effects of lasers and intense pulse light in pregnancy that would take into account the edema and stretching that occurs in pregnancy, using these modalities for cosmetic reasons during gestation is not recommended.

Epilation

Excess hair growth can be treated with safe, albeit temporary, treatment options such as depilatory creams, waxing, and shaving. Electrolysis should be avoided because its safety in pregnancy has not been studied. Concerns have been raised about the type of electrolysis that uses galvanic current because amniotic fluid acts as a conductor of electricity. As aforementioned, the use of laser modalities for cosmetic reasons in pregnancy is not recommended.

Chemical Peels

Salicylic Acid

There is a lack of evidence-based studies on the safety of topical salicylic acid use in pregnancy. Fetal risks associated with the oral intake of salicylic acid (aspirin) are unlikely with topical application of salicylic acid, especially on small areas such as the face (see Ch. 23). However, salicylic acid should not be applied over large surface areas.

Glycolic Acid

Topical application is considered safe during pregnancy due to a minimal dermal absorption and a lack of reports of fetal risks. However, there is a lack of studies during pregnancy.

Trichloroacetic Acid

Use in pregnancy is not recommended because of possible dermal penetration.

Liposuction

Liposuction is not recommended at any stage of pregnancy.[42] Specifically, tumescent liposuction is contraindicated due to unnecessary lidocaine exposure to both the mother and fetus. Because of metabolic changes related to pregnancy, adequate adipose tissue is necessary to maintain the nutritional demands of the fetus. Lidocaine can be excreted in breast milk and, therefore, is not recommended in breastfeeding women. A lipectomy at the time of cesarean section is not recommended, but the decision is based on the discretion of the obstetric physician.

Fillers

Collagen and hyaluronic acid injections have not been extensively studied during pregnancy. However, one report discusses collagen injections for urinary stress incontinence during pregnancy. The patient had no complications during pregnancy.[43] There are no reports of hyaluronic acid use in pregnancy.

Body Art

In most cases, *piercings* and *tattoos* do not interfere with pregnancy. However, navel and abdominal surface piercings may contribute to *striae gravidarum* from gravid distention.[44] Furthermore, a nipple piercing can interfere with breastfeeding, an oral piercing can interfere with airway management, and nasal jewelry can be inhaled or swallowed during orotracheal intubation.[44]

No evidence-based recommendations can be made on tattooing during pregnancy or breastfeeding. However, there are no convincing data on adverse fetal effects from tattoo pigments and dyes in the first trimester.[44] One patient underwent an extensive 5-hour tattoo session during gestational week 6 and a 2-hour tattoo session during gestational week 21 and had an uneventful delivery.[45] No cases of tattooing during breastfeeding have been reported. Because the procedure is lengthy and may be associated with infections and hypersensitivity reactions to tattoo pigments, most authors recommend avoiding tattooing during pregnancy.

POSTPARTUM CONSIDERATIONS

During breastfeeding, the same considerations for the use of antibiotics and anesthesia apply as during pregnancy. Lidocaine should be used with prudence (see Anesthesia). If the location of the surgery is near the breast, the physician should caution the patient that tenderness after the procedure may inhibit the patient from breastfeeding. If the location is near the cesarean section scar, the surgeon should evaluate whether the procedure can be delayed until after the surgical site has healed. The general consensus is that cosmetic procedures are safe postpartum and can be performed as long as they do not interfere with breastfeeding.

MATERNAL RISKS

Delayed diagnosis and/or treatment if surgery is deferred

Risk of bleeding and infection because epinephrine is often omitted from anesthesia

Signs of systemic toxicity from inadvertent arterial injection or large volumes of anesthetics

Symptoms of faintness or light-headedness due to decreased venous return if improperly positioned

Slow healing, postinflammatory hyper- or hypopigmentation, and worsening of hypertrophic/keloid scars

FETAL RISKS

Malformation, miscarriage, intrauterine growth restriction, and mental retardation from radiation exposure

Poor thyroid development related to maternal exposure to povidone–iodine

---

Cardiac or central nervous system toxicity from inadvertent excessive exposure to anesthetics

Spontaneous abortion or preterm labor from fetal distress

Teratogenicity from use of inappropriate antibiotics

KEY POINTS

- A biopsy of suspicious lesions should not be delayed because of pregnancy.
- Defer nonessential surgical procedures until at least the second trimester or postpartum.
- Minimize radiation exposure, especially in the first trimester.
- Use of pregnancy category B medications, such as lidocaine and penicillin family antibiotics, is recommended.
- Position the patient in left lateral decubitus position to prevent aortocaval compression syndrome.
- The removal of benign lesions, such as nevi, skin tags, and seborrheic keratoses, for cosmetic or medical reasons, using procedures such as shaving, electrodessication, cryotherapy, and radiosurgery, is safe in pregnancy.
- Laser treatments for symptomatic lesions, such as *granuloma gravidarum*, and genital warts can be performed with standard safety precautions.

REFERENCES

1. Sweeney M, Maloney ME. Pregnancy and dermatologic surgery. *Dermatol Clin.* 2006;24:205–214.
2. Orlando R, Piccoli P, De Martin S, et al. Cytochrome P450 1A2 is a major determinant of lidocaine metabolism in vivo: effects of liver function. *Clin Pharmacol Ther.* 2004;75:80–88.
3. Kanal E, Borgstede JP, Barkovich AJ, et al. American College of Radiology White Paper on MR Safety: 2004 update and revisions. *Am J Roentgenol.* 2004;182:1111–1114.
4. ACOG Committee Opinion No. 474: nonobstetric surgery during pregnancy. *Obstet Gynecol.* 2011;117:420–421.
5. Adelstein SJ. Administered radionuclides in pregnancy. *Teratology.* 1999;59:236–239.
6. Kaufman G, Guth AA, Pachter HL, et al. A cautionary tale: anaphylaxis to isosulfan blue dye after 12 years and 3339 cases of lymphatic mapping. *Am Surg.* 2008;74:152–155.
7. Broer N, Buonocore S, Goldberg C, et al. A proposal for the timing of management of patients with melanoma presenting during surgery. *J Surg Oncol.* 2012;106:36–40.
8. Wall BF, Meara JR, Muirhead CR, et al. *Protection of Pregnant Patients During Diagnostic Medical Exposures to Ionizing Radiation.* United Kingdom: Health Protection Agency, The Royal College of Radiologists and College of Radiographers; 2009.

9. Center for Disease Control and Prevention. Radiation and pregnancy: a fact sheet for clinicians. www.bt.cdc.gov/radiation/prenatalphysician.asp. Published November 29, 2011. Accessed May 31, 2012.

10. International Atomic Energy Agency. Radiologic protection of patients (RPOP). Pregnancy and radiation in diagnostic radiology. https://rpop.iaea.org/RPOP/RPoP/Content/SpecialGroups/1_PregnantWomen/Pregnancyandradiology.htm. Accessed June 27, 2013.

11. Toppenberg KS, Hill DA, Mill DP. Safety of radiographic imaging during pregnancy. *Am Fam Physician*. 1999;59:1813–1818.

12. Eide MJ, Weinstock MA, Dufresne RG Jr, et al. Relationship of treatment delay with surgical defect size from keratinocyte carcinoma (basal cell carcinoma and squamous cell carcinoma of the skin). *J Invest Dermatol*. 2005;124:308–314.

13. Nahum GG, Uhl K, Kennedy DL. Antibiotic use in pregnancy and lactation: what is and is not known about teratogenic and toxic risks. *Obstet Gynecol*. 2006;107:1120–1138.

14. Tahirovic H, Toromanovic A, Grbic S, et al. Maternal and neonatal urinary iodine excretion and neonatal TSH in relation to use of antiseptic during caesarean section in an iodine sufficient area. *J Pediatr Endocrinol Metab*. 2009;22:1145–1149.

15. Velasco I, Naranjo S, Lopez-Pedrera C, et al. Use of povidone-iodine during the first trimester of pregnancy: a correct practice? *BJOG*. 2009;116:452–455.

16. Van De Velde M, De Buck F. Anesthesia for non-obstetric surgery in the pregnant patient. *Minerva Anesthesiol*. 2007;73:235–240.

17. Ueki R, Tatara T, Kariya K, et al. Comparison of placental transfer of local anesthetics in perfusates with different pH values in a human cotyledon model. *J Anesth*. 2009;23:526–529.

18. Biran V, Gourrier E, Cimerman P, et al. Analgesic effects of EMLA cream and oral sucrose during venipuncture in preterm infants. *Pediatrics*. 2011;128:e63– e70.

19. Taddio A, Ohlsson A, Einarson TR, et al. A systematic review of lidocaine-prilocaine cream (EMLA) in the treatment of acute pain in neonates. *Pediatrics*. 1998;101:E1.

20. Hahn IH, Hoffman RS, Nelson LS. EMLA-induced methemoglobinemia and systemic topical anesthetic toxicity. *J Emerg Med*. 2004;26:85–88.

21. Friedman PM, Mafong EA, Friedman ES, et al. Topical anesthetics update: EMLA and beyond. *Dermatol Surg*. 2001;27:1019–1026.

22. Guay J. Methemoglobinemia related to local anesthetics: a summary of 242 episodes. *Anesth Analg*. 2009;108:837–845.

23. Rosenberg PH, Veering BT, Urmey WF. Maximum recommended doses of local anesthetics: a multifactorial concept. *Reg Anesth Pain Med*. 2004;29:564–575.

24. Philipson EH, Kuhnert BR, Syracuse CD. Maternal, fetal, and neonatal lidocaine levels following local perineal infiltration. *Am J Obstet Gynecol*. 1984;149:403–407.

25. Ralston DH, Schnider SM. The fetal and neonatal effects of regional anesthesia and obstetrics. *Anesthesiology*. 1968;48:34–64.

26. Nacitarhan C, Sadan G, Kayacan N, et al. The effects of opioids, local anesthetics and adjuvants on isolated pregnant rat uterine muscles. *Methods Find Exp Clin Pharmacol*. 2007;29:273–276.

27. Ueki R, Tatara T, Kariya N, et al. Comparison of placental transfer of local anesthetics in perfusates with different pH values in a human cotyledon model. *J Anesth*. 2009;23:526–529.

28. Scarborough DA, Herron JB, Khan A, et al. Experience with more than 5,000 cases in which monitored anesthesia care was used for liposuction surgery. *Aesthetic Plast Surg*. 2003;27:474–480.

29. Klein JA. Tumescent technique for regional anesthesia permits lidocaine doses of 35 mg/kg for liposuction. *J Dermatol Surg Oncol*. 1990;16:248–263.

30. Gatti JE, Bryant CJ, Noone RB, et al. The mutagenicity of electrocautery smoke. *Plast Reconstr Surg*. 1992;89:781–784.

31. Crowner BE, Torres-Russotto D, Carter AR, et al. Systemic weakness after therapeutic injections of botulinum toxin A: a case series and review of the literature. *Clin Neuropharmacol*. 2010;33:243–247.

32. Bakheit AM. The possible adverse effects of intramuscular botulinum toxin injections and their management. *Curr Drug Safe*. 2006;1:271–279.

33. Newman WJ, Davis TL, Padaliya BB, et al. Botulinum toxin type A therapy during pregnancy. *Move Disord*. 2004;19:1384–1385.

34. Morgan JC, Iyer SS, Moser ET, et al. Botulinum toxin A during pregnancy: a survey of treating physicians. *J Neurol Neurosurg Psychiatry*. 2006;77:117–119.

35. Bodkin CL, Maurer KB, Wszolek ZK. Botulinum toxin type A therapy during pregnancy. *Move Disord*. 2005;20:1081–1082.

36. Nussbaum R, Benedetto A. Cosmetic aspects of pregnancy. *Clin Dermatol*. 2006;24:133–141.

37. Abramowitz I. The treatment of varicose veins in pregnancy by empty vein compressive sclerotherapy. *S Afr Med J*. 1973;47:607–610.

38. Rabe E, Pannier-Fischer F, Gerlach H, et al. Guidelines for sclerotherapy of leg veins. *Dermatol Surg*. 2004;30:687–693.

39. Richards KA, Stasko T. Dermatologic surgery and the pregnant patient. *Dermatol Surg*. 2003;28:248–256.

40. Arena S, Marconi M, Frega A. Pregnancy and condyloma. Evaluation about therapeutic effectiveness and laser CO2 on 115 pregnant women. *Minerva Ginecol*. 2001;53:389–396.

41. Ferenczy A. Treating genital condyloma during pregnancy with the carbon dioxide laser. *Am J Obstet Gynecol*. 1984;138:9–12.

42. Mysore V. Tumescent liposuction: standard guidelines of care. *Indian J Dermatol Venereol Leprol*. 2008;74(suppl):S54–S60.

43. Carr LK, Herschorn S. Periurethral collagen injection and pregnancy. *J Urol*. 1996;155:1037.

44. Kluger N. Body art and pregnancy. *Eur J Obstet Gynecol Reprod Biol*. 2010;153:3–7.

45. Kluger N. Can a mother get a tattoo during pregnancy or while breastfeeding? *Eur J Obstet Gynecol Reprod Biol*. 2012;161:234–235.

CHAPTER 25

Dermatoethics in Pregnancy

Zachary Schwager ■ Lionel Bercovitch

INTRODUCTION

Medical ethics is the discipline devoted to the study of the moral obligations of healthcare providers, institutions, and healthcare policies toward patients and each other and how best to promote the interests of patients. Ethical dilemmas arise when clinicians are faced with conflicting and mutually exclusive courses of action that create moral uncertainties.[1] A dilemma can also arise when a course of action may be morally acceptable to some, while being unacceptable to others.

THE PRINCIPLES OF MEDICAL ETHICS

Beauchamp and Childress formulated the concept of four ethical principles that are the foundation of modern bioethics.[1] These are summarized in Table 25.1.

This framework for ethical analysis is the one that is most widely used in contemporary ethics and will be used in this chapter. Beauchamp and Childress[1] state that none of the four principles should be ranked above the others, but the resolution of ethical conflicts often requires prioritizing moral obligations through a process of shared decision making, negotiation, and thoughtful compromise.[2] In the setting of an ethical conflict, the interests of the patient are paramount (autonomy + beneficence + nonmaleficence), but respect for patient autonomy trumps beneficence and nonmaleficence. There are situations in which the interests of others may outweigh respect for patient autonomy (e.g., when requests for treatment are unreasonable or place an undue burden on rare resources, when public health or the safety of another individual is endangered by the patient's actions). If burdens or harms and benefits are equal, nonmaleficence outweighs beneficence.[2] DiGiovanni illustrates this principle with the example of a cesarean section that is done for the benefit of the fetus.[3] In such cases, the amount of risk the surgery poses to the pregnant woman must be weighed against the benefit to the fetus.

OBSTETRIC ETHICS

Maternal–Fetal Ethical Conflicts

Obstetric ethics is complicated by the fetomaternal relationship. The physician has obligations of beneficence and respect for autonomy toward the pregnant patient. The fetus lacks the neurologic development needed to possess values and beliefs and is, therefore, not considered autonomous. The physician, however, has beneficence-based obligations to the fetus once it has become a patient. Exactly when this occurs is open to interpretation, but it is generally accepted to be either at the age of viability, around 24 weeks' gestation, or when the mother confers this status to her fetus, whichever is sooner. Indeed, advances in imaging, prenatal diagnosis, and fetal surgery have served to move this date ever earlier. At this point, the management of the pregnancy must take into account what is beneficent to the fetus and what minimizes harm to the fetus (nonmaleficence). In the majority of cases, maternal and fetal interests are aligned. However, there are situations in which these interests do not coincide. In these cases, navigating maternal–fetal ethical conflicts requires the physician to identify and address the ethical issues regarding patient autonomy, beneficence toward the fetus and the expectant woman, and questions of maternal decision-making capacity and fetal "patienthood." The term *conflict*, in this context, should not imply that the mother and fetus are in any way in conflict but that the healthcare provider's moral choices involving the woman and fetus may be in conflict.

Defining "Patienthood" of the Fetus

Being a patient does not require an independent moral status. The fact that the fetus is under the physician's care by virtue of its relationship to the actual patient, the pregnant woman, and the fact that there are medical interventions that can affect the health of the fetus that is eventually attaining independent moral status, confers at least dependent moral status and, therefore, "patienthood" on the fetus.[4] In general terms, an individual becomes a patient when presenting to a healthcare provider for interventions that can produce clinical benefit that outweigh harm.[5] By extension, and by the generally accepted definition, the fetus is therefore considered to be a patient when it has reached the gestational age of viability (i.e., the ability to survive outside the uterus with technologic support and to achieve independent moral status [approximately 23 to 24 weeks]).[6] However, there is no universally accepted definition of fetal patienthood, largely due to the numerous conflicting religious, theologic, and philosophic approaches to this issue.[5]

TABLE 25.1	The Four Basic Principles of Medical Ethics	
Principle	**Definition of Obligation**[1]	**Working Definition in the Obstetric Setting**
Beneficence	To act in the best interests of the patient	"To protect and promote the pregnant woman's health interests"[3] and those of the fetus
Nonmaleficence	To do no harm—to minimize the risks to the patient	To avoid doing harm to the pregnant woman or the fetus[3]
Respect for Autonomy	To respect the patient's preferences in medical care (assuming decision-making capacity and informed consent)	"To respect the (pregnant) woman's right to choose what happens to her"; because the fetus lacks the neurodevelopment to possess values and to reason, "there is no autonomy-based obligation to the fetus"[3]
Justice	Clinical intervention results in a fair distribution of clinical benefits and burdens in a population	"Individuals should receive equal treatment unless scientific and clinical evidence establishes that they differ from others in ways relevant to the treatments in question"[6]; caregivers need to "explicitly identify biases that distort organizational culture and healthcare policy, and use relevant concepts of justice to advocate for fetal, neonatal, and pregnant patients"[13]

(Adapted from Beauchamp T, Childress J. *Principles of Biomedical Ethics*. 5th ed. New York, NY: Oxford University Press; 2001.)

It is also generally accepted that the previable fetus achieves the status of a patient only by virtue of the pregnant mother's autonomous decision to confer such a status on her fetus, which is based on her personal beliefs and values.[5] In cases of maternal uncertainty and pending a maternal decision, Chervenak et al. recommend conferring *provisional* patient status to the previable fetus as a basis for justification of directive counseling, particularly when maternal behaviors or medical interventions can harm it in significant or irreversible ways.[4] In such situations, the physician caring for the pregnant woman will have acted to promote the well-being of the fetus so that if the pregnant woman later autonomously decides to confer patient status on her fetus, the status of the fetus will have been maximized. Even so, the pregnant woman is only obligated to agree to reasonable interventions that do not threaten to harm her.[5]

The pregnant woman is free to confer, withhold, or withdraw the status of patient from her previable fetus.[5] Appellate courts have ruled that a pregnant woman's decisions regarding medical treatment should take precedence regardless of the presumed fetal consequences of those decisions.[7] Additionally, in common law, the fetus does not have any legal rights or status until it is born alive and has been completely separated from the pregnant woman's body.[8]

Informed Consent

Informed consent is the process of shared decision making between healthcare providers and patients. Legally, as well as ethically, it requires that the patient be provided with sufficient relevant information upon which a reasonable patient might make an informed decision, that the patient be free from coercion, and that the patient has sufficient

decision-making capacity and comprehension to make a decision regarding the proposed intervention. Although such consent is usually obtained in writing for surgery and for treatment in the hospital, in the outpatient nonsurgical setting, such consent is often verbal. However, the mere existence of a signed consent is not *prima facie* evidence of informed consent because the information provided to the patient regarding risks, benefits, and alternatives might not have been adequate. In a life-threatening emergency, the doctrine of implied consent applies. It is presumed that a reasonable patient would want prompt lifesaving treatment to be administered and that treatment not be delayed in order to obtain consent from a surrogate decision maker. In the case of diagnostic or therapeutic interventions for a pregnant woman, the informed consent process should include providing information about the risks, benefits, and alternatives as they apply to the fetus as well as to the patient.

CASE #1

A 30-year-old P_1G_0 was seen in the 16th week of pregnancy for a generalized pustular rash of 2 weeks' duration, fever, and a seizure. Examination disclosed a toxic-appearing pregnant female with a generalized superficial pustular rash, and laboratory tests showed hypoalbuminemia and hypocalcemia. A skin biopsy showed histopathologic features of pustular psoriasis, and a diagnosis of *impetigo herpetiformis* was made. She was started on prednisone 60 mg daily but could not be weaned to a lower dose without flaring. Cyclosporine was not effective and produced a worrisome rise in blood pressure. Because of continued toxicity, seizures, and concerns regarding both the health of the mother and the viability of the fetus, termination of the pregnancy was advised at 20 weeks' gestation. The patient refused, asking to carry the pregnancy until 32 weeks and, if not possible, at least until the age of fetal viability.

CASE #2

A 33-year-old G_3P_2 with a distant history of malignant melanoma of the back presented during the 10th week of pregnancy with a seizure. Magnetic resonance imaging showed evidence of nodular densities in the parietal and temporal lobes of the brain and lungs as well as an enlarged axillary node. A biopsy of this node revealed metastatic malignant melanoma that was positive for a V600E mutation in *BRAF*. She was offered the options of treatment of the cerebral metastasis by gamma-knife surgery and management of her stage IV disease with vemurafenib, a BRAF kinase inhibitor that was felt to offer her the best chance of progression-free survival and prolongation of survival. She was advised that the drug is a pregnancy category D medication, meaning that it carries risk to the fetus, but that the benefits to the pregnant woman in a life-threatening situation may justify the risk. She was also advised that there have been no published reports of fetal toxicity. Despite being advised to start therapy with vemurafenib immediately and begin gamma-knife therapy in the second trimester, she elected to defer all treatment until after delivery. However, she agreed to an elective cesarean section after 32 weeks' gestation, despite the fact that the delay of over nearly 5 months approaches the median survival for stage IV melanoma, which is about 6 months.

ANALYSIS OF CASES

The American College of Obstetrics and Gynecology (ACOG) has presented a useful approach for decision making in the face of ethical dilemmas.[9] This is summarized in Table 25.2.

Case #1

This case involves a severe pregnancy-related skin condition, *impetigo herpetiformis*, which is a variant of pustular psoriasis in pregnancy and which can be associated with significant maternal toxicity and, rarely, even death. The most effective treatment for this condition is the delivery of the infant, but, in this case, we are also dealing with a previable fetus. *Impetigo herpetiformis* can be associated with significant fetal risks, including stillbirth, neonatal death, intrauterine growth restriction, and fetal abnormalities. In the antepartum case that is corticosteroid resistant, the options are to either consider cyclosporine, a biologic drug such as infliximab, narrowband ultraviolet B treatment added to systemic corticosteroids, or, as a last

TABLE 25.2	**The Ethical Decision-Making Process**

1. **Identify the decision makers.**
   a. Assess patient's capacity to make a decision.
   b. Identify a surrogate decision maker in cases in situations in which the patient is thought to lack the capacity to make medical decisions.
   c. In the obstetric setting, the pregnant woman who has decision-making capacity is the appropriate decision maker for the fetus.
2. **Collect data, establish facts, try to recognize personal values and bias in order to remain objective, and use consultants as needed.**
3. **Identify all medically appropriate options, including those raised by the patient, family, and consultants.**
4. **Evaluate options according to the values and principles involved.**
   a. Gather information regarding the values of the primary stakeholders, especially the patient.
   b. Eliminate those options that are morally unacceptable to all parties.
   c. Reexamine the remaining options according to the interests and values of each party.
5. **Identify ethical conflicts and set priorities.**
   a. Define problem in terms of the ethical principles involved (e.g., beneficence, respect for autonomy).
   b. Does one principle appear more important than others in this conflict? Is one course of action better than the others?
   c. Look at similar cases if they exist.
6. **Select the most ethically satisfying option.**
7. **Reassess the decision after it is acted on to determine if the best possible decision was made and what lessons can be learned.**

(Adapted from ACOG Committee Opinion No. 390, December 2007. Ethical decision making in obstetrics and gynecology. *Obstet Gynecol.* 2007;11:1479–1487.)

resort, termination of the pregnancy. In view of the gravity of this case and the urgency to control the disease, cyclosporine is considered to be the best option. Cyclosporine is a pregnancy category C medication. There has been no evidence of teratogenicity, although there is increased risk of premature delivery or low birth weight (risks which already exist in this patient). Because cyclosporine was not effective in rapidly controlling her disease and was not tolerated well, the obstetrician and patient are now faced with the dilemma of whether to terminate the pregnancy, to consider another form of therapy that might not work as quickly as the urgency of the situation necessitates, or to allow the pregnancy to continue until the fetus is considered viable, recognizing that even when delivery occurs at 23 to 25 weeks, there is a strong likelihood of neonatal morbidity and developmental disability or impairment if the infant survives.

Considering the ACOG ethical decision-making framework for the pregnant patient, the first priority is to assess whether this critically ill patient who has recently had a seizure is capable of understanding and processing all the information that is necessary to make an informed decision. If she is too toxic and ill or her mentation is too clouded, a surrogate decision maker will have to be involved. If there is an advanced directive specifying who the surrogate should be, then the choice is straightforward. In the event there is no such directive or if the patient has not previously made her wishes known, then there is a hierarchy for determining who the appointed surrogate should be, usually (depending on the jurisdiction) beginning with the spouse, then an adult son or daughter, then a parent, then an adult sibling, and the lowest priority being an adult close friend. If the father of the fetus is not the legally wedded or common law spouse of the pregnant woman, then he would be considered a close adult friend.[3] Ideally, surrogate decision making should attempt to reach a decision that the pregnant woman would have, if she had decision-making capacity. Otherwise, substituted judgment should try to make such a judgment based on knowledge of the patient's values and, in any event, to arrive at a decision that is in the patient's best interest. This is particularly complicated when the interest of the fetus needs to be considered.

If the patient has decisional capacity, then counseling regarding the previable status of the fetus should be nondirective but should lay out the benefits and maternal and fetal risks of each treatment option. The pregnant woman retains the autonomous right to confer or withhold patient status from the fetus and to decide whether to terminate the pregnancy, and this decision must be respected by the physician. Should she respond somewhat to medical therapy, then her decision to allow the pregnancy to proceed until at least fetal viability, and if possible to fetal lung maturity, appears to align both maternal and fetal interests. If the patient deteriorates further, then the likelihood of maternal death rises and delivering a viable fetus becomes even lower, and directive counseling is warranted. Regardless, the patient with decisional capacity has the autonomy to decide which course she wishes to follow.

In the example of surrogate decision making, the principle of beneficence has priority. In the example of the competent pregnant woman, the principle of autonomy trumps all others. In this case, the most ethically satisfying decision—namely, respecting the woman's autonomous decision—may be the least satisfying in terms of outcome given the severity of the underlying condition. This is something that can only be determined in retrospect.

Case #2

This case can also be analyzed using the ACOG framework (see Table 25.2). The obstetrician and/or oncologist can assess the patient's decision-making capacity by presenting to her the alternatives and ascertaining her understanding of them. Assuming that her intracranial metastasis and recent seizure have not interfered with her capacity to receive, understand, and process these options, the next step would be to collect all the information relative to the treatment decisions. She has stage IV metastatic melanoma, in which the tumor cells carry the V600E mutation in *BRAF*, making her a candidate for therapy with vemurafenib. If left untreated, the median survival for this melanoma is approximately 6 months, whereas the median survival for patients with stage IV melanoma having the V600E *BRAF* mutation treated with vemurafenib is 15.9 months.[10] Additionally, the progression-free survival in the published clinical trials of this drug is 6.8 months.[10] This is an important consideration, because it is possible that, without treatment, the mother might succumb prior to the fetus reaching viability or lung maturity. Although there are treatment alternatives, including interleukin-2 and conventional chemotherapy, these carry significant risks to both the pregnant woman and her fetus. Although vemurafenib is a pregnancy category D medication based on its mechanism of action, there are no published cases of fetal adverse effects or evidence of teratogenicity in animal studies, and there has not been any experience with use of this medication in pregnant patients to date.

This patient also has a cerebral metastasis. Because of the location, it was felt to be unresectable, and gamma-knife radiosurgery was recommended. Because of the potential for rapid growth of a cerebral metastasis, early treatment following a diagnosis is recommended. Although the safety of gamma-knife radiosurgery during pregnancy has not been established, one study showed that extracranial fetal radiation doses were quite low, and the authors felt that gamma-knife radiosurgery could be recommended to carefully selected patients with brain metastases during the second and third trimesters.[11]

Chervenak et al.[4] discussed the ethical framework for directive counseling of the pregnant patient with cancer. Beneficence-based obligations to the pregnant woman and fetus can be considered *congruent* when the treatment reduces the woman's risk of morbidity or mortality without increasing the risk of iatrogenic harm or mortality to the fetus, whereas treatment can be considered *incongruent* for the fetus if it increases the risk to the fetus and *incongruent* for the woman if it increases the risk of future infertility despite reducing maternal mortality or morbidity. In the case of the previable fetus, the woman has the autonomous right to confer patient status or withhold or withdraw previously conferred patient status from the fetus, or to assign greater priorities to the life of the fetus if she wishes. Once the fetus is viable, directive counseling and recommendations should take into account the effect of any decision on fetal health. This should be balanced against autonomy-based and beneficence-based obligations to the pregnant woman. The informed consent process must take all of this into account, including the wishes and values of the pregnant woman and the risks that she is willing to undertake for her own life and health, the health and future of the fetus, and her future fertility.[4]

In this particular case, there are ample data to suggest that treatment can prolong progression-free survival and overall survival in the patient. In addition, the pregnant woman has conferred the status of patient on her previable fetus. Because of the fairly short median survival in untreated patients and the risk of rapid growth of the cerebral metastasis, delaying therapy until the fetus achieves lung maturity risks the life and well-being of the pregnant woman. Although there is no published experience on the use of vemurafenib in pregnancy, there is no hard evidence that it is deleterious to the fetus either, and delaying treatment until the second trimester in this situation probably would not add undue risk to the pregnant patient. Similarly, gamma-knife radiosurgery could be performed fairly shortly, early in the second trimester. In this particular case, it appears that the pregnant woman's priority is the welfare of the fetus, not her own. Through the process of directive counseling and informed consent, it might be possible to present treatment choices that appear congruent for both the pregnant woman and her fetus. If, however, the beneficence-based obligations to both the pregnant woman and the previable fetus are incongruent, counseling should be nondirective, taking into account the woman's autonomy to determine whether the fetus is a patient and to make her own assessment of whether fetal risks should be taken in order for her to benefit from treatment.[4]

In this case, perhaps without full information, the patient has elected to delay treatment until the fetus has achieved lung maturity. There are also the options of delaying therapy until after 12 weeks, when organogenesis is likely complete, and then monitoring the fetus for signs of significant side effects of treatment and considering termination if these develop before viability, or of the immediate termination of the pregnancy. Given the likely low risks of fetal harm from instituting therapy early in the second trimester, as well as the significant risks to the pregnant woman of delaying therapy, instituting therapy with vemurafenib and radiosurgery could be considered to be a beneficence-based course of action that is congruent for both the fetus and the pregnant woman. She should also be informed that malignant melanoma can rarely metastasize to the placenta and fetus. However, because information as to whether the benefits of the options are congruent or incongruent for the woman and fetus can be incomplete, as it is in this case, this needs to be factored into the informed consent process. Furthermore,

utilizing a multidisciplinary approach can enhance the decision-making process in medically complex cases such as this.[12] If, despite being informed of all the options and assuming that she possesses the capacity to make sound medical decisions, she insists on delaying therapy until fetal lung maturity has been achieved, then the physician is ethically obligated to accept the patient's autonomous decision. Should she autonomously decide to begin treatment with vemurafenib and undergo radiosurgery early in the second trimester, this would align the most ethically satisfying course of action with the decision that is most likely to yield the best medical outcome for the pregnant woman and fetus.

KEY POINTS

- A physician treating a pregnant woman has obligations of beneficence and respect for autonomy toward the pregnant woman and of beneficence and nonmaleficence toward the fetus.
- Maternal and fetal interests usually coincide; however, cases may arise where these interests diverge, creating conflicting moral choices for the healthcare provider.
- Navigating a maternal–fetal ethical conflict requires the clinician to identify and address principle-based obligations to the pregnant woman and fetus, issues of maternal decision-making capacity, and issues of fetal "patienthood."
- The fetus becomes a patient at the age of viability (around 24 weeks' gestation) or when the mother confers this status on her fetus; however, the pregnant woman is free to confer, withhold, or withdraw the status of patient from her previable fetus assuming her decision-making capacity is intact.
- If maternal decision-making capacity is impaired and no advanced directives exist, a surrogate decision maker must be appointed to make decisions in the best interest of the pregnant woman and her fetus.
- In the case of interventions for a pregnant woman, the informed consent process should include providing information about the risks, benefits, and alternatives as they apply to the fetus as well as to the patient.
- Beneficence-based obligations can be considered congruent for the pregnant mother and fetus when the treatment reduces the woman's risk of morbidity without increasing the risk to the fetus; it is considered incongruent for the fetus if it increases fetal risks; and it is incongruent for the pregnant woman if it increases the risk of future infertility.

REFERENCES

1. Beauchamp T, Childress J. *Principles of Biomedical Ethics*. 5th ed. New York, NY: Oxford University Press; 2001.
2. Mahowald M. *Bioethics and Women Across the Lifespan*. New York, NY: Oxford University Press; 2006.
3. DiGiovanni LM. Ethical issues in obstetrics. *Obstet Gynecol Clin N Am*. 2010;37:345–357.
4. Chervenak FA, McCullough LB, Knapp RC, et al. A clinically comprehensive ethical framework for offering and recommending cancer treatment before and during pregnancy. *Cancer*. 2004;100:215–222.
5. McCullough L, Chervenak F. *Ethics in Obstetrics and Gynecology*. New York, NY: Oxford University Press; 1994.
6. Chervenak FA, McCullough LB, Levene MI. An ethically justified, clinically comprehensive approach to peri-viability: gynaecological, obstetric, perinatal and neonatal dimensions. *J Obstet Gynaecol*. 2007;27:3–7.
7. ACOG Committee Opinion No. 321: maternal decision making, ethics, and the law. *Obstet Gynecol*. 2005;106:1127–1137.
8. Flagler E, Baylis F, Rodgers S. Bioethics for clinicians: 12. Ethical dilemmas that arise in the care of pregnant women: Rethinking "maternal-fetal conflicts". *CMAJ*. 1997;156:1729–1732.
9. ACOG Committee Opinion No. 390, December 2007. Ethical decision making in obstetrics and gynecology. *Obstet Gynecol*. 2007;11:1479–1487.
10. Sosman JA, Kim KB, Schuchter L, et al. Survival in BRAF V600-mutant advanced melanoma treated with vemurafenib. *N Engl J Med*. 2012;366:707–714.
11. Yu C, Jozsef G, Apuzzo ML, et al. Fetal radiation doses for model C gamma knife radiosurgery. *Neurosurgery*. 2003;52:687–689.
12. Dalton SR, Hicks M, Shabanowitz R, et al. Ethical dilemmas in the management of tumor-stage mycosis fungoides in a pregnant patient. *J Am Acad Dermatol*. 2012;66(4):661–663.
13. Chervenak FA, McCullough LB. Women and children first—or last? The New York Declaration. *Am J Obstet Gynecol*. 2009;201:335–339.

INDEX

NOTE: Page numbers followed by *f* denote figures; those followed by *t* denote tables.